Client-Centered Exercise Prescription

John C. Griffin, MSc

George Brown College

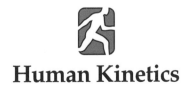

Human Kinetics

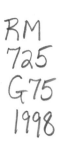
37947167
DLC

1-30-01

Library of Congress Cataloging-in-Data

Griffin, John C.
 Client-centered exercise prescription / by John C. Griffin.
  p. cm.
 Includes bibliographical references and index.
 ISBN 0-88011-707-9
 1. Exercise therapy. 2. Exercises. 3. Physical fitness.
 4. Personal trainers. I. Title.
 RM725.G75 1998   97-45094
 615.8'2--dc21   CIP

ISBN: 0-88011-707-9

See Credits listings on page 263.

Acquisitions Editor: Scott Wikgren; **Developmental Editor:** Elaine Mustain; **Assistant Editor:** Melinda Graham; **Copyeditor:** Brian Mustain; **Proofreader:** Sara Wiseman; **Indexer:** Craig Brown; **Graphic Designer:** Nancy Rasmus; **Graphic Artist:** Yvonne Winsor; **Photo Editor:** Boyd LaFoon; **Cover Designer:** Jack Davis; **Photographer (cover):** Tom Roberts; **Photographer (interior):** Tom Roberts/Human Kinetics, unless otherwise noted; **Illustrators:** Keith Blomberg; K. Galasyn Wright, figures 5.7a, and 10.17a,b; Paul To, figure 10.4; Marge Pavich, figure 10.10; Michael Richardson, figures 12xx.1, 12xx.3, 12xx.5, 11.8, 14.2a,b, 14.13a, 14.20, 14.23 and 15.3. **Printer:** United Graphics

Printed in the United States of America 10 9 8 7 6 5 4 3 2

Human Kinetics
Web site: http://www.humankinetics.com/

United States: Human Kinetics, P.O. Box 5076, Champaign, IL 61825-5076
1-800-747-4457
e-mail: humank@hkusa.com

Canada: Human Kinetics, 475 Devonshire Road, Unit 100, Windsor, ON N8Y 2L5
1-800-465-7301 (in Canada only)
e-mail: humank@hkcanada.com

Europe: Human Kinetics, P.O. Box IW14, Leeds LS16 6TR, United Kingdom
+44 (0)113-278 1708
e-mail: humank@hkeurope.com

Australia: Human Kinetics, 57A Price Avenue, Lower Mitcham, South Australia 5062
(08) 82771555
e-mail: humank@hkaustralia.com

New Zealand: Human Kinetics, P.O. Box 105-231, Auckland Central
09-523-3462
e-mail: humank@hknewz.com

To my wife, colleague, and friend whose values and love are unconditional
   Mary

To my son, whose life is a gift to all of us
   Jay

To my daughter, whose love of life brings joy to those who share
   Laura

To my parents, my loving mentors
   Gord and Ruth

Acknowledgments

I would like to acknowledge my friends and colleagues for their critical and comprehensive reviews of the manuscript. I am grateful for your timely assistance and enthusiastic support. For your unique contributions, I would like to extend special recognition to Dr. Bill McLeod, for his thoughtful review of the first draft of the manuscript; Ruth Hanton, for her insights in the art and science of client communications and her role in coauthoring part of chapter 11; Cathy McNorgan, for walking the line between physiotherapy and fitness and guiding my limits in chapter 14; Paul Sperl, for reminding me about who I was and with whom I was talking; and Mary Griffin, for identifying opportunities to make each chapter and each paragraph more user-friendly and client-centered. Your expertise, care, effort, and time are truly appreciated.

Contents

Client-Centered Exercise Prescription

Reproducible Forms

Exercise prescription is about helping people adopt, enjoy, and maintain an active lifestyle. How well we help our clients do this is the true measure of our success. Knowledge of exercise sciences, technical skills, or having a fit body do not guarantee success in one-on-one prescription. Client-centered relationships empower clients toward self-sufficiency much more effectively than traditional sport-specific prescriptions. *Client-Centered Exercise Prescription* is a significant resource that features this more personalized approach for exercise specialists.

A majority of exercise prescription textbooks take a "component" approach, examining cardiovascular function, body composition, flexibility, muscular strength, and endurance. The automobile industry has discovered that letting a single team build a car from the bottom up produces much better results than sending it down an assembly line and building it by component pieces. In the same way, this book takes clients off the assembly line and establishes them as the center of decision making.

The prescription process model is like a journey taken by the exercise specialist and client along a road leading to a unique program design. Each stage of the journey has its own set of client-centered outcomes. This book will guide you, the exercise specialist, in knowing what questions to ask and what interventions and decisions you must make along the way. This text challenges you to provide far more than a list of exercises. It will guide you through three stages of exercise prescription, each characterized by "counseling"—that is, carefully listening to client feedback, and modifying the path as necessary in response. Even when the journey involves side trips and doubling back, it always moves in the direction of better health for your client. The three stages of this ongoing journey are

- Stage 1—Beginning the journey with counseling,
- Stage 2—Matching your client's needs, and
- Stage 3—Personalized prescription.

The journey begins with an inquiry from someone who needs help. Every time we take on such a client, we encounter a new set of circumstances, a new personality, a new history, and a new journey. The first challenge in stage one is to get a clear picture of the client's **history**, needs, and hopes for achievement. This picture will develop, and perhaps change, as our relationship progresses. The counseling must challenge the client to create clear **priorities** for measurable and progressive **objectives**.

In the **second stage**, we gather more detailed information through the selective **assessment** of physical fitness. Without some physiological parameters to set prescription factors or monitor progress, we can only use broad guidelines that are not specific to our client's needs. A variety of training methods allows us to **match specific benefits to specific clients**. The client's own preferences and availability of equipment will also influence our prescription.

The **third stage** is the design process in which we select appropriate exercises, from a wide menu of choices, according to how they fit our client's goals. The details of the **personalized exercise prescription** are based on two main criteria: the physiological rationale, and the questions of how the decision will interface with the client. The follow-up program demonstration, along with the type of self-monitoring designed into the program, can strongly affect the client's motivation and self-esteem, and ultimately determine the client's adherence to the program.

Parts I through IV of the book follow the above-mentioned three stages. Part V looks at prescription situations that merit special consideration. It focuses on exercise prescription for clients recovering from or having a history of orthopedic injury. The final chapter provides activity recommendations for special populations. Part V also contains specific prescriptions for stretching and strengthening.

In recent years, a number of factors have encouraged a shift to more client-centered exercise prescription. First, understanding of the effects of physical activity on human health has advanced. Secondly, training has undergone a technological revolution—and the interface of client with machine, as well as training methodology using machines, requires close supervision. Thirdly, fitness consumers want specific

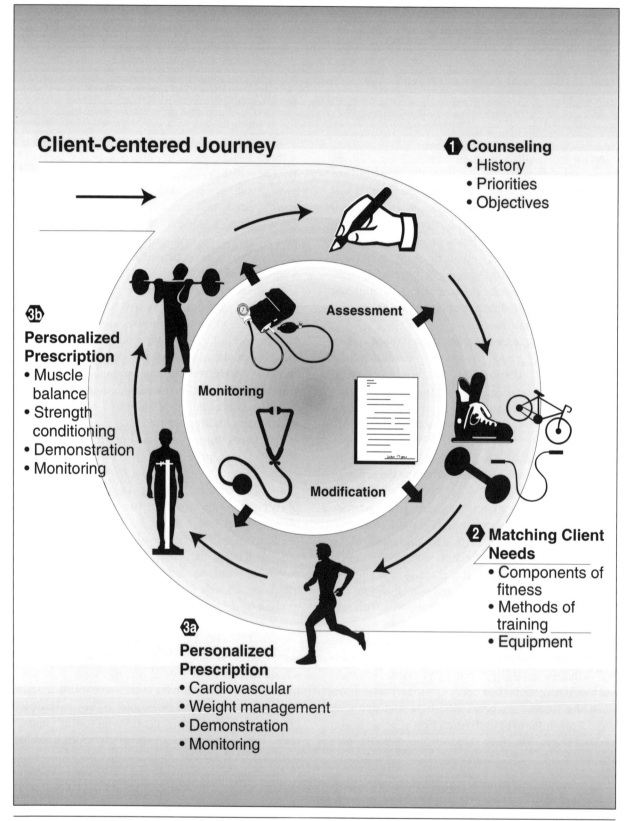

Figure P.1   The three stages of the prescription model are counseling, matching your client's needs, and giving personalized prescription.

results, more choices, and guidance about where and how to exercise; they also want service along with prescriptions. Finally, exercise specialists are growing in numbers and are establishing new employment opportunities in private, clinical, and community sectors.

As one of these professionals—perhaps you are a clinical kinesiologist, a personal trainer, or a fitness specialist in a private or community setting—you no doubt recognize the scarcity of available resources. This text is written for you. Physical therapists, athletic trainers, chiropractors, and physical educators will also benefit from it. Inclusion of practical examples and background scientific knowledge make the text well suited for undergraduate health/fitness courses as well. The text may also be used in conjunction with a traditional exercise physiology course. It provides

- a bridge between industry practices and recent literature,
- a reliable method of matching client priorities with appropriate prescription factors, and
- specific examples and case studies that demonstrate the actual skills of prescription.

As you read, you will discover that "counseling" is a central concern of this book. I do not intend to suggest that the exercise specialist should be a psychological therapist. I use the term to refer simply to the art of listening intently to client feedback and modifying the program appropriately. It is not a simple art, but it is one that is essential to develop if one is to be the best prescriber possible. It is also achievable, and this text makes clear in many ways and on many levels how this type of counseling can be learned.

Of particular note are several learning enhancement features of the text. Many chapters contain "Backgrounders," which are summaries of the scientific basis of the applied material. "Links" highlight matching client priorities with appropriate prescription factors. The text also contains many forms and charts you will find useful to copy and have at hand for direct use.

Client-Centered Exercise Prescription is a front-line resource that will help you focus on the individual in making your prescription. This text draws on applied exercise physiology, the art of counseling, and personal experience to provide skills that will help you prescribe safe, effective, and enjoyable activities for your clients.

What is Client-Centered Exercise Prescription?

The best sales people tell us that the first step in making a sale is to find out what consumers need or perceive themselves as needing. Similarly, a big part of what we do is to help clients "buy into" their exercise. If we act merely as experts, our success will be limited. Preaching the merits of fitness can create a frenzy of activity in our clients that can die out just as quickly as it began. Our first job is not to preach—it is to listen. We must hear what the people we are serving say to us. Our clients need our attention and our guidance, especially at the beginning of their commitment.

Clients constitute the starting point of the prescription process. Rather than trying too early to design a solution, we must help our clients empower themselves by working with them to identify and develop their underused potential. Program designs are not ends in themselves. The skills learned along the way will help our clients stick with the program and become independent exercisers. Our role is to formulate the right questions and choices and to provide the pros and cons from **their** perspective. We cannot help what (or whom) we do not understand. The journey to helping clients has many options for rerouting, and the map is in our clients' hands.

Recently, I invited a colleague of mine to do a guest lecture on counseling skills for exercise prescription. After I introduced her, she said: "For the next 15 minutes, I am your client." This was followed by a very long and awkward silence. Finally, a student said: "But we don't know anything about you." Of course, that was the whole point! Very quickly the question floodgates opened and the students and the guest were well on their way.

Each client represents a new journey. Even if the choices are similar, the perspective of each client is different. This difference creates the challenge, the joy, and the skill inherent in exercise prescription—it is the reason why we all must be client-centered.

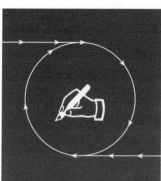

PART I

Beginning the Journey With Counseling

In the first stage of our journey, we create rapport in which our clients learn to trust us and develop confidence in our competence. This is the foundation of "client-centered" prescription.

We must have such a close relationship with our clients that they feel free to frankly discuss their present situation as well as their realistic vision of the future. We can help them clarify their experiences so they can better understand themselves—that is, we filter their experiences through our own and put them in a useful perspective.

The techniques we use for discovery and self-exploration may vary with the client's personality, but they will always include effective questioning and probing to determine the client's **needs**, **wants**, and **lifestyle**. The areas of *overlap*—where a need and a want coincide and the lifestyle is compatible—are the areas of the greatest potential for success. Obtaining proper understanding of our client's history enables us to set priorities and to formulate a motivational strategy.

Getting to Know Our Client: More Than a History

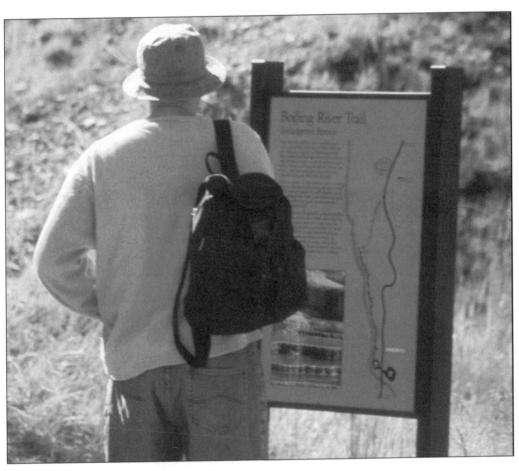

- Where Are the Counseling Opportunities in Client-Centered Prescription?
- Counseling to Help
- Counseling to Discover

Our job as exercise "counselors" is to help clients begin to take charge of their own exercise regimens. We help them pursue their own objectives, whether they be active lifestyles, recovery from injuries, or better athletic performance. We tailor every prescription decision throughout the journey to the clients and to their specific situations.

Where Are the Counseling Opportunities in Client-Centered Prescription?

Our first challenge is to put clients at ease and to develop comfortable working relationships. Next we work together to get a clear picture of their present health, activity and lifestyle history, needs, what they hope to achieve, and potential sources of motivation. In our counseling we challenge the clients to create clear priorities, and then help them fine-tune their goals, making them measurable and progressive. To do this, we need detailed information gathered through assessing the clients' physical fitness.

Designing programs involves helping clients choose which elements of the exercise prescription suit their goals. It is important not only to carefully set objectives but to follow up after the design to verify the validity of the prescription. We must demonstrate every facet of the program to our clients in ways both easy to understand and clearly linked to their ultimate goals. We must teach them how to monitor themselves, and how to make adjustments accordingly—a process that can strongly affect their motivation, their adherence to the program, and ultimately the success of the program.

Counseling permeates the entire prescription journey. However, as the journey progresses, the thrust of the counseling changes. We may find ourselves

- counseling to **help** clients feel comfortable and committed to change,
- counseling to **discover** information related to the clients or the programs, or
- counseling to **focus** on the direction and priorities that emerge.

In this chapter we discuss counseling to help and counseling to discover. Chapter 2 considers counseling to focus.

Counseling to Help

Helping is a client-centered process leading to new behaviors. Building upon a foundation of caring, rapport, and comfort, we lead clients into a commitment to change their habits. We keep our clients at the center of this process by listening more than we talk, and by encouraging them to learn from their own experiences. Counseling must be seen as an opportunity to help clients develop more options. Helping enables clients to learn to open doors, to throw off chains, and to stretch!

To make sure we are approaching our clients effectively for helping, we must learn to

- prepare the environment,
- establish rapport,
- show we care,
- outline the structure,
- establish credibility, and
- establish the clients' level of commitment.

Prepare the Environment

Your clients will be poorly focused if their basic needs for comfort are not met. Be sure there is good lighting, appropriate temperature, good air flow, and comfortable chairs (avoid a desk). Familiarize clients with various facilities, washrooms, and club procedures. If you work within a facility, help your clients feel comfortable and confident around the equipment.

Establish Rapport

A friendly welcome is essential. Create an environment conducive to relaxed conversation, and start a short chat about an area of mutual interest (e.g., home, work, children, sports, etc.). Try to have people fill out most forms before they arrive. In the first few minutes, avoid discussing health/fitness concerns in any detail. Showing new clients around may help them relax, increase their comfort zone, and take the counseling out of the traditional office setting.

Show You Care

Accepting your clients as they are makes it easier for them to accept themselves and therefore to change. Being sensitive to their concerns will build trust and show genuine interest. Listening well shows that you care.

Outline the Structure

Clients want to know what they are "letting themselves in for." When they can see the complete picture, it helps them focus and pace themselves. Outline what will be done and why. Describe options and choices they will have throughout the program. Show them a copy of a sample questionnaire, assessment form, or prescription. Allow enough time for questions. Avoid feeling rushed.

STAGES OF CHANGE QUESTIONNAIRE

Physical activity can include such activities as walking, cycling, swimming, climbing stairs, dancing, active gardening, walking to work, aerobics, sports, etc. Regular physical activity is 30 minutes of moderate activity accumulated over the day, almost every day, or vigorous activity done at least three times per week for 20 minutes each time.

1. Here are a number of statements describing various levels of physical activity. Please select the one that most closely describes your own level:

   (Please pick one)

   I am not physically active and I do not plan on becoming so. ☐ 1

   I have been thinking about becoming physically active, but I haven't done anything about it yet. ☐ 2

   I am physically active once in a while, but not regularly. ☐ 3

   I have become involved in regular physical activity within the past six months. ☐ 4

   I participate in regular physical activity and have done so for more than six months. ☐ 5

2. (Answer if not currently active)

   I was physically active in the past, but not now. ☐ Yes
   ☐ No

Reprinted, with permission, from *The Canadian Physical Activity, Fitness & Lifestyle Appraisal: CSEP's Plan for Healthy Active Living.* Published by the Canadian Society for Exercise Physiology, 1996, p. 8-19.

Establish Credibility

Without sounding boastful, explain your qualifications and level of experience. Not only does this establish your own credibility, it also evokes in your clients feelings of confidence and shows them what expertise there is to draw upon. For example: "You mentioned some previous back stiffness. . . . I had an opportunity to be part of the Healthy Back program staff at the YMCA while finishing off my kinesiology degree. . . . I'm looking forward to helping you with that problem."

Discover the Client's Level of Commitment

Early discussions should clarify what clients hope to gain or learn and why they are there. Determining their level of commitment to change will help you choose the best strategy for helping them change. The Canadian Society for Exercise Physiology (1996) has developed a Stages of Change Questionnaire designed to establish the stage of motivational readiness of clients (see page 5).

LINKS:

Helping a Client Develop Options

Don, an automotive worker and avid lacrosse coach, suffered a heart attack during a father-son game. At first, he was devastated, feeling that his identity and role in life had been taken away. Feelings of "Why me?" progressed to frustration and helplessness. Medical and corporate counseling helped Don readjust to a modified work environment, however his doctors set lacrosse out of bounds. Then a lacrosse friend of Don's became a "helper." He had Don take a closer look at different roles he could take on with the team. He helped Don discover that his years of experience were invaluable as a strategist and advisor, and that being on the floor was not the only option for a coach. His friend also introduced Don to an exercise specialist who showed him how to build his cardiovascular stamina and monitor his exertion levels and symptoms. Today, Don is co-coaching and providing a service to the team that goes beyond what he provided before the heart attack.

The questionnaire identifies five stages of change corresponding to the number of the statement selected:

1. Precontemplation—Not intending to make changes
2. Contemplation—Considering a change
3. Preparation—Making small changes or ready to change in the near future
4. Action—Actively engaging in the new behavior
5. Maintenance—Sticking with the behavior change

Matching Your Client's Frame of Reference

Once you know your client's stage of change, you can choose strategies that are effective for that specific stage (Prochaska et al. 1992). Becoming client-centered requires that you match your frame of reference to that of your client. Consider one of my clients, who was rehabilitating from a motor vehicle accident and had not previously been active. He had never considered what regular exercise would be like, and had taken no voluntary steps toward doing it—and therefore the "cons" to regular exercise outweighed the "pros" in his mind. If I had simply assigned him an exercise prescription, I would have set him up for failure. Recognizing that he was back at a precontemplative or contemplative stage, I knew that he had not yet made a commitment to take action. I therefore first helped him over his negative perceptions, and highlighted the personal benefits. Providing positive feedback merely for his attendance at the sessions, for example, and giving encouragement for reaching even a small goal, showed him that his behavior was worthwhile and acceptable. Such positive experiences confirmed in his mind the relationship between the rehab effort and feeling better.

Another client was considering an increase in her physical activity, but seemed to be putting it off because of a lack of self-confidence. If I had presented her with a program featuring a wide variety of activities and detailed self-monitoring, I probably would have scared her off. She was at the preparation stage: small changes were within her abilities, but large, complex changes would have set her back. Working together, we established a step-by-step plan that helped build her confidence.

Find out what your clients know, think, and feel about physical activity before actively engaging them. The more information you discover about your clients, the better able you are to determine the right combination of strategies for them.

Use Strategies Appropriate to Clients' Stages of Change

Table 1.1 illustrates how different strategies can help clients at different stages of changing habits of physical activity.

The previous examples show how, in the earlier stages, you should build self-confidence and motivation, and highlight benefits specific to your client. Provide all possible kinds of feedback that can increase positive emotions and help resolve any problems created by change.

Precontemplative Stage

A client comment at the precontemplative stage may be, "Exercise may be fine for young people but I'm too old to start." Your strategy here should be to focus on the "why" and increase his awareness of the importance of appropriate exercise at any age.

Here is a typical conversation between a client (Cl) and an exercise specialist (ES):

(ES): Were you active when you were younger?

(Cl): Oh, yes. I was always involved in sports and activities in the neighborhood.

(ES): Why were you so active at that time?

(Cl): Well, it was fun and the better shape I was in, the more competitive I was in sports.

(ES): That's great! Sounds like being active suited your goals at that time. For that matter, having fun at any age is a worthwhile goal.

(Cl): Yes, but I can't still do those activities, and why would I want to?

Table 1.1   Stages of Change: Characteristics & Strategies

STAGE	CHARACTERISTICS	STRATEGIES
Precontemplation	• not intending to change • low awareness • never considered it • 'cons' outweigh 'pros'	• increase awareness of importance • start a dialogue • increase 'pros' for activity
Contemplation	• intending to change in next 6 months • may be ambivalent • self-confidence may be low	• increase intention to action by addressing ambivalence, highlighting personal benefits, and building self-confidence
Preparation	• intending to take action in next 30 days • making some small changes • may have tried in past year	• help client plan, e.g., set date • focus on the 'pros' • provide helpful resources • strengthen self-confidence
Action	• has changed behavior in last 6 months • risk of relapse is high • needs support—challenging time mentally	• support client to prevent relapse • teach how to deal with lapses • deal with lapses • promote social support
Maintenance	• lasts 6 months onwards • confidence is high • has learned strategies to deal with lapses • may not get support any more	• refine/add variety to program • prepare in case of relapse • support in maintaining behavior to prevent relapse

Adapted from *The Canadian Physical Activity, Fitness & Lifestyle Appraisal: CSEP's Plan for Healthy Active Living.* Published by the Canadian Society for Exercise Physiology, 1996. pp. 2-11. Reprinted by permission.

(ES): Good question. You certainly aren't training for the Olympic games, but the training effects from even light exercise at your age can be very substantial. Your interests have changed, but activity can help you reach new goals.

(Cl): Can it help my tired feet or give me more energy?

(ES): It sure can. Let me tell you a bit about what it can do . . .

Contemplative Stage

The most common excuse of contemplative clients is, "I know I should exercise, but I just don't have time." Try to help the client examine things that will keep her motivated; discuss what might make it hard for her to stick with exercise. Your goal is that she will decide for herself that the gains outweigh the losses. Here is another typical conversation between a client (Cl) and her exercise specialist (ES):

(Cl): I just never seem to have enough time to take up a regular fitness program.

(ES): I'm amazed at how much you accomplish in a day. You are very organized.

(Cl): Sometimes I feel like too many things are pulling in too many directions.

(ES): You seem to enjoy much of what you do.

(Cl): Yes, I just need more hours in the day and more energy to last.

(ES): Well, I can't change the hours in a day, but with your skill for time management, I think we could come up with a strategy for rejuvenation. You already have your priorities well established—a convenient activity break can actually help you meet your commitments.

(Cl): You've got my ear and 20 minutes of my time . . .

Preparation Stage

"I play baseball once a week but I think I'll start doing more," may be a comment from a client in the preparation stage. Now you must seek a commitment. Booking an assessment at this stage may still be too threatening: rather, schedule a consultation to find out what the client really wants to achieve, and establish short-term goals like learning a baseball warm-up routine or getting a few stretches for an old groin pull. A check-off log incorporated into the prescription reinforces every positive action taken in the early activity stages.

Action Stage

The client in the action stage may be a new club member who says, "I started six weeks ago at three to four times a week but I'm not out as often now. Perhaps I need a personal trainer?" These clients have made some very positive actions and need to hear the praise. Rewards that come from reaching goals, along with support from family or from ourselves, can help prevent relapse. The following have been effective with clients at this stage, both one-on-one and in club settings.

- Set a time to update goals and reinforce the goals already achieved.
- Post achievements on their workout logs or on the club bulletin board.
- Look for an opportunity to create "workout buddies" with friends or other clients.
- Organize a novelty activity, perhaps with a new social group.
- Get involved with the clients to refine or add variety to their programs.

Maintenance Stage

Once at the maintenance stage, your clients must work to prevent relapse and to consolidate their gains—especially if they are involved in rehabilitation (Sotile 1996). Remind these clients of their prior state of health, and encourage activities that might help their transition from clinical exercise to active lifestyle: increase their awareness of an exercise technique, for example, or of a method for self-monitoring. The technique of *reframing* helps clients avoid negative self-talk that can eat away at their motivation. For instance, reframe guilt about time away from the office as an earned time-out and an investment in future energy.

Clients often have long periods of time when other priorities preclude regular physical activity, leading to feelings of guilt and a drop in self-esteem. Emphasize to these clients that they are not failures, and help them seize this opportunity to refocus on some start-up strategies. The Relapse Planner (page 9) is useful for those who have discontinued their regular activity (CSEP 1996).

Relapse is almost inevitable, and you should be prepared for it. Refining or adding variety to a prescription may not work—you may need to adopt a strategy from the previous stage. You must help the client resume the process of change, since his confidence will be bolstered by the success that comes with small changes. Don't let new enthusiasts skip a stage, lest they miss a mechanism of support and be less

RELAPSE PLANNER

How confident are you that you'll keep your physical activity during the next three months?

Not confident at all _____ **1**   **Confident** _____ **4**

Not very confident _____ **2**   **Very confident** _____ **5**

Somewhat confident _____ **3**

If your score was less than 4, complete the following exercise:

Many people have periods of inactivity. Sometimes these breaks can last for just a few days and sometimes a few years. Planning ahead for the "tough" times may help you stay active.

1. Have you ever had trouble keeping your physical activity going before? If so, write down the reasons why.

   _____

   _____

2. If you have had trouble, what has helped you get back on track (e.g., support from friends, joining a class, setting goals)?

   _____

   _____

3. What situations do you think would make it tough to keep your physical activity routine? How will you handle these situations to increase your chances of being successful?

   _____

   _____

High-risk situations

(e.g., people at work asking me to go for drinks after work, my usual workout time)

Solutions

1. Tell everyone my regular workout schedule so they will consider it when they are choosing a time.
2. Join them later.
3. Schedule a make-up time every week to cope with any unplanned changes.

4. What will help you get started again if you do have a "break"? Write down your ideas.

   _____

   _____

Start-up strategies

   _____

   _____

Reprinted, with permission, from *The Canadian Physical Activity, Fitness & Lifestyle Appraisal: CSEP's Plan for Healthy Active Living.* Published by the Canadian Society for Exercise Physiology, 1996. p. 8-55.

successful in the long run. Success requires stage-to-stage transitions. The challenge is to match your strategy with natural progression through the stages of change (table 1.1).

Counseling to Discover

The storytelling through which we discover a view of the past and a vision for the future requires that our clients trust in our empathy, personal reliability, and professional competence. But it also requires that we learn the skills of good listening and effective questioning.

The Skills of Listening

Asking good questions is useless if you are not actively listening. The following skills will make you a more effective listener.

Adopt the Appropriate Listening Style

Adopt a style of listening to fit the situation and content of the message being conveyed. For example, if your client just wants to get something off his chest, adopt a passive style and act as a sounding board. If your client is describing his first workout with a new program, listen actively, placing equal emphasis on both what and how things are said.

Check the Feeling

Repeat or reflect a client's feelings. Match her depth of meaning, whether light or serious. Give clues that you are trying to be empathetic. For example, a client recovering from a motor vehicle accident or a work-related injury may harbor pent-up feelings that emerge during her exercise rehabilitation. You might say, "I sense that you are frustrated by the speed of recovery from your injury." You should not assume that you know accurately how a client feels, of course; but you should acknowledge feelings and communicate empathy. Verifying feelings and not assuming immediately that you understand can build trust and reduce negative feelings.

Never judge the merits of what your clients say in terms of good-bad, right-wrong, relevant-irrelevant, etc. The following exchange took place between one of my student trainers and a member of our employee fitness program:

(Member):

> Well, the knee is still a little sore. The exercises are good, but I played hockey with my children over the weekend and it flared up again.

(Student):

> That's the problem, isn't it? Why don't you stick to your program and forget the hockey?

This might well be sound counsel, but the student responded in his "advice-giving mode," with little empathy and no acknowledgement of the person's feelings. An alternate approach for the student may have been as follows:

(Student):

> It sounds like fun with your children. Do you think there is a way we can modify your play to avoid the flare up, or is rest the best at this stage? I am pleased to hear that the exercises are good. Keep it up.

Check the Nonverbal Cues

Nonverbal skills involve your own "attending" behavior and your ability to perceive your client's nonverbal messages. Effective attending does two things: it tells clients that you are with them, and it puts you in a position to listen. Posture and gestures may be a starting point that show you are interested. Egan (1990) suggests a series of nonverbal skills that are summarized by the acronym S-O-L-E-R.

- **S**: Face the client *Squarely*. It may be at a slight angle—what is important is the quality of the attention.
- **O**: Adopt an *Open* posture. Avoid crossed arms or legs, as they are seen as defensive postures.
- **L**: At times *Lean* toward the client. The upper body is on a hinge; leaning forward shows involvement, while leaning backward may be interpreted as a lack of interest.
- **E**: Maintain good *Eye contact*. The level of reluctance or comfort level may be revealed by the consistency of eye contact.
- **R**: Try to be *Relaxed*. Your being natural helps put the client at ease.

These are only guidelines, as your clients differ individually and culturally.

Reading your client's nonverbal communication can increase rapport and improve the effects of your listening. Watch the whole body, not just the face and eyes. Hand gestures, body movement, the use of touch, and the way the person occupies space can be very expressive. Observe shifts in your client's body posture, facial expressions, vocal tone, or rate of speech. Are the verbal and nonverbal messages telling you the same thing (Jones 1991)? A client may say that he understands how to start up the treadmill; but squinting, perplexed looks, and the cocked head provide another message when he is standing on the treadmill. It is important, of course, to check the accuracy of your interpretation with the client and avoid jumping to conclusions.

Check for Clarity or Accuracy

Clarifying is an attempt to verify your understanding of what your client is saying. "Would you describe that again, please?" and "I'm a little unsure about . . ." are examples of phrases useful in clarification.

Restate the client's basic ideas, emphasizing the facts. Although a check for factual content, restatement can serve as a form of encouragement to invite the client to continue with her thoughts. For example, you might say: "Uh huh, so it sounds like it's hard to find time with your new schedule. Is that right?"

A check like this is also valuable as a method of summarizing major ideas and feelings at the end of a session. It pulls important ideas and facts together and may offer a springboard for further discussion. Try to use the client's own words and phrases: "Let's see now, the main points as I heard them are . . ."

The Skills of Questioning

Questionnaires, inventories, and checklists can increase the efficiency of counseling. They may be filled out in advance, allowing time during the counseling to discuss and clarify the most relevant information. See pages 42 and 44 for sample questionnaires. You should develop the techniques of questioning detailed below.

Open or Broad Question Strategy

Start questions with a broad framework, narrowing to specifics later. For example: "Where do you see your fitness and health needs in the next few years?" Open-ended questions are used to gather information, and are increasingly effective as your client feels more comfortable with you. Use them to learn how your client thinks or feels about something. For example: "I'd like to hear more about your past experience with health clubs," or "How did you come to be involved in old-timers baseball?"

Closed or Narrow Question Strategy

After obtaining general information, use a series of narrow questions to focus the client's attention on a specific topic. Closed-ended questions provide detailed information, check accuracy, and clarify understanding. They may help the client recall facts or choose options from a list. For example, "You mentioned that you wanted to start weight training—would you prefer free weights, machines, or calisthenics?" They are also effective in getting agreement or commitment. For example, "How many days per week do you think you can devote to this part of your prescription?" Be careful, however, not to overuse narrow questions, lest the conversation become too centered on your concerns rather than on the client and her concerns.

Probing Strategies

Probing techniques help your clients think more deeply about the issues. When initial responses to questions are superficial, use probing questions to prompt clients to provide more information, meaning, critical awareness, or reflective thinking. Listen carefully, then proceed from "where the client is at." Acknowledge previous responses before presenting the next probe. There are several types of probes:

- **Clarification.** These probes ask for more information or meaning. "Can you give me an example of . . .?" "What do you mean by muscle tone?"

- **Critical Awareness.** These probes analyze, justify, or evaluate a response. They usually deal with values and attitudes. "Why do you think that is the best way to get in shape?" "How does the old diet compare to the new one?"

- **Perception.** The intention of these probes is to anticipate a cause and effect or probable consequences. "If you sprinted without warming up, what do you think would happen?" "How do you think you would feel if . . .?"

- **Refocusing.** Often the discussion needs to shift back to the main issue. "How does that relate to your fitness goals?" "That's right, and how can that time be managed to allow . . .?" (Orme 1977).

Softening a Question

Questions can be threatening. Use of a lead-in statement can soften the impact of an open-ended question, particularly if clients are being asked about their values or lifestyles. For example, "There has been a lot written recently about the effects of smoking—how do you feel about your own smoking habits?" or "Many people have trouble starting an exercise program—what would help motivate you?" Note that the softening statements that introduce the questions are in the third person.

Highlights

- The prescription journey begins with development of a comfortable working relationship. The rapport and confidence gained with your client will ensure that you are able to gather valuable information about her needs, wants, and lifestyle.

- Helping is a client-centered process leading to new behavior. You help clients by increasing their options and by creating situations that allow the clients to take advantage of the options.

- The following are six methods of helping a client during the counseling process: preparing the environment, establishing rapport, showing that you care, outlining the structure of the help, establishing credibility, and establishing commitment.

- The five stages of change are

    1. **Precontemplation**. Not intending to make changes.

    2. **Contemplation**. Considering a change.

    3. **Preparation**. Making small changes or being ready to change in the near future.

    4. **Action**. Actively engaging in the new behavior.

    5. **Maintenance**. Sticking with the behavior change.

- The effectiveness of your counseling depends on your ability to target the needs at specific stages of change.

- Use the following techniques of effective listening: adopting a listening style that fits the situation; checking for clarity or accuracy; checking for your client's feelings; and checking for nonverbal language both in yourself and in your clients.

- In the client-centered approach, the following skills of questioning are critical to discovery: open or broad question strategy, closed or narrow question strategy, probing strategies, and softening a question.

Chapter 2

Setting Priorities and Measurable Objectives

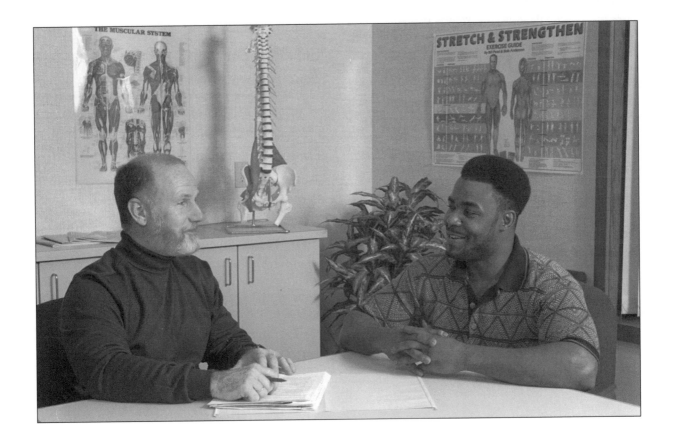

- Counseling to Focus
- Helping Clients Focus on Priorities
- Maximizing Benefits: From Our Client's Perspective
- Goals and Objectives

By careful listening and questioning, we have encouraged our client to tell her story. We have discovered sufficient information and understood her feelings well enough to assemble a history. The counseling process now moves from discovery to focus. The value of the final prescription will depend on how well we empower her to set priorities for her actions—priorities that will satisfy her needs and wants within the limitations of her lifestyle.

Counseling to Focus

Needs are not the same as wants (Trottier 1988). *Needs* originate in human biology and in the human social condition. In the case of our clients, needs are basic requirements related to an injury, a specific weakness in a fitness component, a health risk factor, or some other personal situation such as participation in a sport or a problem with motivation. *Wants* are desires to meet these needs in specific ways; or they are perceptions of value for things that may not be related to needs at all. Wants often determine our clients' choices about how to address their needs; wants, of course, are influenced by social forces. *Lifestyle* includes time, facilities, partners, travel, employment, etc. The areas of overlap—where a need and a want coincide and the lifestyle is compatible—are the areas of the greatest potential for success. It is on these overlapping areas that we should focus.

Figure 2.1 depicts the client history as a Venn diagram showing the "focal" overlap of three primary areas of that history: needs, wants, and lifestyle.

Focus on Needs

Once you feel fairly confident you understand what your client is telling you about her needs, restate your interpretation and ask if it is correct. Word questions in a way that invites an affirmation. For example, "Let me summarize what I understand to be your key needs: _____. Is this accurate?" If your client does not agree or agrees hesitantly, return to your probing for clarification.

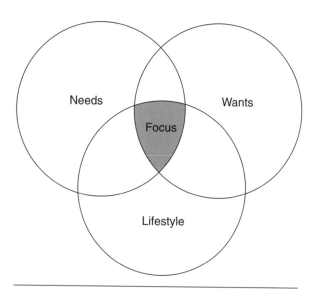

Figure 2.1   The areas of the greatest potential for success are where needs and wants coincide with a compatible lifestyle.

Medical Needs

A questionnaire can identify medical issues and help determine if you need clearance from a health care specialist. Gather information on past medical history, present symptoms, medications, and existing medically prescribed limitations to exercise.

Clients may be quite general in their comments ("I'd like to feel more healthy or have more energy"); or they may be specific ("My doctor says I've got to lower my blood pressure and reduce my cholesterol"). If they believe that exercise will produce the desired health effects and are willing to commit to realistic goals, these health needs will be effective motivators.

High Risk Needs

Always evaluate coronary heart disease risk factors such as smoking, high blood pressure, obesity, inactivity, and poor diet. Age, previous injuries, or low back pain may present special limitations.

Fitness Component Needs

Starting with a fitness assessment provides an indication of your client's fitness component needs. However, if you first determine the client's priorities—*before* doing the fitness assessment—you will be able to select only those test items that relate to those priorities. The prescription model is flexible, allowing you to loop back and verify needs through selective assessment. No matter when it is done, fitness assessment is a vital source of information for both writing the prescription and monitoring progress.

Self-Esteem Needs

Good self-esteem can help people adopt more healthful lifestyles. Physical self-esteem needs may include how a client feels about his appearance, his perception of personal skill levels, or his realistic expectations of an ideal self (CSEP 1996). The value of physical activity for mental health is widely recognized (Quinney et al. 1994).

Motivation to continue physical activity usually comes from the sheer pleasure of the experience. But positive feelings about oneself as an active, fit person can also be powerful motivators.

Special Design Needs

Special design needs include

- specific equipment (e.g., special shoes or orthotics needed for running),
- focus on a specific sport or skill for training (e.g., energy systems and anatomical demands), and

■ limitations of the venue or facility (e.g., the lack of resistance equipment in a home program may require bi-weekly visits to the Y).

Educational or Informational Needs

Whether a client actually changes his lifestyle often depends on well-timed sharing of specific information. Literature is readily available for exercise and diabetes or asthma, and a compendium for medications is a valuable resource. Referrals to clinics specializing in hyperlipidemia, hypertension, or obesity can provide credible supplements to exercise guidance.

Special Motivational Needs

Depending on their reasons for participation and their stage of change, clients may have specific motivational needs. Your strategies can include self-testing, logging, supervision, and support systems. I recently had a client returning to exercise after almost 15 years. At that earlier time he had religiously followed the Cooper aerobics point-based exercise system, and wanted to use it again with the new equipment in our facility. Using the physiological value of an "aerobic point," I prescribed a program of cardiovascular cross-training that allowed him to continue using a system of motivation with which he was comfortable.

Focus On Wants

Wants relate to clients' preferences. They may include what your clients enjoy, their special interests, or their expectations or aspirations. Marketing trends and other societal influences shape your clients' wants, which in turn will affect the way you address their needs.

To focus on your clients' wants, you need to examine their activity preferences, interests, and expectations:

■ **Activity preferences.** You may want to present clients with a list of possible activities and ask them to check which ones they most enjoy. They may also enjoy a particular method of training, type of equipment, training partner, or location.

■ **Special interests.** Clients may be interested in something old or new, a specific challenge, or background information.

■ **Expectations.** The desire for a more muscular body or one with less fat brings huge numbers of people to the doors of fitness clubs and exercise specialists. But be careful not to encourage the pursuit of the fashion industry

ideal. The desire to change body image and appearance can be positive, but you must exploit that desire responsibly by helping your client establish realistic goals.

Let's pursue a number of questions that we may use to probe your client's "wants". You can use the form on page 16 for gathering the necessary information.

Elements of a healthy life style include a positive attitude toward self and others, a love of life, and the practice of healthy habits. But circumstances such as economic status, educational background, cultural or ethnic factors, and home or work environment may make it difficult to adopt a healthy lifestyle. You must develop a sense of empathy and good problem-solving skills in order to find practical ways to help clients change lifestyles.

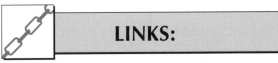

LINKS:

Convenience Brings Compliance

A new employee learns of a small fitness center in her building. She almost never used her previous club membership because of its inconvenience. She wants to "tone-up" and lose some weight, but the center has only resistance machines and one bike, and cycling holds limited attraction for her. She has slightly elevated blood lipids and some motivational needs. Where do her needs, wants, and lifestyle *overlap*?

Working out at her place of employment should ensure better compliance. A "workout buddy" would provide additional support. This client will benefit from a special program design. If the machines using large body parts are set up in a circuit with low resistance and high reps (see chapter 7, Circuit Training, page 101) and every other station is designed as an aerobic calisthenic, the training results should include weight loss, muscular endurance, and re-duced blood lipids (Goldfine et al. 1991).

Her needs, wants, and lifestyle may change; but for the time being she must feel good about her start in the corporate fitness center.

Helping Clients Focus on Priorities

Our clients usually have several concerns, and we must help them establish which is to be dealt with first.

WHAT DOES THE CLIENT WANT?

Activity preferences

What mode of training (e.g., jog, cycle, hike, ski) do you prefer? _____

_____

What method of training (e.g., interval or continuous) do you prefer? _____

_____

Do you prefer group or personal training? _____

_____

Do you enjoy competitive or non-competitive activities? _____

_____

What type of location do you prefer? _____

_____

What is your favorite type of equipment? _____

_____

What aspects of a past prescription did you enjoy? _____

_____

Is there anything in your type or level of current activity that you want to maintain?

_____

_____

Special interests

Do you have any current or past skills that you want to pursue? _____

_____

Do you want more information or resources on particular activities, health, or lifestyle
topics? _____

_____

Do you definitely want to avoid anything? _____

_____

Are you interested in accomplishing something specific or being challenged?

_____

_____

Are you looking for something new or some variety in your prescription?

_____

_____

Expectations

Do you have any objectives that are particularly important? _____

_____

How will we know when you have reached your objective (be specific about measurable areas of improvement)? _____

_____

Are there major behaviors that you wish to change (e.g., eating habits)? _____

_____

Do you have expectations for changes in a medical condition? _____

_____

Do you have any performance or sport-specific expectations? _____

_____

Do you want to know your status or improvement with respect to population standards, or in comparison with your own previous efforts? _____

_____

Can you set priorities for your expectations? _____

_____

FOCUS ON LIFESTYLE

One way to adjust lifestyle is by altering daily routines to encourage more exercise. Which of the following aspects of the client's lifestyle can you target in order to provide the best prescription?

_____ current work routine

_____ current leisure routine

_____ most convenient times

_____ most convenient facility/location

_____ most convenient equipment

_____ other family members and their agendas

_____ degree of support (including child care)

_____ ability to be independent or to work with others

_____ ability to balance a hectic pace

_____ need for structure

_____ ability to make exercise a regular habit

_____ high risk lifestyle habits (other than exercise)

_____ ethnic variances to lifestyle

_____ personality type and learning style

_____ time management: "fitting it in"

_____ positive vs. negative forces regarding exercise

_____ cost/payment options

_____ special considerations (e.g., rehab, seasonal changes, emerging factors, etc.)

For example, if an overweight office worker comes to us suffering from hypertension, stress, and muscular tension, we may need to address his work environment before becoming too specific with an exercise prescription.

It is our task to help clients see the issues before them in more focused and concrete ways. Clients will see priorities as important if they can picture the benefits and imagine what things will be like once their underlying need is met. The final commitment to action will be based on clear analysis of the benefits of your prescription. It is your job to provide this clear analysis.

Our Priorities vs. Our Clients' Priorities

You must not confuse what is important to you with what is important to your clients. For example, not everyone places the same priority on fitness that you do, and you cannot expect all of your clients to immediately buy into your enthusiasm for exercise. For many people, four 30-minute workouts at 60%-85% $\dot{V}O_2$max is too much to add into a hectic week. For these clients, suggest less demanding alternatives that will still result in significant improvements.

The Benefits of Alternatives

DeBusk, et al. (1990) examined an alternative to the traditional prescription. They showed that three 10-minute jogging workouts a day, five days a week for eight weeks at moderate intensity increased $\dot{V}O_2$max by 8% in healthy middle-aged men. Another group, who performed the standard 30-minute jogging workout, increased their $\dot{V}O_2$max by 14%. More vigorous exercise is not necessary for initial conditioning in more sedentary clients.

How Do We Focus on What Counts?

You must define the important issues in your clients' histories. You can help them identify the right priorities by using two techniques: "summarizing" and "clarification."

Summarizing

Judicious summarizing—helping clients combine their thoughts and feelings into a single focus—can enable them to see the "bigger picture," or at least to see their options from a new frame of reference. This new viewpoint can also empower them to make key decisions.

Summaries are particularly useful at certain times. For example, it may seem initially that much of a client's history lies outside your area of focus—yet if you summarize after taking the history, you can emphasize its positive aspects and allow your client to add to or modify what was said.

In the following example, the client (Cl) is a 48-year-old man who has described to the exercise specialist (ES) a number of unsuccessful attempts at regular exercise, and who at this point is quite pessimistic.

(ES): Let's take a look at what we have so far. After almost 20 years of "singles living"—I think those were your words—your body and health are feeling the toll. Most of your married friends have different lifestyles and, as you say, it is a struggle to stay young. Your experiences in school with physical education and sports were not positive and at times embarrassing. In the last three years, you have joined two different health clubs who appeared to welcome you initially, but there was little follow-up assistance. You want to look and feel better, but you appear to have little support.

(Cl): (Pauses) Not a rosy picture, but that about sums it up. Maybe I wasn't thinking straight for a while, but until lately, I haven't wanted to stop and look at my situation. Maybe the time has come for a serious change. I do feel anxious that I need to turn things around.

(ES): One way of doing that is to take a look at what you have accomplished and enjoyed in the last few years. Let's work together on a general vision of where you would like to be, and we can build on these things as we create some short-term objectives.

This client, during the exploratory phase of the history taking, revealed some frustration and even despair about his condition and his past experiences. The summary provided by the exercise specialist not only stated the facts, but also suggested an approach to turn things around one step at a time. This helped refocus the client's feelings.

Clarification

Particularly if an issue is complex, you need to determine which aspect of the issue has the highest priority. For example, your client's lack of commitment and poor time management have led to a number of failed starts on a diet and exercise program. Through a combination of careful listening, empathetic responding, and judicious probing, you help her realize that her efforts have been scattered with no clear action plans or measurable outcomes. The client, seeing the problem more rationally, is now in a position to generate possible solutions or at least to make a genuine commitment to find solutions.

Clarify, Don't Interpret

Clarification involves exploring your clients' feelings as well as behaviors. By clarifying emotions, you help clients understand them. It is important that you catch the meaning of a message without interpreting or analyzing the meaning. The following two responses illustrate this difference:

(Cl): The XYZ Club said they would do a fitness assessment and design a personalized program for me. They took a few measurements and gave me the same program card as everyone.

(ES response #1): Do you feel cheated and angry that they have not provided the services they promised?

(ES response #2): So you think you were ripped-off for your money and feel embarrassed that you were taken in by the club.

Response #1 reflects what the client said and clarifies the feelings of the client. By clarifying the client's feelings, the exercise specialist has begun to establish empathy and is in a better position to understand what the client wants. Response #2 may be true, but it is not what the client said and may not be an accurate interpretation of how he feels. It is critical that the client feels understood, not analyzed.

Many clients will say they are displeased with an aspect of their health, fitness, or well-being; but when you try to clarify their feelings, the responses are vague or ambiguous. There is no single correct way to verify their exact feelings. For some clients, your subsequent conversation will build the trust that is essential before they will make a commitment. Other clients, however, are very solution-oriented: if they see something amiss, they want to fix it right away. Using the wrong approach may lead to failure and a frustrated, inactive client. In his bestseller, *Men Are From Mars, Women Are From Venus*, Dr. John Gray suggests that such differences are sometimes gender specific. Don't assume anything, but be aware that your method of clarification must be client-centered.

Clarification as the Bridge to Commitment

The first challenge is to get your clients to clarify the issues before them; the second is to have them commit to appropriate plans of action. The process of clarification can help them determine what needs to be changed and have them poised to move forward.

In the following example, a young woman talks to her exercise specialist about her difficulties with her weight. The specialist helps the client clarify how she feels about her weight.

(Cl): My problem is that I am overweight. I just don't like how I look.

(ES): How does this make you feel?

(Cl): I'm frustrated with myself and embarrassed . . . It just makes me so angry because I do more to watch my weight than a lot of my skinny friends!

(ES): You sound disappointed by the results of your efforts to lose weight.

(Cl): Yeah . . . but I don't know what to do about it.

(ES): The causes of overweight are different for different people. Could you tell me why you think you have put on the weight?

(Cl): Well, I don't think I eat that badly, but I've never been very active. I think it has been my avoidance of exercise that is the main reason.

(ES): So, regular exercise causes you some difficulty. Any examples of an attempt that has gone astray?

(Cl): Yes, I bought an exercise bike last year and used it regularly for three weeks, but after about six weeks it was out in the garage. I got bored easily, and the seat was very uncomfortable.

(ES): You want to do something about your weight, but stationary cycling didn't keep your interest. Besides biking what sort of other exercise choices do we have?

(Cl): Well, I don't like sports or jogging, but I like to walk if the scenery is pleasant or I'm with a friend. I'm pretty much a homebody in the winter except to walk the dog, but I like to garden in the nicer weather. I have been thinking about buying an exercise video.

(ES): Oh, great ideas! We've come a long way. That is a good list that we can work from. Which do you think are the most likely combination of choices from that list that you can see yourself doing on a regular basis?

The exercise specialist established early trust by avoiding judgment and premature advice. The specialist's reflective listening, probes, and clarification helped the client get a clearer picture of the problem. The specialist then moved into the analysis step of decision making. We leave the pair as they are about to select the best combination of options (priorities) and the most effective strategy for achieving those priorities.

Maximizing Benefits: From Our Client's Perspective

Because health and fitness comprise so many dimensions, we often are faced with the problem of where to start. Most people wrongly set priorities in terms of comfort—that is, they are concerned with experiencing less effort, risk, and pain, and they want things to go smoothly (Egan 1990). We, however, should set priorities for the biggest benefits, where the resources of both parties are invested for a reasonable return.

How Do We Set Priorities That Make a Difference in Our Client's Life?

Your client has come for guidance and consultation. She has expectations but is looking to you for help with a plan that will produce results. What is most important? What should you tackle first? What will make a difference in her life?

The following three principles can serve as guidelines to help you set those priorities:

- Begin with client concerns.
- Choose manageable issues that can show improvement.
- Highlight the client's health concerns.

Begin With Client Concerns

Begin with concerns (needs or wants or lifestyle issues) that the client sees as important. You may feel that her focus should be broadened; but beginning at this point will send an important message: "Your interests matter to me."

For example, a sedentary client with elevated blood lipids wants to start a weight training program to tone up. You soon see that she is more interested in her appearance than in the health issue. For the present, however, you address the client's chief concern: with appropriate prescription precautions and monitoring, she begins light weight training. Later you will look for opportunities to address the lipid problem.

Choose Manageable Issues That Can Show Improvement

If you first help your client manage a relatively simple prescription, the reinforcement he experiences may empower him to attack more difficult tasks. Clear and measurable results that show up early in the training can magnify commitment. Intervention and monitoring (chapters 7 and 11) provide feedback, and help the client to focus on his gains.

For example, Jay, a young athlete, is brought to you by his parents. He is part of an active family with a very full agenda. Jay enjoys sports, but his parents have noticed some fatigue and anxiety about meeting all his obligations, including doing homework and spending time with friends. Your first conversation with Jay is about how he manages all the demands on his time. You identify the areas where he is doing well, and also those that show a lack self-discipline. He enjoys "checking off" accomplishments and seeing progress. You suggest that Jay maintain a monthly calendar that lists all his sports activities, school assignments, and blocks of free time when he could schedule in advance to have his friends come over. You also give Jay's parents a list of symptoms of overtraining for which they are to be watchful.

Highlight the Client's Health Concerns

Consider seriously any health issues the client wants to change. Determine the client's primary goal: overall fitness, performance-related fitness (e.g., for athletic competition), or health-related fitness (chapter 6). If he is open to modifying his behavior in any health-related area, cautiously seize the opportunity. He may expect immediate and tangible results, however, so educate him while still sympathizing with his impatience.

For example, effective screening will reveal any cardiovascular or metabolic problems the client may have. If necessary, work closely with other health care practitioners and consider other "lifestyle" approaches (e.g., diet, reducing stress, eliminating smoking, etc.) along with the exercise prescription. Many clients with fitness or performance goals have a limiting musculoskeletal problem. Determine the stage of the injury, its seriousness, and the original or ongoing cause. Address this hurdle first or at least in parallel with other prescriptions. Chapter 14, "Exercise Prescription for Injury Recovery and Prevention," is a valuable resource for such clients.

Moving the Client From Choice to Commitment

Value is determined by your clients, not by you. Value is the consumers' estimate of the service's capacity to satisfy what they need and want (Trottier 1988). Most exercise specialists know well the positive effects of exercise. But clients select their program priorities based on the benefits they see from their own perspective ("What does it do for me?" [Weylman 1995]). The challenge is knowing how to describe benefits in a way that will clearly demonstrate their value to clients. Benefits become valuable to your clients when they fill the clients' needs and wants.

Come Up With Options

Analysis involves processing the information to best suit the client. During this phase, you discuss with your client the possible choices and the consequence of each.

For example, a client wants to develop a flatter stomach and increased muscular support for a lower back problem, all in a home program (lifestyle). After brainstorming with the client, you present her with the following prescription choices:

- Perform sit-ups.
- Reduce body weight and body fat.
- Stretch muscles that pull the back into lordosis.
- Join an aerobics or aquafit class specializing in abdominal work.
- Use a video that teaches abdominal exercises and/or prevention of low back problems.
- Perform a variety of abdominal strengthening exercises.

- Introduce sitting abdominal exercises at her work desk or standing exercises at the bus stop.
- Do a short routine before bed each night and first thing in the morning.

Analyze the Options

The next step is to weigh or rank the options. You can eliminate some options immediately because they are impractical or do not meet criteria required by the client. Your client may discard the aquafit class suggestion, for example, because it cannot be done at home. Working with your client, you rank the rest of the options according to interest, time, availability, etc.

One way to analyze options is to make a simple table (see table 2.1) that clearly describes the benefits of any given feature.

Lead the Client to Commitment

Finally, help your client commit to an action based on the analysis—select the highest priority, the best combination of options, and the most effective strategy for your client at this time. For example, the client above may choose to work at home with a prescription that includes stretching the back muscles, a variety of abdominal strengthening exercises, and some aerobic work to burn calories. You can also provide a list of appropriate home videos to provide variety in the workouts.

A cautionary note: At this crucial point of commitment and implementation, a host of things can happen to challenge this rational process. Guard against these potential pitfalls:

- Skipping or ignoring the analysis stage and moving quickly to a decision.

Table 2.1   Describing the Benefits of a Prescription Feature

FEATURE	BENEFITS
The prescription is designed to suit the space and equipment within your home	• suits your busy schedule • no time wasted waiting for equipment or commuting • less expensive in the long run • will produce desired results • provides a personalized approach • your space and equipment allow you to circuit train

- "Defensive avoidance" (Egan 1990); that is, rationalizing a delay in choice or commitment.
- Seizing upon a comfortable short-term option.
- Being swayed by a highly recommended or popular course of action.
- Pushing before the client is ready to change a lifestyle habit (see discussion of stages of change in chapter 1, including table 1.1).
- Translating the decision into action half-heartedly.

Goals and Objectives

Goals provide visualization of a future outcome. The history, assessment results, and priorities of one of my clients centered around cardiovascular improvement. Her goal was "to feel less tired and to last longer when doing aerobic activities." That specific goal permitted me to propose specific objectives, and to describe the desired outcome more precisely. Objectives are action-oriented. They tell how well and under what conditions the outcome should be performed. One objective for my client was "to complete 10 walk-jog sessions within three weeks at her training heart rate, increasing her duration by 10% each week." Working in small, measurable chunks gives people more frequent successes in the journey to their goal.

The Importance of Goals

Goals are broad, general (usually long term) statements that describe overall intentions (Strachan and Kent 1985). They translate priorities into action. Working with your clients to write the goals down, you clarify your own thinking and make sure that you are using the same vocabulary as your clients use. The act of writing down goals sometimes triggers a design idea that opens up new ways of approaching a problem.

Helping clients develop goals can have a number of advantages (Egan 1990):

- It can focus attention. Clients with clear goals are less likely to engage in aimless behavior, such as walking down a row of weight machines wondering which one to try.
- Setting goals mobilizes energy and effort. It is not just a mental exercise but often arouses in clients a need to act.
- Setting goals seems to increase persistence. Clients with clear goals work harder and don't give up as easily.
- Setting goals motivates clients to search for strategies to accomplish them.

How Do You Write an Effective Goal?

Write each priority as a goal statement that includes an action verb. For example:

- To lose weight and body fat.
- To improve my poling action in cross-country skiing.
- To reduce my blood pressure.

Try this simple checklist to judge the quality of each of your client's goals:

____ Is it a broad statement based on a single priority?

____ Does it describe the client's intentions?

____ Is it easy to understand?

____ Is it good for the client's overall health?

Moving Beyond Goals to Measurable Objectives

The vagueness of many goals makes them easy to ignore. "I'm going to become more active this year" is a common New Year's resolution, yet it rarely leads to action. People need specificity. Ask the question, "What will you be doing or what will be different when you make the change?" The answer may be, "I'm going to spend three days a week in an exercise class at my health club and ride my bike to work each day." Notice how specific this statement is. It describes a pattern of behavior that will be put in place, not a vague concept of greater activity.

A goal is often defined by a series of objectives that break the strategies down into a number of distinct and sometimes progressive steps. Here are some sample objectives:

Goal: To learn more about my personal diet.

Objectives:

1. To attend a weekly seminar this semester and keep a binder of all the course notes.
2. To have my diet analyzed before and after the course and calculate the improvements.

Goal: To improve my ability to work with free weights.

Objectives:

1. To attend a second program demonstration session next week with my exercise specialist to get personal feedback.

2. To ask my friend, who has more experience, to be a training partner one day per week.

3. To keep a training log that records my performance and my subjective feelings of improvement.

How Do You Write a Good Objective?

Objectives provide the specific directions that make goal statements a reality. They are precise statements of specific commitments to produce measurable results. The structure of an objective includes

1. **outcome**—what your client will do and how success will be measured, and
2. **activity**—the action(s) taken to accomplish the outcome.

Here's an example of an objective: "to run three days a week, adding 5 minutes to the length of my run each week, until I am running 40 minutes non-stop." The *activity* is running three days a week. The successful *outcome* is being able to run 40 minutes straight.

Setting objectives can take as little as 10 minutes and can provide an improved awareness of your client's "future vision."

A simple technique recommended by experts in the field of self-improvement is the SMART system of creating objectives (CSEP 1996; Francis 1990). In this system, exercise objectives have five criteria. They must be

- specific,
- measurable,
- accomplishment-oriented,
- realistic, and
- timed.

Use SMART to help clients develop objectives that have some probability of success. For one client, this may mean focusing on being clear and specific. You may help one client devise a way to measure improvement, and another to develop realistic time frames. Most clients need some help with at least one of the five criteria. SMART not only helps to devise objectives, it also provides a menu for intervention.

Specific

Objectives should be clear and specific enough to drive action. Effective use of questioning, probing, and paraphrasing can help your client articulate the level of specificity he needs in order to act.

A client whose goal is to get in shape, but who does not state for what reason or in what component area(s), makes it impossible to for you to prescribe an exercise program—let alone be client-centered. By contrast,

the goal of "running 40 minutes non-stop" is a specific and measurable outcome.

Measurable

For many clients, being able to measure progress is an important incentive. If the objective is not specifically measurable, how will the client know when it is accomplished? Always have your clients ask themselves, "What will I be doing or what will be different when I make the change?"

You can easily measure many specific exercise objectives. For example, you can selectively assess changes in cardiovascular fitness, body composition, strength and endurance, flexibility, posture and muscle balance, and performance-related fitness. Conducting fitness assessments and providing periodic evaluations are two important motivational strategies known to help improve exercise compliance (Francis 1990).

Not all objectives, however, are easy to measure. It is difficult to objectively quantify a goal such as, "To feel better about exercising." Outcomes should be verifiable in some way. One suggestion is to construct a rating scale from 1-10, with 1 representing the poorest and 10 the best (Clark and Clark 1993). The client estimates where on the scale he thinks he is at a given time, and logs any trends. Another method is to describe, in advance, what is meant or implied by the objective. For example, your client who wants to feel better about exercise might verify this accomplishment if he ". . . looked forward to each workout; saw activity as a break in the day; enjoyed the social aspect of the activity, and felt much more relaxed and energized after exercise . . ." If you can't quantify, measure, rate, or otherwise describe an objective, then you should forget it, because your client will never be able to attain it!

Accomplishment-Oriented

Help clients state objectives in terms of outcomes or accomplishments. It helps if a client can visualize each accomplishment. "I want to start doing some exercise" is a non-specific activity, whereas, "Within six months, I will be running three miles in less than 30 minutes at least four times a week" is a specific outcome that your client can visualize. Stating objectives as accomplishments helps a client avoid leaping into action without knowing where she is going. Gently probing for outcomes encourages her not just to work hard but also to work SMART.

Realistic

Many people quit exercising because they are disillusioned when their program fails to accomplish the anticipated results. The exercise objective might have been unrealistic to begin with. An objective is realistic if

- the resources necessary for its accomplishment are available (exercise non-compliance is often related to inconvenience of location or inaccessibility of equipment),
- it is under the client's control (her genetic background may never allow her to look like a thin fashion model), and
- it has a high priority (i.e., it is something your client wants to do because it will satisfy her most important needs in a way that accommodates her lifestyle) (Egan 1990).

An objective is most realistic when these three elements coincide. Objectives are unrealistic if they are set too high, but they are inadequate if they are set too low. They must be relevant to the goal, painting a manageable picture of what success looks like while challenging the client.

Use the SMART criteria as a checklist to evaluate the objectives below.

___ specific ___ measured ___ accomplished
___ realistic ___ timed

Goal: To improve my cardiovascular fitness.

Objective(s):

1. To walk briskly in the evenings for 40 minutes, four days per week.

2. To monitor weekly my time and heart rate over a measured distance and to have my CV fitness remeasured at three and six months—targeting a 10% increase every three months.

S ___ Walk for CV fitness improvement

M ___ Forty minutes, four days/wk; duration, heart rate, and distance monitored

A ___ Ten percent increase in fitness every three months.

R ___ Accomplishment has been demonstrated repeatedly in research and in personal experience; commitment and resources of the client are unknown.

T ___ Ten percent improvement every three months for one-half year is a realistic time frame.

Timed

A timed objective provides a powerful motivation for following an exercise program. To set realistic target dates, consider each objective from a time perspective.

An objective can be long-term (several years) or short-term (perhaps within a day). Losing 25 pounds in four months may be realistic, but a short-term objective of losing 1.5 pounds per week may seem more manageable. Short-term objectives, successfully completed early in your client's program, can start a cycle of challenge and achievement that enhances his self-confidence.

The Objective-Setting Worksheet on page 26 is designed to guide the process of setting objectives following the SMART criteria.

Highlights

- Needs originate in human biology and in the human condition. Wants are desires to meet needs in specific ways. Lifestyle factors include time, facilities, partners, travel, employment, etc. We focus on the areas of overlap, where a need and a want coincide and the lifestyle is compatible, for these hold the greatest potential for success.

- Client **needs** may be related to medical, high risk, educational, or motivational factors; they also can be defined by results of fitness assessments, by lack of self-esteem, or by special designs necessitated because of physical limitations.

- **Wants** relate to our clients' areas of enjoyment, their interests, expectations, and aspirations; wants are often influenced by social factors.

- **Lifestyle** factors such as economic status, education, cultural or ethnic background, and home/work environment may make it difficult to maintain optimal patterns of exercise or diet.

- Setting priorities helps clients determine what should be changed. It involves

  1. **focusing** on what our clients want to do that will satisfy their most important needs within the boundaries of their lifestyles;

  2. **summarizing** to help them explore problems in a more focused and concrete way;

  3. **clarifying** their feelings and behaviors;

  4. **setting priorities** according to their importance in improving the clients' health; and

OBJECTIVE-SETTING WORKSHEET

Goal #1:	
Objective: 1	Time:
Success Indicators:	
___ Specific ___ Measured ___ Accomplished ___ Realistic ___ Time	
Objective: 2	Time:
Success Indicators:	
___ Specific ___ Measured ___ Accomplished ___ Realistic ___ Time	
Objective: 3	Time:
Success Indicators:	
___ Specific ___ Measured ___ Accomplished ___ Realistic ___ Time	

5. **differentiating choices** in terms of features (what they are), and benefits (what they mean to the client).

- **Choice** involves selecting the highest priority, the best combination of options, and the most effective strategy for your client at this time.

- **Goals** are broad, usually long-term statements of overall intentions. Goals focus clients' attention, mobilize their efforts, and increase their persistence; when clients have concrete goals, they tend to search for strategies to accomplish them.

- **Objectives** emerge from a goal, describing its outcome more precisely. Objectives are action-oriented and tell how well and under what conditions the outcome should be achieved. The structure of an objective includes the *outcome* (what the client will do and the measure of success) and *activity* (the action(s) taken to accomplish the outcome). Exercise objectives have five criteria (SMART): They should be Specific, Measurable, Accomplishment-oriented, Realistic, and Timed.

Chapter 3

Client-Centered Motivation: Case Studies

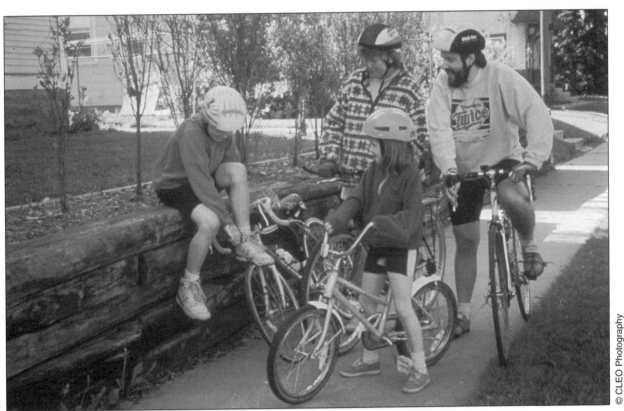

© CLEO Photography

- Determining Clients' Motivators
- Linking Compliance With Real Life
- Motivation and Commitment
- Case Study #1: Motivating a New Client
- Case Study #2: Motivating an Intermittent Exerciser

We can cajole, encourage, or threaten, but in the long run clients become active only because they think it is good for them. They will stick with it because they enjoy it and believe they are achieving something. The heart of effective motivation is learning what drives a particular client at a particular time.

Determining Clients' Motivators

Motivation is a dynamic process. When we initially create exercise programs, we must assess our clients' motivational status from their point of view.

Questions to Ask Yourself

Begin by asking yourself the following questions:

1. **Is the client a beginner or an advanced exerciser?** Beginners need more intervention to be certain that they clearly understand the program, and to insure their safety. Beginning adults may fear looking foolish as they learn new tasks, and they may be uncomfortable taking risks. Are there opportunities for the client to feel successful immediately? Advanced exercisers may just want to change their program, and they feel comfortable continuing by themselves; or they may have hired a personal trainer to provide regular motivation.

2. **What are the client's specific goals?** These may already be clearly stated by the client, or they may be goals you have picked up from interactions with the client. Consider, for example, mastery of a skill: have parameters been included for the client to determine his level of success? Or social interaction: will you be present for each session, or does the program include ending at a local coffee shop? Or family approval: does the program include family as well as individual activities? Or health benefits: are these measurable as part of the program design?

3. **Is the client motivated intrinsically or extrinsically?** Clients tend to have a preference for either intrinsic or extrinsic motivators. If you pay careful attention during assessment stages, you will pick up on the client's preference (see chapter 2 for additional information).

4. **Is the program designed to stand alone?** Are specific progressions included on the prescription? Can the client record data on the written prescription, such as heart rate or energy level? This would provide immediate, visual feedback.

5. **What are you realistically able to provide?** Consider your own needs regarding commitments of time, energy, finances, and emotions as you plan a follow-up system.

Potential Motivators

For most programs to be successful, you must understand how best to motivate your client. You may find it helpful to use a combination of intrinsic and extrinsic motivators.

Potential intrinsic and extrinsic motivators include the following:

- **Motivation through supervision** (e.g., a personal trainer, or staff monitoring within a facility). This is the most effective because it involves personal contact.
- **Motivation through a partner.** If the partner is reliable, the ongoing commitment is very helpful. People are more likely to exercise if they know someone is waiting for them.
- **Motivation through music.** If your client enjoys the music, it may help to prolong his energy during a cardiovascular workout.
- **Motivation through a phone call.** If your client knows you will be calling, he may work out just so he can honestly tell you he did it.
- **Increased knowledge through reading monthly publications or specific related articles.** Knowing good reasons for exercise and for correct diet may encourage your client to make additional changes in his lifestyle. Some of your clients will be very interested in the technical side of the exercise process.
- **Scheduled time for a retest and program modification.** If your client knows you will be retesting him in three weeks, it may encourage him to continue faithfully with the program.
- **Visual recording.** Some clients will want to see concrete changes attributable to their fitness programs. For example, your client may want to see if his heart rate is decreasing with the same amount of work over a period of two months.

Ask your clients how they are motivated, and what kind of rewards they are most likely to want. Show them the list above to give them an idea of some options.

Linking Compliance With Real Life

Table 3.1 suggests some client-centered approaches to increasing adherence.

When clients are not compliant with your exercise prescriptions, review their behavior over the previous weeks. In a non-threatening manner, ask them why they are not following the program. Listen carefully to what they tell you. Here are some questions to ask yourselves as well as your client:

Table 3.1   Client-Centered Strategies for Improving Adherence

CLIENT INFORMATION	CLIENT-CENTERED STRATEGIES
• Smokers have difficulty sticking with exercise	• Give permission to feel winded and less energized after exercise • Avoid making smoking a big issue, but have literature available
• Overweight clients may have to struggle harder and may have unrealistic expectations about what can be accomplished	• Be honest and help client form realistic goals • Provide monitoring techniques that clearly show their progress • Avoid positive feedback that is undeserved, but look for opportunities for progress recognition • Social support systems such as 'buddies' or a personal trainer are often helpful if good rapport is present
• A client's personality problems or mood may affect attendance	• Don't assume that you are responsible for how your clients feel or that they often miss sessions due to mood disturbances
• Improvement of health is often given as a reason for initiating exercise	• Point out the specific health benefits that may be expected from their type of prescription • Screening tools (e.g., PAR-Q or FANTASTIC) can assure clients they are ready for exercise and increase their health-related awareness
• Clients need to be aware of the benefits and costs of their fitness program	• Help your clients list the benefits they hope to experience and also the inconveniences and difficulties they may encounter. Discuss how they will deal with these
• Satisfaction with you as an exercise specialist is an important issue for many clients	• Seek your clients' input on many aspects of goal setting, techniques of training, variations in routines, satisfaction, etc. • Personal one-on-one feedback can work both ways: to your clients and from them • Your support and availability will affect attendance
• Clients often have trouble getting past common road blocks	• Project PACE (Patrick, et al. 1994), a new physician-based assessment and counseling for exercise programs, suggests the following responses: a) If time is the barrier: "We're only talking about three thirty-minute sessions each week. Can you do without three television shows a week?" b) If enjoyment is a problem: "Don't exercise. Start a hobby or an enjoyable activity that gets you moving." c) If exercise is boring: "Listening to music during your activity keeps your mind occupied. Walking, biking, or running can take you past lots of interesting scenery."

- Does the program meet her specific needs? Does the client clearly understand the link between your prescription and her goals?

- Is the program at an appropriate level for her current levels of fitness and self-esteem?

- Has the client grown in her understanding? What is her stage in the learning process?

- Is the program's time frame realistic?

- Has there been a change in the client's life (work or home)? Are the changes appropriate to the priorities you've set?

- Are the program and follow-up consistent with the client's preferred reinforcement system?

- Have rewards been delayed because results are not immediate? Were there too many rewards initially, and too few now? Is the client inclined toward intrinsic or extrinsic rewards?

We initially assume that our clients have good intentions to start or maintain an exercise program. There will be times, however, when they discontinue the program for various reasons. We may hear a wide range of excuses.

I recall a female client who worked outside the home and had two children ages six and eight. She had a low estimation of her physical capabilities and had even expressed doubts about her need to exercise. She exercised with me two times a week for three weeks, but did not work out at all during the fourth week. Her reason was that she had deadlines at work. On the weekend I happened to meet her in the neighborhood park. She gave me the following reasons for stopping her exercise program. Determine how you would respond to them.

1. I want to exercise, but by the time 5:00 quitting time comes around, I am not able to leave. I have too many things left to do.

2. I don't have the time. I have too many other responsibilities: I work, I have to do grocery shopping, pick up the kids, take them to lessons, help with their homework, cook dinner, make lunches . . . Get the picture?

3. It will take too long to make a dent in my weight gain. I am so heavy, why even bother?

Of the reasons cited above, what do you feel is the main issue and how would you address it?

Remember: *program adherence is not an all-or-nothing situation. We need to be flexible to allow for real life.*

Motivation and Commitment

You can expect resistance from your clients when they need to make decisions, and when they need to move from discussion to action. Making decisions and moving into action involve a commitment of the client's physical and psychological resources. There is both the initial commitment to exercise objectives and an ongoing commitment to the full strategy. With the latter, there must be steady progress toward the objectives; but the client must also get up and move forward during lapses.

Several factors can help our clients commit to, then follow through on, their objectives:

- **Ownership.** Make sure the objectives are the client's, not yours. Jogging is still one of the most popular suggestions for a start-up activity. However, it also has the highest attrition rate—particularly when it was someone else's choice.

- **Options.** Provide a choice of activities that can produce similar training results.

- **Reinforcement.** Provide encouragement for any action taken toward the client's objective. Teach clients how to monitor themselves (chapter 7), as this will show them their progress and help build self-confidence.

- **Appeal.** Look for ways to increase the appeal of the exercise program or to change the source of interest. A training partner, new exercises, a change of equipment, even a change of workout time can make the workout more pleasant.

- **Obstacle Management.** Help clients see how to manage disincentives. One of the appeals of personal trainers is the expectation that they will help to remove obstacles, or at least to work around them.

- **Challenge.** Help clients set not just substantive objectives but challenging ones. Small, measurable victories toward an objective can feed the drive to achieve.

- **Contracts.** Use contracts to help clients commit themselves to their choices.

The worksheet on the next page will help guide your clients through a self-contracting process of commitment to their exercise objectives (CSEP 1996).

Working with personal trainers can increase exercise adherence by 40% over a 24 week period (Pronk, Wing, and Jeffery 1994). Trainers have become a primary source of motivation for many clients and a fixture in most fitness centers. To be most effective, a trainer must use motivational techniques that are client-centered—working with the clients, following their

SELF-CONTRACT

1. My physical activity goal is: _____

_____

_____

2. To achieve my goal, I would need to change the following: _____

_____

_____

3. I am willing to do the following to make it happen: _____

_____

_____

4. Others will know about the change I am making when:_____

_____

_____

5. I might sabotage my plan by: _____

_____

_____

6. Therefore, my contract to myself is: _____

_____

_____

7. Check-up dates:_____

_____

_____

Signed: _____

Client

_____

Appraiser

From *The Canadian Physical Activity, Fitness & Lifestyle Appraisal: CSEP's Plan for Healthy Active Living.* Published by the Canadian Society for Exercise Physiology, 1996. p. 8-47. Reprinted by permisison.

priorities and objectives within the context of their lifestyles.

In the two case studies to follow, consider how you would apply appropriate client-centered motivating tactics. It may be helpful to think of yourself in three distinct roles—as a leader, a designer, and as an educator. **Leadership** involves the way in which you approach and support your client. **Design** includes developing creative programs, devising incentives, and meeting goals. **Education** relates to how you provide information in a client-centered way, how you engender feedback, and how you create autonomy in your client.

Case Study #1: Motivating a New Client

Trent was a young, single accountant who had just joined a local club. Audrey worked at the club as a personal trainer and met Trent for the first time during his appointment for an assessment. Audrey sensed some apprehension and so spent time listening carefully until Trent was more comfortable sharing his feelings.

Assessment

"When people come into the center for the first time, Trent, they nearly always feel overwhelmed with the new equipment and protocols. I'll guide you through all of this, and we'll have a chance to talk about each stage of the assessment."

The assessment was a good time to build rapport through the telling of a personal story:

"I really can appreciate how hard it is to make the changes in your lifestyle that you'd like to make. There are many obstacles. I've struggled with some of them myself. When I first came to work at this club, Trent, all the state-of-the-art machines were terribly intimidating. I jumped right into the most intriguing ones. They were appealing, but very specific to individual muscle groups. What we'll do is start with more simple exercises using your own body weight, and each week we'll introduce a new piece of equipment, OK?"

Audrey's feedback during and after the assessment was both specific and encouraging.

(A): I don't very often see someone as flexible as you in the shoulders, Trent—especially when you have such good strength in your pectoralis and other chest muscles.

(T): I didn't realize that these tests provided that degree of detail.

(A): Yes, in fact, your aerobic capacity places you in an above-average category. You scored better than 75% of other men your age.

(T): That's encouraging, but I'm not about to run a marathon tomorrow.

(A): Maybe not, but we'll set some smaller goals that will still be pretty challenging.

Trent had remarked on the professional quality of the test result information. Audrey was pleased at how the test results led to discussion about goals and possible outcomes. In addition to his exercise prescription, Trent was keen to get some squash lessons and to avoid the type of high-intensity running he remembered ten years earlier in high school.

(T): About these goals: I hope you won't be like my high school P.E. teacher—he was brutal!

(A): Well, Trent, the good news is that you'll set your own objectives. I'll help you make them measurable, but the commitment will be to yourself.

(T): I want to be able to finish a squash game as strongly as I started it.

(A): Trent, that's both realistic and challenging. It will help us plan your exercise prescription; and if we monitor your perceived exertion during the squash, we can keep track of your progress.

Because Trent was unfamiliar with the equipment, Audrey scheduled her time to be with him for his entire workouts during the first week. This gave her time to improve Trent's technical skills and to share many personal anecdotes about her own training. At the end of the week, Audrey presented Trent with a club tee shirt and her phone and e-mail numbers in case of problems.

Overcoming Problems

Things went well for a few weeks, but Audrey started to notice that Trent was not out as often. She set up a meeting and learned that Trent's new career was demanding and his commitment to his program was slipping. Recognizing how important the first three months of a new habit are, Audrey helped Trent set up an exercise diary with a copy for his office and one for his refrigerator at home. Trent appreciated a 10%

discount incentive on his squash lessons that Audrey arranged if he checked in with her on his squash days. Audrey also set more short-term objectives that allowed Trent to perceive progress in his program more easily. Trent found a squash partner and now, after one full year of club membership, he meets with Audrey every four months for a fitness assessment or a prescription update.

"Questions to Think About"

- How did Audrey's support of Trent change after the first few weeks?

- What adjustments to Trent's program did Audrey make because of the demands on his time?

- How did feedback in the early encounters differ from that at the end of the year? Was the change necessary?

Case Study #2: Motivating an Intermittent Exerciser

Jane, a single mother of two, had a busy schedule that found her on and off exercise for many years. The community fitness center had asked Tony, an exercise specialist, to work with her because both still played some competitive baseball. Jane was just returning to the center after her second child and wanted to get in shape before the baseball season. Tony realized that Jane's yo-yo pattern of exercise occurred when it was crowded out by her work schedule, home duties, or vacations. She also admitted that her exercise routine would take a downward spiral when she couldn't see any results, it wasn't fun, or it was boring.

Assessment

"I know at times you don't see the type of progress you'd like, but you are very effective when you do come out more regularly. Everyone I work with goes through short relapses for various reasons. I appreciate that it's hard to make an ongoing commitment. I've struggled with this myself. We can take a look at your overall approach to an exercise habit."

Jane always felt that she was taking time from someone or something else when she exercised. Tony started their second meeting by discussing these feelings. He wanted to help Jane realize that slippage in attendance did not imply failure and that the time spent exercising would more than pay back benefits and quality of time to job and family.

"Jane, I've noticed how concerned you are about your family and about the time you spend away from them. I admire your devotion and care. They are rare qualities. Your support and encouragement is important. In working with many single parents, I've found it important to remember that the better care you take of yourself—physically and emotionally—the better you will be able to care for the people you love."

He worked with Jane on some positive self-talk. They developed some questions that highlighted the benefits of regular workouts. Whenever Jane started to feel guilty about taking time to exercise, she reviewed these questions in her mind:

- "How does exercise make me feel later in the day?"

- "How do I feel after completing a workout that I originally had planned to skip?"

- "What are some of the positive feelings I get with a good workout?"

Dealing With Time Commitments

Tony's second approach tackled the problem of not enough time. He introduced Jane to the concept of *active living* whereby, during hectic weeks, she could substitute walking to work, taking the stairs, and doing manual chores for her formal workout. Since Jane's exercise pattern was usually irregular (less than six workouts per month), Tony discussed the benefits of adding only a few more sessions per month, and of slightly increasing the intensity of her workouts.

Knowing that injury can be a major reason for dropping out, Tony adjusted her previous prescription and introduced some interesting cross-training variety in her new program. Subsequent progressions were regular and became more specific to baseball. Jane felt she now had the right attitude and approach to maintain a more regular, healthy, and balanced lifestyle.

Questions to Think About

- What leadership qualities did Tony demonstrate that were well-suited to helping Jane?

- Select one feature of Tony's exercise prescription and explain why it was appropriate for Jane.

- Education is not just learning facts. How did Tony influence Jane's attitude toward regular exercise?

==== **Highlights** ====

- It is not enough to determine what, in your mind, would be the best approach for your client. You must determine how you can motivate your client to aggressively pursue the appropriate goals and behaviors.

- Your exercise prescription must be based on your client's needs as well as her desires. Only in this way will you be able to create the proper motivation that will lead to ongoing compliance with your prescriptions.

PART II
Matching Our Client's Needs

The prescription journey has provided us with a picture of our client's history, needs, and hopes, as well as potential sources of motivation. We have helped our client to clarify priorities by refocusing on what is important.

We are now able to intelligently select assessment items that best match our client's priorities. Without some physiological parameters to set prescription factors or monitor progress, we would be restricted to acting within broad guidelines that are less specific to our client's needs.

By gathering more detailed information through assessment of selected physical fitness components, we will be able to fine-tune the goals, making them measurable and progressive (chapter 2). We will create exercise strategies based in large part on our interpretation of the assessment results.

Chapter 4

Client-Centered Cardiovascular and Body Composition Assessment

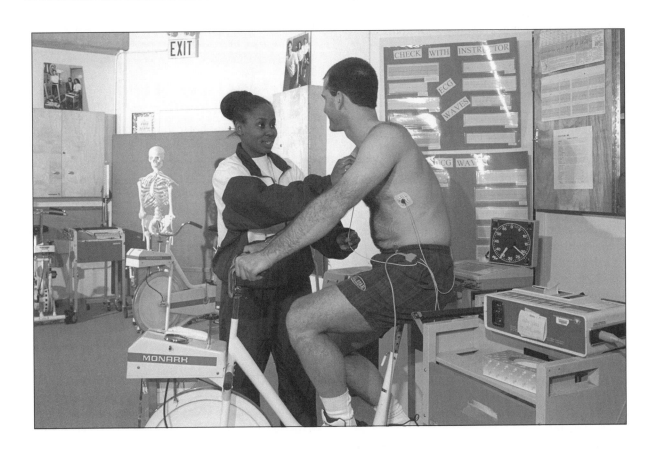

- What Is Client-Centered Assessment?
- Health and Lifestyle Appraisal
- Screening
- Choosing Laboratory or Field-Based Tests
- Cardiovascular Assessment
- Body Composition Assessment

In client-centered assessment, we look for things our clients *want* to do that will satisfy their most important *needs* in ways that compliment or at least accommodate their *lifestyles*. By so doing, we deviate from two rather standard practices: (1) We do not perform assessments before establishing priorities; (2) We do not use a predetermined battery of tests that cover most of the components of fitness. Both of these popular practices appear to be sound, so why would we want to deviate?

What Is Client-Centered Assessment?

First impressions are strong and lasting. If the first thing we do is probe and prod and induce fatigue, clients without good self-esteem may leave with less resolve to change than when they entered. Even if we have established some rapport, we have not taken sufficient time to establish the clients' commitment, to question them carefully, and to focus on their emerging areas of concern.

Test Item Selection

Beginning an exercise prescription with a fitness assessment is a shotgun approach to gathering information about a client's needs. By waiting until you have determined the client's priorities, you can select specific test items that relate to those priorities. Before testing, you should understand your clients' fitness, health, educational needs, and any special needs (chapter 1); you also must learn about their areas of enjoyment, interests, expectations, and specific aspirations. The client-centered prescription model is flexible, allowing you to loop back and verify needs through selected assessment items. It's OK to use certain tests, such as standard screening tools, for all first time clients. But when your client has expressed a specific interest or need, be sure to include test items for that component. There may also be other information you can gather from simple field-based tests that can help you design an initial prescription that best suits your client's capabilities.

Re-test sessions need not include all of the initial test items, especially if you used a generic battery of tests. Select only the components that your client has been working on or those in which you anticipate a change. Accurate monitoring throughout the program can often suffice both to show improvement and to indicate when progressions should be made. This may also decrease the need for regular, formal reassessment in areas such as muscular strength. The closer an assessment comes to simulating your client's training activities, the greater will be the tests' sensitivity and validity.

Every client is at a different stage of readiness to make changes in his or her lifestyle (chapter 1). Learn to view assessment in terms of stages. Many first-time clients will not be ready to move much beyond an initial counseling and lifestyle appraisal: pushing on to a full battery of exhaustive tests can destroy what little motivation they have. On the other hand, athletes after preseason training may be very anxious to challenge their limits.

Case Histories

For each new client, you must learn to determine what should be assessed and how it should be measured. The following examples trace these decisions about assessments. More details about the individual assessments are described throughout the chapter, and you will find further case histories in chapter 9.

Case History #1

Your first client is a 55-year-old man, moderately overweight. He has been doing some outdoor cycling so he is already in an "action" stage of behavioral change (chapter 1). His doctor has recently encouraged him to get more exercise, and so he has come to your fitness center for guidance.

Is any screening necessary? A number of risk factors become evident in the preliminary counseling, so you select a series of items from the health and lifestyle appraisal (e.g., RISK-I and PAR-Q on pages 46 and 47).

Your client has been cycling outdoors. Considering your preferred mode of assessment, a bicycle ergometer has the added advantage of being non-weight bearing, with no balance concerns. Which method of assessment is most appropriate? There is no need to push your client to exhaustion. You want to determine his response to various intensities of cycling. Your selection is a three-stage submaximal bike test (figure 4.3, page 50) with the results graphed, allowing you to estimate his heart rate at a large range of workloads (figure 7.2, page 94).

Since your client's concern about weight is primarily from a health perspective, your choice for body composition is the sum of trunk skinfolds (page 54), an area of fat distribution more directly associated with metabolic disorders. You will relate the results to a health benefits rating.

Case History #2

Your second client is a previously sedentary 33-year-old woman whose main objective is weight loss. She appears to be moving from a preparation stage to an action stage of behavioral change. She has made it clear that she does not want to be poked and prodded with "those fat pinchers."

How do you proceed with this level of reservation? A health and lifestyle appraisal is a non-invasive way to gain useful information and to continue building rapport. The FANTASTIC Lifestyle checklist (page 42) takes a holistic approach to weight management; the Inventory of Lifestyle Needs and Activity Preferences (page 44) gives her some choices.

Can you evaluate body composition without skinfold calipers or invasive equipment? Body Mass Index (BMI) (page 54) utilizes height and weight measures to provide an indication of relative overweight. You can examine the pattern of fat distribution through the waist girth measure (page 54), which in itself is a barometer for improvement.

If no significant health risks exist and your client does not want a formal cardiovascular assessment, do you even need to do an assessment? You can use a Heart Rate Reserve calculation (page 95) to determine your client's training zone based on her age, resting heart rate, and desired training level. If you regularly monitor heart rate and compare it to measures of perceived exertion, you can initiate a safe program.

Health and Lifestyle Appraisal

We need to understand the links between physical activity, health, and physical fitness (chapter 6). It is preferable to assess a client's health status and lifestyle during the early phase of counseling, before other fitness assessments. We also can use this information for pre-assessment screening.

The human body does not function optimally when it is abused. The major causes of disability and death are no longer infectious diseases but rather diseases of lifestyle. Behaviors that contribute to various chronic illnesses include alcohol and drug abuse, smoking, inappropriate diets, and insufficient physical activity. Elements of a healthy lifestyle include positive attitude toward self and others, ability to cope with stress, a zeal for life, and the practice of healthy behaviors. Early recognition of and empathy with our clients' lifestyles helps us set priorities and plan well-rounded fitness programs.

A health risk appraisal or, more positively, a health and lifestyle appraisal may be a client's first step to behavior change. It may be just the extra nudge that a client "preparing" to take some action needs. Its greatest value is as a tool that leads to healthy lifestyle

intervention. Inactivity is so common in many lifestyles that we have a critical role to play as providers and promoters of health care. In the next sections we will examine some sample lifestyle appraisal tools.

FANTASTIC Lifestyle Checklist (Wilson, 1984)

The FANTASTIC Lifestyle Checklist (page 42) allows clients to understand the effects of various habits and attitudes on the health of their lifestyle. Most lifestyle behaviors can be modified: activity, nutrition, tobacco or alcohol use, sleep, stress, and personality. The scoring system provides a straightforward interpretation of associated health benefits. The structure of the Checklist makes it easy to discuss results with clients. The Checklist directs clients to their lifestyle areas that need attention; it also provides tips to help people make the appropriate changes.

Inventory of Lifestyle Needs and Activity Preferences (CSEP 1996)

This Inventory (page 44) helps people identify their three most important lifestyle needs from a list of 35 suggestions. Use the Inventory to help your clients identify activities that will satisfy their three lifestyle needs. This is an excellent counseling tool that can bridge clients to the next stage and help them choose activities that can be part of their prescription.

RISK-I

Risk-I (pronounced risky) can be self-administered and involves selecting the appropriate numerical value in each of the risk categories on the chart (CSEP 1996; Getchell and Anderson 1982; Pollock, Wilmore, and Fox 1978). The first five categories (age, family history, smoking, body mass index, and exercise) are risk factors for coronary heart disease (CHD). The last two categories (back and knees) are areas of musculoskeletal risk. You can use the total score, which represents overall risk, to screen clients toward a medical referral. RISK-I's application is broader than most tools because of the inclusion of the musculoskeletal risk. Although the scoring is not precise, it opens the opportunity to talk to clients about a broad spectrum of issues that may need attention in their exercise prescription. RISK-I

FANTASTIC LIFESTYLE CHECKLIST

Instructions: Unless otherwise specified, place an 'X' beside the box that best describes your behavior or situation in the past month. Explanations of questions and scoring are provided on the next page.

Family Friends	I have someone to talk to about things that are important to me	almost never	seldom	some of the time	fairly often	almost always
	I give and receive affection	almost never	seldom	some of the time	fairly often	almost always
Activity	I am vigorously active for at least 30 min per day (e.g., running, cycling, etc.)	less than once a week	1-2 times/ week	3 times/week	4 times/ week	5 or more times/week
	I am moderately active (gardening, climbing stairs, walking, housework)	less than once a week	1-2 times/ week	3 times/week	4 times/ week	5 or more times/week
Nutrition	I eat a balanced diet (see explanation, page 43)	almost never	seldom	some of the time	fairly often	almost always
	I often eat excess: (1) sugar, or (2) salt, or (3) animal fats, or (4) junk foods	four of these	three of these	two of these	one of these	none of these
	I am within _____ kg of my healthy weight	not within 8 kg (20 lb)	8 kg (20 lb)	6 kg (15 lb)	4 kg (10 lb)	2 kg (5 lb)
Tobacco Toxics	I smoke tobacco	more than 10 times/week	1-10 times/ week	none in the past 6 months	none in the past year	none in the past 5 years
	I use drugs such as marijuana, cocaine	sometimes				never
	I overuse prescribed drugs or 'over the counter' drugs	almost daily	fairly often	only occasionally	almost never	never
	I drink caffeine–containing coffee, tea, or cola	more than 10 times/week	7-10/day	3-6/day	1-2/day	never
Alcohol	My average alcohol intake per week is _____ (see explanation, page 43)	more than 20 drinks	13-20 drinks	11-12 drinks	8-10 drinks	0-7 drinks
	I drink more than four drinks on an occasion	almost daily	fairly often	only occasionally	almost never	never
	I drive after drinking	sometimes				never
Sleep Seatbelts Stress Safe sex	I sleep well and feel rested	almost never	seldom	some of the time	fairly often	almost always
	I use seatbelts	never	seldom	seldom	most of the time	always
	I am able to cope with the stresses in my life	almost never	seldom	seldom	fairly often	almost always
	I relax and enjoy leisure time	almost never	seldom	seldom	fairly often	almost always
	I practice safe sex (see explanation, page 43)	almost never	seldom	seldom	fairly often	always
Type of behavior	I seem to be in a hurry	almost always	fairly often	fairly often	seldom	almost never
	I feel angry or hostile	almost always	fairly often	fairly often	seldom	almost never
Insight	I am a positive or optimistic thinker	almost never	seldom	seldom	fairly often	almost always
	I feel tense or uptight	almost always	fairly often	fairly often	seldom	almost never
	I feel sad or depressed	almost always	fairly often	fairly often	seldom	almost never
Career	I am satisfied with my job or role	almost never	seldom	seldom	fairly often	almost always

Step 1   Total the X's in each column → ☐ ☐ ☐ ☐ ☐

Step 2   Multiply the totals by the numbers indicated (write answers in box below) →   0   ×1   ×2   ×3   ×4

Step 3   Add your scores across bottom for your grand total → ☐ + ☐ + ☐ + ☐ = ☐

Grand total
(see explanation)

Adapted with permission from the "Fantastic Lifestyle Assessments." © 1995, Dr. Douglas Wilson, Department of Family Medicine, McMaster University, Hamilton, Ontario, Canada L8N 3Z5

▼ A balanced diet:

According to Canada's Food Guide to Healthy Eating (for people four years and over):

Different People Need Different Amounts of Food

The amount of food you need every day from the four food groups and other foods depends on your age, body size, activity level, whether you are male or female, and if you are pregnant or breast feeding. That's why the Food Guide gives a lower and higher number of servings for each food group. For example, young children can choose the lower number of servings, while male teenagers can select the higher number. Most other people can choose servings somewhere in between.

Grain products	Vegetables & fruit	Milk products	Meat & alternatives	Other foods
Choose whole grain and enriched products more often.	Choose dark green and orange vegetables more often.	Choose lower fat milk products more often.	Choose leaner meats, poultry and fish, as well as dried peas, beans, and lentils more often.	Taste and enjoyment can also come from other foods and beverages that are not part of the 4 food groups. Some of these are higher in fat or calories, so use these foods in moderation.
recommended number of servings per day:				
5-12	5-10	Children 4-9 yrs: 2-3 Youth 10-16 yrs: 3-4 Adults: 2-4 Pregnant and breast-feeding women: 3-4	2-3	

▼ Alcohol intake:

1 drink equals:

		Canadian	Metric	U.S.
1 bottle of beer	5% alcohol	12 oz.	340.8 ml	10 oz.
1 glass wine	12% alcohol	5 oz.	142 ml	4.5 oz.
1 shot spirits	40% alcohol	1.5 oz.	42.6 ml	1.25 oz.

▼ Safe sex:

Refers to the use of methods of preventing infection or conception.

What does the score mean?

85-100 Excellent	70-84 Very good	55-69 Good	35-54 Fair	0-34 Needs improvement

Note: A low total score does not mean that you have failed. There is always the chance to change your lifestyle—starting now. Look at the areas where you scored a 0 or 1 and decide which areas you want to work on first.

Tips:

❶ Don't try to change all the areas at once. This will be too overwhelming for you.

❷ Writing down your proposed changes and your overall goal will help you to succeed.

❸ Make changes in small steps towards the overall goal.

❹ Enlist the help of a friend to make similar changes and/or to support you in your attempts.

❺ Congratulate yourself for achieving each step. Give yourself appropriate rewards.

❻ Ask your physical activity professional, family physician, nurse, or health department for more information on any of these areas.

Adapted, with permission, from the "Fantastic Lifestyle Assessment," 1985. Dr. Douglas Wilson, Department of Family Medicine, McMaster University, Hamilton, Ontario, Canada L8N 3Z5.

INVENTORY OF LIFESTYLE AND ACTIVITY PREFERENCES

Lifestyle needs

I feel it is important to me to

____ like the people I'm with

____ be in a group

____ be independent

____ get to know other people well

____ meet many new people

____ be a leader

____ feel confident

____ learn something

____ be in pleasant, attractive surroundings

____ be alone

____ have a structured activity

____ be able to do things at the last minute

____ follow rules

____ be praised

____ have fun and enjoy myself

____ release frustration

____ release energy

____ have common interests with other people

____ improve my health

____ be able to contribute something to a group

____ have other people like me

____ be physically active

____ use my imagination

____ create something

____ find the activity challenging

____ feel safe and secure

____ try something new and different

____ be myself

____ use my talents

____ improve myself and my skills

____ accomplish something

____ relax

____ spend time with my family

____ take a risk

____ enjoy the outdoors

Once you have checked the lifestyle needs that are important to you, list the *three* most important and identify which activities would most probably satisfy these needs.

Lifestyle needs	Activity preferences
1. _____	_____ _____ _____ _____
2. _____	_____ _____ _____ _____
3. _____	_____ _____ _____ _____

From *The Canadian Physical Activity, Fitness & Lifestyle Appraisal: CSEP's Plan for Healthy Active Living.* Published by the Canadian Society for Exercise Physiology, 1996. p. 8-27. Reprinted by permission.

Screening

We can use information from the health/lifestyle appraisals (e.g., FANTASTIC and RISK-I) to classify and screen individuals by health status prior to exercise as-sessment or prescription. The American Council of Sports Medicine (1995) suggests that, for apparently healthy individuals of any age, submaximal exercise testing up to 75% of age-predicted maximal heart rate can be done by a well-trained and experienced exercise specialist.

PAR-Q and Medical History

Older individuals and people with high risk symptoms should obtain medical permission before proceeding with vigorous exercise. All maximal exercise tests should include supervision by a physician.

The Physical Activity Readiness Questionnaire (PAR-Q) can help determine whether a client should provide a detailed medical history before entering an exercise program. You can use PAR-Q (see page 47) as a screening instrument both for submaximal aerobic assessment and for beginning moderate and progressive exercise programs (CSEP 1996; Shephard 1988).

PAR-Q helps to identify clients for whom certain physical activities might be inappropriate, or who should receive medical advice concerning the type of activity most suitable for them. In order to assure the validity of the test as well as to protect yourself legally, administer the PAR-Q without providing any interpretation to your clients. All judgments must be their own. If they give one or more "Yes" responses, direct them to their doctors for a review of their medical history before permitting them to complete active test components such as aerobic or strength or endurance tests.

Personal Observation

The questionnaires discussed above will identify most concerns that can make a fitness assessment inappropriate. It is advisable, however, that you make some general observations within the screening process (CSEP 1996). Cancel or postpone the appraisal if clients

- demonstrate difficulty in breathing at rest;
- are ill or have a fever;
- have swelling in their lower extremities;
- are pregnant and do not have the consent of their physicians;
- cough persistently;
- are currently on medication for cardiovascular or metabolic problems;

- have clearly ignored instructions about eating/drinking/smoking before arrival;
- exhibit any other trait that you believe may predispose them to unnecessary discomfort or risk.

For some of these observations (e.g., coughing, swelling), you should direct clients to their physicians; for others (e.g., illness, eating/drinking), instruct them to return once the concern no longer exists.

Informed Consent

Any client who is exposed to possible physical, psychological, or social injury must give informed consent prior to participation in an assessment or exercise program. The informed consent form should provide the client with an adequate explanation of the tests and program, the potential risks and discomforts that may be involved, and their rights and responsibilities. It should be read, understood, and signed prior to the administration of the active appraisal. Questions that arise provide an opportunity for dialogue and a chance to gather information and build rapport.

Informed consent does not absolve you from negligence in the administration of an assessment or the prescription of exercise. Although the form should be individualized for each facility or business, the following basic components should be in every informed consent form (Nieman 1990):

- A general statement of the background and objectives of the program.
- An explanation of the procedures to be followed.
- A description of any risks or discomfort that may be experienced.
- A description of the benefits that can reasonably be expected.
- An offer to answer any of the client's questions.
- An instruction that the client is free to withdraw consent and to discontinue participation at any time.
- An explanation of the procedures to be taken to ensure the confidentiality of the information requested.

Choosing Laboratory or Field-Based Tests

Before we can develop an exercise prescription, we must assess baseline values for selected components of fitness. Sometimes we sample all the components of

Select the number that best describes your situation for each of the following and compare the total score for an overall risk rating.

RISK-I

	1	2	3	4	5	Score
Age	20s	30s	40s	50s	60s	
Family history	No known heart disease	One relative over 50	Two relatives over 50	One relative under 50	Two relatives under 50	
Smoking	Non-user	User < 5 yrs ago	< 10/day	10-20/day	> 20/day	
Body mass index	19-22	23-26	27-30	31-34 or < 19	> 34	
Exercise	Active > 2 times/wk	Active 1-2 times/wk	Moderately active 1-3 times/month	Stopped activity < 3 months ago	Sedentary	
Back	Healthy	Minor problems in past	Aches occasionally or after activity	Problems in past or current discomfort	*Frequent problems/ diagnosed condition	
Knees	Healthy	Minor problems in past	Occasional pain after vigorous activity	Problems in past or current discomfort	*Frequent problems/ diagnosed condition	
					Total score =	

Family History. Count parents, grandparents, brothers, and sisters who have had a heart attack or a stroke.

Smoking. If you inhale deeply or smoke a cigarette right down, add one to your score.

Body Mass Index (BMI). This is a measure of body proportion and a better indicator of risk than just weight (CSEP 1996). It is the ratio of body weight (in kilograms) divided by the square of height (in meters).

Example:

Weight = 75 kg   Height = 1.72 m

$$BMI = 75/1.72^2$$
$$= 75/2.96$$
$$= 25.3 \text{ (RISK-I score = 25)}$$

For more information on BMI, see page 54.

Interpretation:

Total score	Rating
7-10	Very low risk
11-15	Low risk
16-20	Average risk
21-25	High risk
26-30	*Dangerous risk
31-35	*Extremely dangerous risk

*Medical clearance necessary.

PAR-Q & You

(A Questionnaire for People Aged 15 to 69)

Regular physical activity is fun and healthy, and increasingly more people are starting to become more active every day. Being more active is very safe for most people. However, some people should check with their doctor before they start becoming much more physically active.

If you are planning to become much more physically active than you are now, start by answering the seven questions in the box below. If you are between the ages of 15 and 69, the PAR-Q will tell you if you should check with your doctor before you start. If you are over 69 years of age, and you are not used to being very active, check with your doctor.

Common sense is your best guide when you answer these questions. Please read the questions carefully and answer each one honestly: Check YES or NO

YES	NO		
❑	❑	1.	Has your doctor ever said that you have a heart condition <u>and</u> that you should only do physical activity recommended by a doctor?
❑	❑	2.	Do you feel pain in your chest when you do physical activity?
❑	❑	3.	In the past month, have you had chest pain when you were not doing physical activity?
❑	❑	4.	Do you lose your balance because of dizziness or do you ever lose consciousness?
❑	❑	5.	Do you have a bone or joint problem that could be made worse by a change in your physical activity?
❑	❑	6.	Is your doctor currently prescribing drugs (for example, water pills) for your blood pressure or heart condition?
❑	❑	7.	Do you know of <u>any other reason</u> why you should not do physical activity?

If you answered

YES to one or more questions

Talk to your doctor by phone or in person BEFORE you start becoming much more physically active or BEFORE you have a fitness appraisal. Tell your doctor about the PAR-Q and which questions you answered YES.

- You may be able to do any activity you want—as long as you start slowly and build up gradually. Or, you may need to restrict your activities to those which are safe for you. Talk with your doctor about the kinds of activities you wish to participate in and follow his/her advice.
- Find out which community programs are safe and helpful for you.

NO to all questions

If you answered NO honestly to <u>all</u> PAR-Q questions, you can be reasonably sure that you can:

- start becoming much more physically active—begin slowly and build up gradually. This is the safest and easiest way to go.
- take part in a fitness appraisal—this is an excellent way to determine your basic fitness so that you can plan the best way for you to live actively.

Delay becoming much more active:
- if you are not feeling well because of a temporary illness such as a cold or a fever—wait until you feel better; or
- if you are or may be pregnant—talk to your doctor before you start becoming more active.

Please note: If your health changes so that you then answer YES to any of the above questions, tell your fitness or health professional. Ask whether you should change your physical activity plan.

<u>Informed Use of the PAR-Q:</u> The Canadian Society for Exercise Physiology, Health Canada, and their agents assume no liability for persons who undertake physical activity, and if in doubt after completing this questionnaire, consult your doctor prior to physical activity.

> You are encouraged to copy the PAR-Q but only if you use the entire form

NOTE: If the PAR-Q is being given to a person before he or she participates in a physical activity program or a fitness appraisal, this section may be used for legal or administrative purposes.

I have read, understood and completed this questionnaire. Any questions I had were answered to my full satisfaction.

NAME _____

SIGNATURE _____ DATE _____

SIGNATURE OF PARENT _____ WITNESS _____
or GUARDIAN (for participants under the age of majority)

©Canadian Society for Exercise Physiology
Société canadienne de physiologie de l'exercise

Supported by: Health   Santé
                 Canada   Canada

Reprinted, with permission, from the Canadian Society for Exercise Physiology, Inc. Copyright 1994.

fitness (i.e., cardiovascular, body composition, flexibility, muscular strength, and endurance). At other times, we may assess only high-priority components. Where appropriate, we may use less expensive and more easily administered field-based tests as supplements to or even as substitutes for laboratory tests.

You can readily find details of a variety of assessment protocols (CSEP 1993; Heyward 1998; Kendall et al. 1993; Nieman 1990; Skinner 1987). Table 4.1 categorizes a number of assessment tools into laboratory and field-based measures.

The very process of administering a fitness assessment draws attention to the "client-centered" nature of our relationship. The test process and the test results help to educate, motivate, and stimulate interest in exercise and other health-related issues. However, the primary function of measurement is to determine status.

Any fitness assessment protocol should meet the following criteria:

- **Validity:** It accurately measures what it is supposed to measure.
- **Reliability:** It gives consistent results when used by different testers or when repeated by the same tester.
- **Economy:** It is relatively inexpensive, time efficient, and easy to administer.

Test results are a means to an end. They should not distract from the purpose of serving our clients. It is better to undertest than to overtest, so that we can devote more time to counseling and to the demonstration phase of the program.

Cardiovascular Assessment

Your own experience and educational background will affect the type of test you select. The following section will help you in your selection of laboratory protocols.

Client Considerations in the Selection of Laboratory Tests

Table 4.2 compares the four major assessment devices for a number of criteria. You must be able to select an exercise mode and test protocol that is suitable for your client's age, gender, anticipated mode of exercise, and health and fitness status.

Although step testing offers an inexpensive alternative to treadmill and bicycle ergometry testing, it has some technical limitations, such as the client's size and ability to maintain good form. Arm ergometry offers a suitable means for testing clients with lower extremity impairment.

Treadmill Protocols

Treadmill protocols are best suited to clients who

- want a walking, jogging, or running prescription;
- want to achieve their highest measurable oxygen uptake; or,
- are familiar with running on a treadmill.

Table 4.1   Laboratory and Field-Based Assessment Tools

	LABORATORY	FIELD-BASED
Cardiovascular	• treadmill (e.g., Bruce, Balke) • bicycle ergometer • arm ergometer	• Åstrand-Ryhming bicycle test • 1.5/2.0-mile run • Canadian Aerobic Fitness Test • Physical Activity Index
Body composition	• hydrostatic weighing • bioelectrical impedance	• skinfolds • circumferences • height/weight • body mass index

Table 4.2   Client-Centered Selection of Assessment Method

PERFORMANCE FACTOR	TREADMILL	BICYCLE	STEP	ARM ERGOMETER
Familiarity and skills not required	****	***	**	*
Adjustment of workload	****	** (friction)	*	** (friction)
Instrument calibration	**	*** (friction)	****	*** (friction)
Ability to achieve highest oxygen uptake	****	**	***	*
Obtaining blood pressure	***	****	**	*
Obtaining VO$_2$	***	****	*	**
Obtaining ECG	***	****	**	*
Obtaining heart rate (stethoscope)	***	****	*	**
Least local muscle fatigue	****	**	***	*
Cost and maintenance	*	***	****	**
Client compliance	****	**	***	*

Each mode is rated from * (lowest) to **** (highest) in the various performance factors.

The Bruce Protocol

The Bruce protocol (figure 4.1) is an accurate maximal test for normal and high risk clients (Heyward 1998). It may underestimate men under 29 years. The sharp grades may cause calf fatigue and may be a limitation for sedentary or older clients.

The Balke Protocol

The Balke protocol (figure 4.2) provides a quick, convenient method to assess exercise tolerance where the speed is constant and small grade changes are made each minute (Heyward 1998). It is particularly suitable for sedentary adults who may have difficulty jogging (e.g., knee problems). The length of the test and steep grades at a walking speed may be limitations for fit clients.

Bicycle Ergometer Protocols

Bicycle ergometer protocols are best suited to clients who

- want a cycle or stationary bicycle prescription;
- already cycle frequently;
- prefer less joint trauma; or
- are overweight and unfamiliar with the treadmill.

Predictive maximal cycle ergometer tests estimate maximal oxygen uptake from the highest power output completed. These tests are better measures of exercise tolerance than those that simply measure aerobic power, because anaerobic capacity can significantly contribute to performance during the final workload. Submaximal tests, such as the Åstrand protocol (figure 4.3),

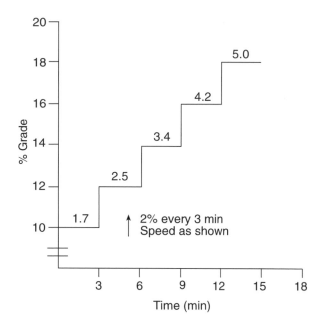

Bruce et al. (1973)
For: normal and high risk
Initial work load: 1.7 mph, 10%, 3 min = normal

1.7 mph, 0-5%, 3 min = high risk

Figure 4.1 Bruce treadmill protocol.

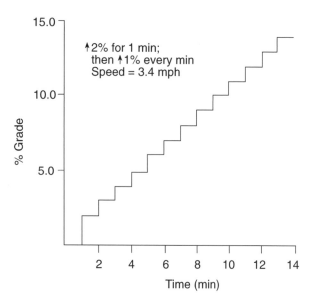

Balke and Ware (1959)
For: normal risk
Initial work load: 3.4 mph., 0%, 1 min

Figure 4.2 Balke treadmill protocol.

are useful tools for tracking training programs and for monitoring blood pressure and heart rate. This added control is suited for older clients. Although the standard error may be about 15%, the measured responses to reproducible workloads provide information for the

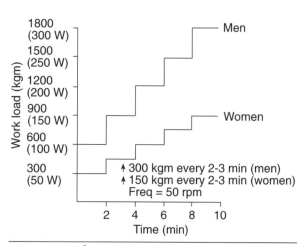

Figure 4.3 Åstrand protocol.

prescription of cardiovascular intensity (Heyward 1998).

Submaximal or Maximal?

Submaximal tests on the treadmill, bicycle ergometer, or with bench stepping are similar to maximal tests but are terminated at a predetermined heart rate. The submaximal test assumes a linear relationship between oxygen uptake, heart rate, and work intensity. In other words, as the workload increases, the oxygen cost of the activity and the heart rate will rise at the same time. Variability in maximal heart rates and mechanical efficiencies usually results in overestimation for highly trained individuals and underestimation for untrained, sedentary clients (Heyward 1998).

Modifying Tests

It is a challenge to select suitable assessment items for many clients. Conditions such as musculoskeletal problems, overweight, lack of conditioning, advanced age, or high health risks may require that you modify the tests.
  Consider the following modifications:

- It is more appropriate to use a bicycle than a treadmill, step, or arm ergometer with clients who need increased monitoring of heart rate or blood pressure.
- Reduce total test time to under 15 minutes for clients who are easily fatigued.
- For clients with poor leg strength, a treadmill is preferable to a bike or step; for those with poor balance, a bike is better than treadmill or step.
- Start at a lower intensity for clients suspected to have a low oxygen uptake; start at high intensity for those who are regularly active.
- Longer warm-ups and smaller increases in workloads are appropriate for those requiring more time to reach steady state.

Field-Based Tests

Results from relatively simple field-based tests may be adequate to identify and quantify your client's needs. Field-based tests are usually less expensive and more easily administered than lab tests. For the personal trainer or small facility director, they may be the only option. They can be very helpful if the regular method of monitoring is similar to that used for the field tests (e.g., waist girth, skinfolds, or heart rates—all quickly measured—can be quick indicators of progress).

Field-Based Test #1:
Physical Activity Index (PAI)

Physical activity and fitness reinforce each other. Just as the most fit tend to be the most active, the most active are frequently the most fit; and the components of fitness are determined by patterns of habitual physical activity (more detail in chapter 6).

The Physical Activity Index (page 52) can help determine the health benefits of an activity. Earlier appraisal tools, such as the FANTASTIC Lifestyle Checklist or RISK-I, may have identified lack of physical activity as a habit in need of change. Yet an intense cardiovascular appraisal may not be appropriate for some clients. The PAI will help you assess the activities in which your client already participates.

For example, if your client exercises at a moderate intensity (3 points) for 40 minutes (5 points) four times per week (4 points), then her physical activity index is $3 \times 5 \times 4 = 60$. This "good" rating is a level of physical activity with considerable health benefits, such as lowering blood lipids, blood pressure, and body fat. You can administer the PAI periodically to show improvements and help motivate your client.

Field-Based Test #2:
Walking Test

Use this test for relatively inactive clients who are comfortable with walking but for whom jogging is inappropriate. If they are overweight, older, or have scored less than 40 on the PAI, the following walking test (Getchell 1982) may be a useful alternative to laboratory assessments.

All you need for this test is a timing device, a track or measured distance of 1, 1.5, and 2 miles, and appropriate weather. Have your client do warm-up stretches, then walk as briskly as she can. If she begins to tire early, encourage her to slow down. If she cannot complete the mile or cannot complete it in under 20 minutes, terminate the test. If she reaches the mile in less than 20 minutes, have her keep going for another half mile. If she reaches the 1.5 mile point in less than 30 minutes, have her keep going. Her goal now is to reach 2 miles in less than 40 minutes. Of course, if any signs of intolerance to the exercise start to appear, terminate the test and have your client cool down. Table 4.3 will help you determine a safe and reasonable starting point for exercise prescription, based on the results of the walking test.

Body Composition Assessment

The most popular laboratory techniques to assess body composition are hydrostatic weighing, bioelectrical impedance, and skinfold measures. These analyses are based on measuring the ratio of fat to fat-free mass.

Client Considerations in the Selection of Tests

Underwater weighing is the laboratory standard for assessing body composition; but the time, expense, and expertise needed are often prohibitive. As better equations are developed and appropriate pre-test conditions are followed, bioelectrical impedance should prove to be a most convenient, safe, accurate, and rapid method.

Skinfold measurement correlates well with underwater weighing. Done by an experienced exercise specialist, the method has several advantages:

- The equipment is inexpensive and portable in comparison with popular laboratory tests.
- Measures are made quickly and easily.
- Measures correlate highly with body density and provide more accurate estimates of body fat than height-weight ratios (Nieman 1990).

Any skinfold protocol's predictive formula is specific to the population with which it was developed. To be more effective and fair to your client, select a protocol suited to her. Many equations have been developed for specific types of people. For example, the American Alliance for Health, Physical Education, Recreation and Dance (1988) promotes the use of triceps and medial calf skinfold sites. Heyward and Stolarczyk (1996) discuss the major methods of assessment, including "decision trees"—charts that direct the decision process for choosing the most appropriate skinfold equation. The recent trend has been to use generalized rather than population-specific equations. These equations, such as those developed by Jackson and Pollock (1985), apply to a large range of people with little loss in predictive accuracy. The error associated with generalized skinfold equations is only slightly greater (3.7% v. 2.7%) than that of the hydrostatic weighing technique (Nieman 1990). A major source of error in skinfold measurements is the

PHYSICAL ACTIVITY INDEX (PAI)

Instructions:

Select the appropriate points for each of the following three parts.

Part #1—When you engage in sport, fitness activities, or active leisure, which description is most appropriate?

Intensity descriptions		Points
Very heavy:	Continuous intense effort resulting in rapid heart rate or heavy breathing for the length of the activity.	5
Heavy:	Bursts of effort that cause rapid heart rate or heavy breathing.	4
Moderate:	Requires moderate effort and works up a sweat.	3
Light:	Requires light effort and is often intermittent.	2
Minimal:	Requires no extra effort.	1

Part #2—When you participate in the activity described in Part #1, how long do you keep at it?

Duration descriptions	Points
35 minutes or more	5
25-34 minutes	4
15-24 minutes	3
5-14 minutes	2
Less than 5 minutes	1

Part #3—How often do you participate in the activity described in Part #1?

Frequency descriptions	Points
Daily	5
3-6 times per week	4
1-2 times per week	3
1-3 times per month	2
Less than once per month	1

PAI scoring:

Multiply your "intensity" points times your "duration" points times your "frequency points to obtain your "health benefits" score.

Physical Activity Index = Intensity pts. _____ × Duration pts. _____ × Frequency pts. _____

Health benefit rating for PAI scores:

PAI score	Rating	Significance
100 or more	Excellent	This level of physical activity is associated with optimal health benefits.
60-99	Good	This level of physical activity is associated with considerable health benefits.
40-59	Average	This level of physical activity is associated with some health benefits. Increased activity will provide increased health benefits.
20-39	Fair	This level of physical activity is associated with some health benefits and some health risks. Duration or frequency of activity should be increased.
Less than 20	Needs improvement	This level of physical activity is associated with considerable health risks.

From *Client-Centered Exercise Prescription* by John C. Griffin, 1998, Champaign, IL: Human Kinetics. Copyright 1998 by John C. Griffin.

Table 4.3   Walking Test Scoring

TEST PERFORMANCE	FITNESS LEVEL (max METs)	RECOMMENDED WALKING PROGRAM
1 mile in more than 25 min.	4 METs* or below	0.5 to 0.8 miles in 15-20 min.
1 mile in 20-25 min.	4.5 METs	1.1 to 1.2 miles in 24 min.
1.5 miles in 26-30 min.	5 METs	1.4 to 1.6 miles in 32 min.
1.5 miles in 23-26 min.	5.5 METs	1.9 to 2.0 miles in 40 min.
2.0 miles in 35-40 min.	6 METs	2.3 to 2.4 miles in 48 min.
2.0 miles in 30-35 min.	6.5 METs	3.0 miles in 58 minutes

*MET is the energy cost at rest. During a vigorous workout, a fit person may reach 10-15 times this resting value (10-15 METs).
Adapted, by permission, from Getchell, B., 1982, Determining Your Level of Fitness, *Being Fit. A Personal Guide.* John Wiley and Sons, Inc. 78.

variability among technicians. Good training in standardized procedures can reduce this significantly (Heyward 1998).

Several studies (e.g., Larsson et al. 1984) have shown that a centralized (trunk area) versus a generalized pattern of subcutaneous fat distribution is more directly associated with metabolic disorders and possibly hypertension. CSEP (1996) uses the sum of two trunk skinfolds (subscapular and suprailiac) to establish a health-benefit rating.

Table 4.4 compares three methods for cost, ease of use, and accuracy in measuring body fat.

Simple Field-Based Tests

Field-based tests provide different, and often supportive, information from that obtained in lab tests (see "Using BMI, Skinfold Measures, and Waist Girth Measure," page 55). The body mass index (BMI) and the waist girth measure are estimates of body composition and, along with skinfold measures, can provide additional useful information.

Field-Based Test #1:
Body Mass Index (BMI)

The body mass index (BMI) is an indicator of proportional weight or obesity. It is more precise than weight tables, is simple to do, and allows for comparisons of large groups. Calculate BMI by dividing body weight (in kilograms) by the square of height (in meters).

For example:

Weight = 80 kg; height = 175 cm = 1.75 m

$BMI = wt/ht^2 = 80/1.75^2 = 80/3.06 = 26.1$

The BMI has the following recommended classifications (Jequier 1987):

- 20-25—Desirable range for adult men and women
- 25-30—Grade I obesity (overweight)
- 30-40—Grade II obesity (medically significant)
- >40—Grade III obesity (morbid obesity)

In the example, the client would be classified as "overweight." BMI is most useful when used in conjunction with skinfold measures. A high BMI could be the result of elevated muscle mass, as with a football player, or excessive body fat. If the skinfold measures are high, this is a definite indication of too much body fat and corresponding health risk.

Field-Based Test #2:
Waist (Abdomen) Girth

Excessive fat in the trunk area is associated with increased morbidity and mortality. Some sources (CSEP 1996) have suggested that waist girth measure provides a valid representation of this pattern of fat distribution.

Table 4.4 Body Composition Assessment Methods

METHOD	SKINFOLD	HYDROSTATIC WEIGHING	ELECTRICAL IMPEDANCE
Cost	*	***	**
Ease of use	**	*	***
Accuracy	**	***	**

*Low; ** moderate; *** high

To measure waist girth, hold the tape horizontally at the level of noticeable waist narrowing and take the measurement at the end of a normal expiration. When narrowing is not apparent, take the girth just below the level of the lowest (12th) floating rib. Maintain tension but do not indent the skin.

Some sources (CSEP 1996) describe waist girth "health-benefit zones" based on age and sex. Getchell and Anderson (1982) suggest that men generally should have a waist measure 5 to 7 inches (12 to 18 cm) less than chest or hips and women should be 10 inches (25 cm) less than bust or hip measures. Monitoring changes to this measure is simple and can be very encouraging, particularly at the start of an exercise program.

Using BMI, Skinfold Measures, and Waist Girth Measure

If your client has a high BMI, use skinfold measures to determine if it is high because of muscle mass or because of excessive body fat. Next, examine the pattern of fat distribution by measuring waist girth or trunk skinfolds. Even with an acceptable BMI and moderate skinfold measures, there may still be health risks if the waist girth is high and the trunk skinfolds are excessive (CSEP 1996).

Highlights

- Select test items that specifically relate to your client's priorities.
- Your assessment should closely simulate the existing training activity of your client.
- A **health and lifestyle appraisal** may be your client's first step to a change in behavior. It will help you to set priorities and plan a well-rounded fitness program.

- The *FANTASTIC Lifestyle Checklist* can help your clients assess how their habits and attitudes affect their health.
- The *Inventory of Lifestyle Needs and Activity Preferences* can help your clients identify lifestyle needs that are important to them.
- *Risk-I* assigns numerical values within each of the five risk categories for coronary heart disease (CHD) and within two categories (back and knees) for musculoskeletal risk.
- The need for a detailed medical history questionnaire before entering an exercise program may be determined by a briefer screening device called the *Physical Activity Readiness Questionnaire (PAR-Q)*.
- Any client who is exposed to possible physical, psychological, or social injury must give **informed consent** prior to participation in an assessment or exercise program.
- Before you develop an exercise prescription for a client, first determine **baseline values** for selected components of fitness by using appropriate laboratory or field-based assessment tools.
- **Treadmill** protocols are best suited to clients who
  1. want a walking, jogging, or running prescription,
  2. want to achieve their highest measurable oxygen uptake, or
  3. are familiar with running on a treadmill.
- **Bicycle ergometer** protocols are best suited to clients who
  1. want a cycle or stationary bicycle prescription,
  2. already cycle frequently,
  3. prefer less joint trauma, or
  4. are overweight and unfamiliar with the treadmill.

- The *Physical Activity Index* analyzes your client's current activity and can help determine the health benefits derived therefrom.

- The **walking test** can provide a useful alternative to laboratory assessments. Use it for inactive clients who are comfortable with walking but for whom jogging is inappropriate.

- Assess body composition by using **hydrostatic weighing, bioelectrical impedance,** and **skinfold measures**. These analyses measure the ratio of fat to fat-free mass.

- The **body mass index (BMI)** is an indicator of proportional weight and is more precise than weight tables; it permits comparison of populations, and is most useful when used in conjunction with skinfold measures.

- The **waist girth** measures the approximate amount of fat in the trunk area.

Chapter 5

Client-Centered Musculoskeletal Assessment

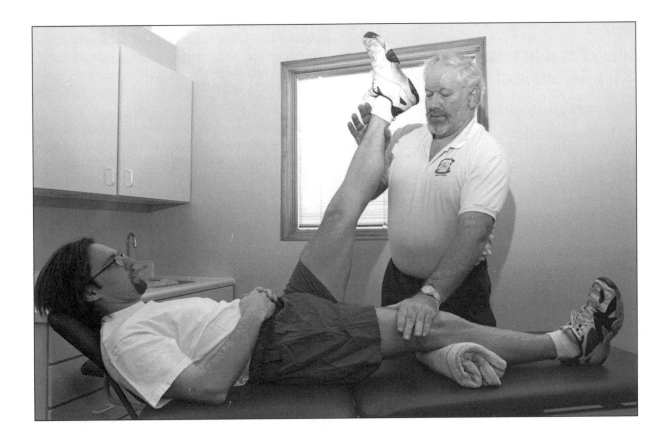

- ■ Muscular Strength and Endurance Assessment
- ■ Flexibility/Muscle Tightness Assessment
- ■ Shortcomings of Muscular Fitness Tests
- ■ Postural Assessment

This chapter introduces laboratory and field-based tests under each of the major musculoskeletal components of fitness: muscular strength and endurance, flexibility/muscle tightness, muscle balance, and posture. We will discuss client issues in the selection of test items and describe specific field tests for determining the distinct needs of the client.

Muscular Strength and Endurance Assessment

We measure strength and muscular endurance using dynamometers, cable tensiometers, electromechanical devices, and constant-resistance and variable-resistance exercise machines. To assess static and dynamic strength, endurance, and power, we use electromechanical and hydraulic devices (such as force platforms) as well as *Cybex* and *Omni-tron* dynamometers. Because these instruments are quite sophisticated and relatively expensive, they typically are found only in research laboratories.

Client Considerations in the Selection of Tests

When selecting tests, consider seven factors:

1. **Joint-muscle relationships**. Strength and endurance are specific to the muscle group, the type and speed of contraction, and the joint angle or range of motion. Always consider how your client is/will be training, the nature of any primary sport participation, the demands of her work environment, or her stated priorities. For example, if your client would like to significantly improve her squash game, you may wish to establish base-line levels of

- dynamic strength for shoulder medial rotators through a full range of motion (the power of a forehand shot comes from a rapid contraction of the shoulder medial rotators);
- static grip strength (a general indicator of strength and important for racquet stability); and
- dynamic endurance of the knee and hip extensors (extension from a partial crouch position is a movement pattern repeated at high intensities throughout a squash match).

2. **Degree of effort.** Most tests require maximum effort. Your client may not be at a stage where this will be accurate or safe. Factors such as time of day, sleep, drugs, and anticipation may also affect a maximum performance. Use caution in "pushing" clients to their maximum. Flaws in technique usually precede fatigue: watch clients carefully, and stop the test when they start to struggle.

3. **Strength level.** Performance on some endurance tests is highly dependent on strength. Use tests that are proportional to the client's body weight or to a percentage of her maximum strength. An example of this technique can be seen in field-based test #1 on the next page.

4. **Normative values.** Although some age- and gender-based norms exist, many tests lack up-to-date norms against which you can compare your client's results—especially for adults over 25 years. However, test results may serve other functions: use them to establish base-line levels for measuring improvement (especially if the test resembles the training), or to determine starting points for exercise prescriptions.

5. **Specificity, reliability, and validity.** Some very reliable laboratory methods have limited usefulness because they are too specific. For example, the sophisticated isokinetic dynamometers normally measure only one joint action. Yet compound movements involving two joints, such as a leg press action, are commonplace in sports. Another example is the cable tensiometer. It is a good measure of isometric strength, but is specific to the angle of contraction and may not reflect dynamic strength.

6. **Body weight test items.** Calisthenic tests produce highly variable results. People with high body fat have relatively less muscle and therefore a lower strength level for their body weight. Since the resistance is the client's weight or a portion of that weight, these clients are lifting a relatively higher load (expressed as a percent of their maximum strength). Distribution of body weight affects the results of sit-up tests, since those with relatively more weight in their lower bodies have less resistance with their lighter upper body. On a positive note, calisthenics are cheap, they usually require no equipment, and they can be modified to vary the resistance by changing body and limb positions.

7. **Client needs.** Strength testing can effectively monitor rehabilitation after injury and provide objective criteria for the resumption of activity. Many nonathletes use strength training for aesthetic as well as functional reasons. Testing can provide a guideline for prescription, and provide a means of monitoring progress.

A variety of assessment tools can be used to measure musculoskeletal fitness. Table 5.1 categorizes a number of such tools into laboratory and field-based measures. Because laboratory tests are expensive and more complex to administer, we will deal in depth here only with field-based tests. Details of the laboratory protocols can be obtained elsewhere (CSEP 1993; Heyward 1998; Kendall et al. 1993; Nieman 1990; Skinner 1987).

Field-Based Tests

Unlike laboratory-based tests for muscular strength and endurance, field-based tests often closely simulate the training activity of your clients, thereby increasing

Table 5.1 Laboratory and Field-Based Musculoskeletal Assessment Tools

	LABORATORY	FIELD-BASED
Muscular strength and endurance	• Isokinetic dynamometer (e.g., Cybex, Kin-Com) • Cable tensiometer	• Grip dynamometer • 1 repetition maximum (1-RM) • Percent 1-RM • Calisthenics (e.g., sit-ups, push-ups, etc.)
Flexibility	• Leighton flexometer	• Goniometer (e.g., ankle, hip) • Sit and reach • Indirect measures (e.g., back hyperextension, shoulder flexion)
Muscle balance		• Postural assessment • Muscle tightness tests • Back fitness test

the validity and sensitivity of the assessments. The tests are usually cheap and easy to administer, and often can be modified to suit desired resistance levels. They can help you establish starting prescription levels if the tests closely resemble the exercise.

Field-Based Test #1: Five Level Sit-Up

With calisthenics, you can use simple biomechanics to change the position of certain body segments and create changes in loading. The Five Level Sit-Up test utilizes a modified arm position to change the resistance. The knee is at 90 degrees to minimize the involvement of the hip flexors. Figure 5.1 illustrates the procedures for the five levels from least difficult (level 1) to most difficult (level 5). The client executes each level one at a time starting with level one. If the execution is appropriate, allow a brief rest and then attempt level two, etc.

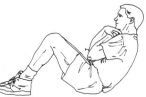

Level One

Hand position for level one has arms at the side just above the surface of the floor.

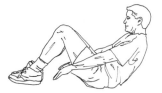

Level Two

Cross arms on the chest with hands resting on the top of the shoulders. Do not raise arms from the chest during the sit-up.

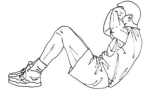

Level Three

Place fists at the temple of your head. Extend arms out from the side of the head. Do not move the arms forward at any point during the sit-up.

(continued)

Figure 5.1 The five level sit-up test uses modified positions and changing resistance to test strength and muscular endurance (level 1 is the least difficult and level 5 the most difficult).

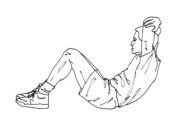

Level Four

Extend arms up and behind the head. Place forearms on top of one another with hands touching your elbows. When performing the sit-up the arms are required to maintain this position and not move forward in front of the head.

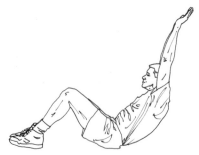

Level Five

Place arms behind the ears and extend to form a straight line from the shoulder to your hands. Place hands so that they are touching one another. When sitting up, maintain your arms behind your ears and do not move them forward.

Figure 5.1   *(continued)*

Scoring: If your client visibly strains on the attempt but does manage to perform it correctly, this is considered her "strength level." If she has to modify her technique to complete the sit-up (such as extending her legs or using momentum), the previous level is considered her strength level. To assess her "endurance level," select the sit-up one level below her strength level. To test for muscular endurance, have your client complete as many repetitions as possible for one minute or to the point of fatigue. The test may also be terminated when she performs a second technical flaw (any flawed repetitions are not counted).

Before using the results of the tests to prescribe an exercise program, first determine your client's objectives: strength, strength-endurance, or endurance. From the results of the strength and endurance tests, you can prescribe the level of sit-ups and the number of repetitions to suit her objective (also see chapter 11). By having her move her heels 2 to 4 inches closer to the buttocks, you can make the level slightly more difficult and fine-tune her prescription.

Field-Based Test #2: Relative Muscular Endurance Weight Lifting

When measuring strength with weights, increase the load to find a weight the client can lift only once (1 RM). To test for relative muscular endurance, assign a submaximal load—that is, a percentage of a repetition maximum (1 RM). The load should be specific to the objective of the client: a particular sport, a work task, a rehabilitative goal, etc. The exercise used for the test should also reflect the client's objective. More easily standardized exercises include bench press, latissimus dorsi pull-down, leg curl, leg extension, leg press, and arm curl. If you use a metronome to establish a desired cadence, terminate the test when the client completes the maximum number of repetitions before falling behind the cadence.

Figure 5.2 (Sale and MacDougall 1981) illustrates the average number of repetitions possible when compared with 1 RM. Use this graph to evaluate results of relative load tests. It shows the percentages of the 1 RM that you can try with your client when prescribing at an 8-10 RM level or a 1-3 RM level.

Flexibility/Muscle Tightness Assessment

Although flexibility is often defined as a range of motion of a joint, it is not a simple matter: it involves both the length and strength of muscles. A short muscle restricts the normal range of motion. Muscles that are too short are usually strong and hold the opposite muscle in a lengthened position. Excessively long muscles are usually weak and allow adaptive shortening of antagonists. When prescribing to increase flexibility, use exercise movements that

■ lengthen short muscles by increasing the distance between the muscles' origin and insertion opposite to the direction of the muscle action, and

■ strengthen weak muscles that have been elongated by strong antagonist muscles.

You will encounter a large number of clients, particularly middle-aged, with musculoskeletal injuries or low back problems. Most low back problems are due to postural misalignment and a lack of muscle balance. The highest incidence of aerobic and running injuries are those of the lower leg precipitated by muscle tightness and poor range of motion around the ankle.

A preoccupation with instrumentation has left many in our profession feeling inadequate when faced with the measurement of flexibility. It is ironic that other health care professionals, such as physiotherapists,

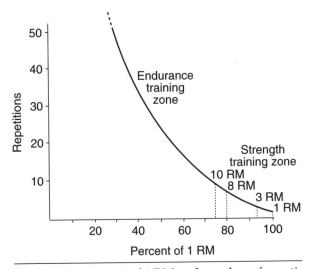

Figure 5.2 Percent of 1 RM and number of repetitions.

Reprinted from: *The Canadian Journal of Applied Sports Sciences,* Vol. 6. Published by the Canadian Society for Exercise Physiology, 1981. p. 87-92.

athletic trainers, and physicians, rely successfully on their skills of manual assessment.

You can determine flexibility directly by measuring the range of motion of a joint or series of joints in degrees with devices like goniometers or flexometers. The Leighton flexometer has a test-retest reliability ranging from .90 to .99 (Heyward 1998). With goniometers, locating the true joint center is critical to obtain true readings. Indirect assessment methods, using measuring tapes, are often criticized as crude and lacking normative data. Examine each assessment to determine if it reliably measures what it says it should measure. Because the length or width of body segments can affect the results of some tests, such as the sit-and-reach, comparing individuals may not be highly valid with these tests. They nevertheless can be effective monitoring tools for individuals. There is no single test that predicts overall body flexibility. The range of motion of each joint is unique.

Client Considerations in the Selection of Test Items

Examine the needs and demands of your client. Has a joint area been overworked, possibly causing muscle tightness? For example, clients who plan a weight bearing or locomotor activity should have ankle flexibility assessed. Clients who sit for long periods of time should be checked for tightness of the hip flexors and trunk extensors. Many manual workers tend to have tight anterior chest muscles such as the pectoralis major and minor. Overuse or underuse of back muscles may leave them tight and the joints inflexible.

Specific Field-Based Tests

Test muscle length to determine if it is limited or excessive. For this component of flexibility, it is particularly important to be client-centered. Each joint and muscle is unique. Careful counseling can help you focus on the areas of potential concern.

A summary of the results of the Flexibility/Muscle Tightness Field-Based Assessments on page 65 provides a convenient reference.

Field-Based Test #1: Length of Pectoralis Minor (figure 5.3a)

1. Have the client lie supine, knees bent and lower back flat.
2. Look from above the head; are the shoulders touching the table?
3. Gently push the shoulders to see if muscle tightness is slight, moderate, or marked.

Field-Based Test #2: Length of Pectoralis Major (Sternal figure 5.3b)

1. Have client lie supine, knees bent and lower back flat and arm straight upward.
2. Have client slowly lower arm at 135 degrees abduction.
3. Be sure shoulder is laterally rotated and elbow is straight.

Normal: arm should rest, relaxed on the table.

Field-Based Test #3: Length of Shoulder Internal Rotators (Subscapularis, figure 5.3c)

1. Have client lie supine, knees bent and lower back flat.
2. Position client's shoulder at 90 degrees, elbow at 90 degrees.
3. Secure shoulder to table to avoid scapular movement.
4. Have client keep the elbow on the table and lower the posterior forearm to the table.

Normal: 90 degrees with forearm flat on table.

Field-Based Test #4: Length of Shoulder External Rotators (Infraspinatus, Teres Minor, figure 5.3d)

1. Same standardized position as internal rotators.
2. Have client lower anterior forearm to the table.

Normal: 70 degrees with forearm 20 degrees off the table

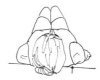

(a) Pectoralis minor

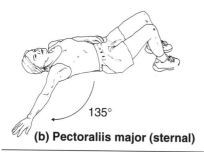

135°

(b) Pectoraliis major (sternal)

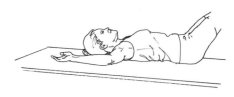

(c) Shoulder internal rotators

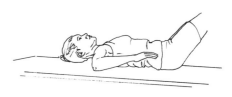

(d) Shoulder external rotators

Figure 5.3 Muscle length assessments—shoulder.

Field-Based Test #5:
Length of Hip Flexors (Figure 5.4a)

1. Have client lie supine on long table (horizontal bench press bench may substitute).
2. Have client hang knee of the test leg just over the edge of the table and flex it freely.

Note: If significant space remains below lower back, there is usually some hip flexor shortness.

3. Have client pull the opposite thigh toward the chest only enough to flatten the lower back and sacrum to the table.
4. Note the angle of thigh and knee.

Normal 1-joint hip flexor (e.g., iliopsoas): thigh remains on the table (any lift is measured in degrees).

Normal 2-joint hip flexor (e.g., rectus femoris): knee flexion of 80 degrees.

Note: If the hip abducts and internally rotates with the flexion, the tensor fascia latae is probably tight.

Field-Based Test #6:
Length of Hamstrings (Figure 5.4b)

1. Have client lie supine on the table or floor.
2. See that client's legs are extended, with low back and sacrum flat on table.

If low back is not flat (short hip flexors), use a rolled towel under the knees just enough to flatten the back.

3. Hold one thigh down and assist client to gently raise the test leg.
4. Be sure the knee is straight and the foot is relaxed.
5. Raise leg until restraint is felt.

Normal: 80 degrees.

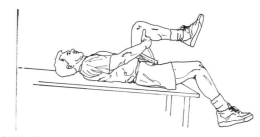

(a) Hip flexors

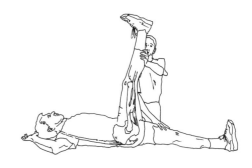

(b) Hamstrings

Figure 5.4 Muscle length assessments—lower body.

Field-Based Test #7: Forward Trunk Flexion (With Flexometer) (Figure 5.5)

1. Client should sit, legs extended, with soles of feet (bare) vertical against the flexometer, 2 cm apart.
2. Have client bend and reach forward gradually with arms even, palms down, and knees straight.
3. Have client lower the head and hold at a comfortable distance near maximum for 2 sec.

Normal: This test does not indicate *where* limitation or excessive motion has taken place (Alter 1988). Various combinations of short hamstrings, back muscles, shoulder muscles, or gastrocnemius may be the cause of poor performance.

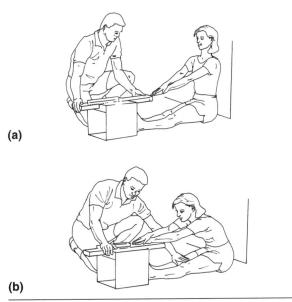

(a)

(b)

Figure 5.5 Muscle length assessments—forward trunk flexion.

Field-Based Test #8: Ankle Range of Motion (Figure 5.6)

The full range of motion for the ankle is conservatively 65 degrees. These field-based tests are more sensitive to where the muscle tightness may be restrictive. Armed with this information, you can be more client-centered with your prescription.

Length of Dorsiflexor (Shin Muscle)

Have client sit on the edge of a table with knees at 90 degrees and legs dangling. Align the center of the goniometer with the center of the lateral malleolus. Next, align one arm of the goniometer with the head of the fibula, and set the other arm at 90 degrees. The neutral position of the ankle has the lateral sole of the foot parallel to the lower arm of the goniometer. Ask your client to actively plantarflex the ankle. An average range of motion should be 45 degrees (Kendal et al. 1993).

A range of motion much less than 40 degrees may affect your client's ability to buffer the trauma of bearing weight—particularly when running or engaging in other locomotor activities.

Length of Plantarflexor (One-Joint) (Deep Calf Muscles)

Client and instrument are set up as previously described. Ask the client to actively dorsiflex the ankle. An average range of motion should be 20 degrees (Kendal et al. 1993). Clients with a range of motion less than this have tight soleus or tibialis posterior muscles. Runners and other aerobic exercisers may experience lower leg rotation or overstretching of the Achilles tendon if these muscles are tight.

Length of Plantarflexor (Two-Joint)

Have client sit on a table or floor with knees straight. Align the goniometer as above. Ask client to actively dorsiflex the ankle. An average range of motion should be 10 degrees (Kendal et al. 1993). Clients with a range of motion less than this have a tight gastrocnemius muscle. This muscle crosses over the back of the knee; when the knee is extended, the gastrocnemius pulls tight and further restricts the ankle in dorsiflexion.

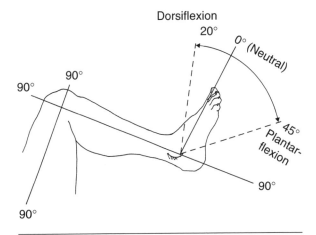

Figure 5.6 Ankle range of motion.

Field-Based Test #9:
Calf Tightness (Griffin 1989)

 Observe the extended leg for this assessment. Extend one leg behind you as far as you can go until you are unable to bear weight with the straight knee. The heel should remain in contact with the ground while the knee bends toward the ground.

 If the angle at the knee looks like this, then the calf muscles are tight.

If the angle at the knee looks like this, then the calf muscles may be moderately tight.

If the angle at the knee looks like this, then the calf muscles allow adequate ankle dorsiflexion.

Field-Based Test #10:
Wall Dorsiflexion (Griffin 1989)

 Sit facing the wall with your legs fully extended, heels placed against the wall with your knees soft. Place your hands behind you for support. Your partner places his finger(s) side by side between the wall and the base of your little toe.

If there is only room for one finger width between the wall and the base of the little toe, then the gastrocnemius is tight and the shin muscles may be weak.

If there are two finger widths between the wall and the base of the little toe, then the gastrocnemius may be moderately tight and the shin muscles may lack strength.

If there is a three-finger width between the wall and the base of the little toe, then the gastrocnemius is not tight and the shin muscles have reasonable strength.

Shortcomings of Muscular Fitness Tests

Many traditional physical fitness tests have long been accepted as measures of muscular strength, endurance, or flexibility. Unfortunately, these tests have become evaluations of performance rather than measures of physical fitness. Emphasis is on excesses, speed of performance, number of repetitions, or extent of stretching, rather than on quality and specificity of movement. For example:

1. **Trunk Flexion.** One of the most common tests for flexibility is forward trunk flexion, or *sit-and-reach*. Sitting with knees extended, the subject reaches forward toward or beyond the toes. Designed to measure flexibility of the lower back and hamstrings, the test focuses on how far the subject can reach.

The test fails to consider variables that can affect the results:

- there may be limitations due to imbalances between length of back and hamstring muscles;
- poor flexibility in the lower back may go undetected if hamstrings have excessive flexibility.

Clients with such imbalances may do well on the test, while people with normal flexibility may not do well. Moreover, some specialists would wrongly prescribe therapeutic exercise to increase spinal flexibility or stretch hamstrings when they are unnecessary or contraindicated.

2. **Push-Ups.** Properly executed push-ups involve scapular abduction during the up phase. When the serratus anterior is weak, the scapulae do not move—and yet the push-up may still be performed. Because other muscles can compensate for this weakness, you may fail to note small changes in body mechanics, such as incomplete flexion of the elbow or an unacceptably wide hand position.

The purpose of push-ups is to test the strength or endurance of arm muscles. Winging and lack of abduction of the scapula reveal a weak serratus anterior. If such weakness is not noticed, the test's validity is reduced, and push-ups are not a good index of muscular endurance of the arms.

3. **Bent Knee Sit-Ups.** Exercise specialists often measure endurance of abdominal muscles by having clients perform as many bent knee sit-ups as possible in sixty seconds . The curled trunk requires a strong contraction of the abdominals to hold this position. Many people start the test with the trunk curled, but their backs begin to arch because their abdominals are not strong enough to maintain the position. Since the speed and length of the test magnify the problem, the lower back is strained. The result is that clients with weak abdominals may pass this test using poor mechanics of the lower back and possibly assistance from the hip flexors.

Postural Assessment

Good posture involves all body parts in a state of balance and the muscles holding the body erect against gravity without fatigue. A misaligned human body does not collapse—rather it twists out of shape to compensate for imbalances, and requires extra muscular energy and tension to hold itself up.

Assessment of posture is a very effective screening tool. By carefully observing alignment, we can detect strain produced by faulty relationships of various body

FLEXIBILITY/MUSCLE TIGHTNESS FIELD-BASED ASSESSMENTS: SUMMARY OF RESULTS

Test	Results
Pectoralis major (sternal) length	
Shoulder internal rotators (subscapularis) length	
Shoulder external rotators (infraspinatus, teres minor) length	
Hip flexors (1-joint) length	
Hip flexors (2-joint) length	
Tensor fascia latae length	
Hamstrings length	
Forward trunk flexion (with flexometer)	
Ankle range of motion	
Dorsiflexor length	
Plantarflexor (1-joint) length	
Plantarflexor (2-joint) length	
Calf tightness	
Wall dorsiflexion	

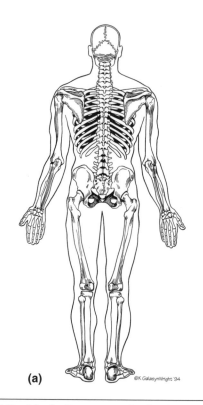

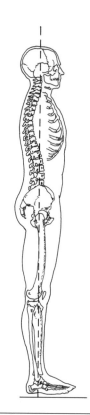

(a)   ©K GalasynWright '94   (b)

Figure 5.7   Ideal alignment—back view, side view.

parts. By keeping the postural assessment simple, we increase the speed of assessment and can go directly to the next stage of muscle balance assessment: muscle testing.

Alignment While Standing

Have your clients remove shoes and socks. Women should wear a two piece bathing suit, and men should wear trunks, to allow a clear view of landmarks. You will find a plumb line and a horizontal line grid very helpful, but not necessary for screening purposes. A brick or cement block wall also is helpful. Assess your client in a standing position from three positions—side, back, and front. Ask your client to stand in an upright, relaxed position, looking forward. Figure 5.7 shows the anatomical structures that coincide with the line of reference.

Side View

The following points coincide with a vertical line of reference in a lateral view:

- Slightly anterior to lateral malleolus
- Slightly anterior to axis of knee
- Slightly posterior to axis of hip
- Bodies of lumber vertebrae

- Shoulder joint
- Bodies of most of cervical vertebrae
- Mastoid process
- Slightly posterior to apex of coronal suture (Kendal 1993)

Observe: alignment of knees, hyperextended or flexed; position of pelvis; curves of the spine, exaggerated; head position; chest position.

Front View

Observe the following: position of the feet, knees, and legs; height of the longitudinal arch; pronation or supination of the foot; rotation of the femur as revealed by the patella; knock knees, or bow legs; rotation of the head; or prominence of the ribs. Have client stand with heels three inches from the wall; place your cupped hand behind the neck, to approximate normal cervical lordosis. Place your fist behind the lower back as a check for excessive lumbar lordosis.

Back View

Start by observing alignment of the Achilles tendon; angle of the femurs; height of the posterior iliac spines; lateral pelvic tilt; spinal deviations; position of shoulders and scapulae.

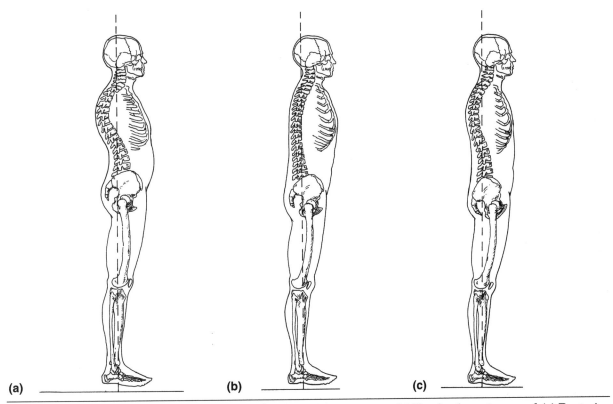

Figure 5.8 Common postural faults (a) Kyphosis-lordosis posture, (b) Flat-back posture, and (c) Posterior pelvic tilt.

Postural Faults

Figure 5.8 illustrates common postural faults. Practice in judging good and faulty posture will quickly improve your skill levels.

The "standard posture" (Kendal 1993) represents an ideal skeletal alignment that minimizes stress and maximizes efficiency. No one will match the standard in every respect.

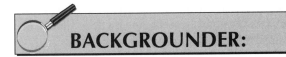

BACKGROUNDER:

Good and Poor Alignment

Joint: Foot

Good alignment

- Half dome arch
- Feet slightly toe-out
- Walking: feet parallel, weight transferred from heel along outside to ball of foot

Poor alignment

- Low arch/flat foot
- Weight borne on inside or outside of foot
- Walking: toeing in or toeing out

Joint: Knees and legs

Good alignment

- Kneecaps face straight ahead
- Lateral view: knees straight, not locked

Poor alignment

- Knees bowed or knocked; kneecaps inward or outward; rotated femur
- Flexed or hyperextended knee

Joint: Spine and pelvis (back view)

Good alignment

- Weight even on feet; hips level
- No lateral curve to spine; slight left deviation in right-handers is ok

Poor alignment

- One hip higher—lateral pelvic tilt; hips rotated, forward one side
- C- or S-curve scoliosis

Joint: Spine and pelvis (side view)

Good alignment

- Front of pelvis and thighs vertically aligned
- Buttocks not prominent
- Natural curves for lumbar, thoracic, and cervical

Poor alignment

- Thigh forms angle at pelvis
- Lordosis—forward tilt of pelvis
  Flat back—pelvis tilts backwards
- Thoracic rounding: kyphosis
  Forward head: cervical lordosis

Joint: Trunk

Good alignment

- Flat abdomen
- Chest slightly raised, normal back

Poor alignment

- Lower or entire abdomen protrudes
- Hollow chest, ribs prominent one side, flared lower ribs

Joint: Arms and shoulders

Good alignment

- Arms relaxed, palms facing body
- Shoulders level, not forward
- Shoulder blades: flat of rib cage about 4" apart

Poor alignment

- Arms stiff, away from body; palms facing backwards
- One or both shoulders up, down, or rotated
- Scapulae: too close or far apart; prominent-winged scapulae

Joint: Head

Good alignment

- Erect and balanced

Poor alignment

- Protruding forward, tilted, or rotated; chin too high

Field-Based Test #11: Postural Assessment Chart

The Postural Assessment Chart on page 70 lists key body areas to be examined. Four or five alignment checks are listed in the rows opposite the body area. For example, you would start at the feet checking for pronation/supination; toeing in/out; and the condition of the arch. In the small box in front of the item, mark "L" for problems on the left side and "R" for problems on the right. Mark items for the pelvis, spine, chest, or head with an "X" or a brief description (e.g., "forward").

Field-Based Test #12: Longitudinal Arch (Griffin 1989)

Observe the arch for this assessment. While client is standing, feet shoulder-width apart, have him lift one foot off the floor to observe the arch. This assessment may also be done in a sitting position if it is more comfortable. The idea is to assess the arch in a non-weight bearing position.

 If the foot appears flat with little or no arch, the client should not be encouraged to pursue weight-bearing activities.

 If the arch looks small it may be supple and will require extra support.

 If the arch looks full it is probably healthy, mechanically sound, and able to support trauma.

Field-Based Test #13: Static/Dynamic Foot Alignment (Griffin 1989)

Observe the back of the ankle for the degree of rolling inward while walking or jogging. This assessment is best analyzed without shoes on.

 If the heel rolls inward, flattening the arch while client is walking or jogging lightly, the client pronates.

 If the heel rolls inward somewhat while the client is walking or jogging lightly, the client should take precautions to avoid overuse.

 If the heel remains stable and the achilles tendon is vertical while client is walking or jogging lightly, then the ankle is aligned.

When postural screening reveals faulty body mechanics, confirm those results using the muscle tests. The postural analysis will help you determine which muscle length tests you should perform.

Highlights

- Measure **strength and muscular endurance** with dynamometers, cable tensiometers, electromechanical devices, and constant-resistance and variable-resistance exercise machines.

- Use these seven factors to help you determine which strength and muscular endurance tests to employ: joint-muscle relationships; degree of effort; strength level; normative values; specificity, reliability and validity; body weight test items; client needs.

- The **Five Level Sit-up** test utilizes a modified arm position to change the relative load and determine both a "strength" and an "endurance" level.

■ **Relative muscular endurance** is tested by assigning a submaximal load as a percentage of a repetition maximum (1 RM).

■ Measure **flexibility** directly by testing the range of motion of a joint or series of joints in degrees with devices like goniometers or flexometers.

■ Because the range of motion of each joint is unique, always examine the needs and demands of your client. For example, you should assess ankle flexibility of clients who plan a weight bearing or locomotor activity. If clients sit for long periods of time, check for tightness of the hip flexor and trunk extensor muscles.

■ **Muscle length testing** involves standardized movements which increase the distance between origin and insertion opposite to the direction of the muscle action. The chapter presents ten field-based tests for muscle tightness.

■ **Analysis of posture** permits you to select appropriate muscle length tests, and to devise a personalized prescription.

POSTURAL ASSESSMENT CHART

Feet

☐ Pronated ☐ Supinated ☐ Arch ☐ Toe in/out

Knees

☐ Rotation–patella ☐ Hyperextended ☐ Flexed ☐ Bowlegs ☐ Knock knees

Pelvis

☐ Anterior tilt ☐ Posterior tilt ☐ Lateral tilt ☐ Rotation

Spine

☐ Lumbar lordosis ☐ Flat ☐ Thoracic kyphosis ☐ Cervical lordosis

☐ Scoliosis

Chest

☐ Depressed ☐ Elevated ☐ Rotation–ribs ☐ Abdomen protruding

Shoulder

☐ Low ☐ High ☐ Forward ☐ Rotation–palms

Head

☐ Forward ☐ Tilt ☐ Rotation ☐ Chin

Scapulae

☐ Abducted ☐ Adducted ☐ Winged ☐ Elevated

Chapter 6

Matching Components, Methods, and Equipment With Our Clients

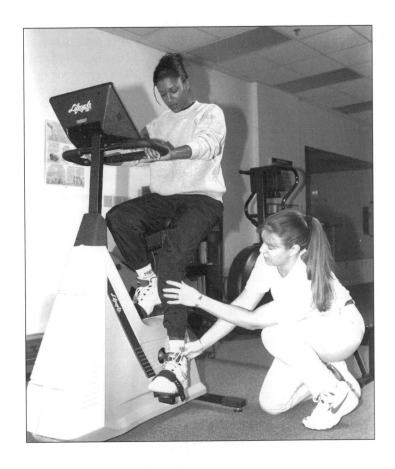

- Traditional and Emerging Components
- Physical Activity, Fitness, and Health
- How Much Exercise Is Enough?
- How the New Look at Fitness Affects Prescription

- Training Methods: Matching the Client
- Client-Centered Equipment Selection
- Home Equipment

Clients today want more than just aerobic fitness and weight control. We must offer more than just the physiological components of fitness!

What has recent research told us about the effectiveness of various types and quantities of exercise? How much do the benefits of exercise depend on the type of client? This chapter discusses these questions, especially as they touch on another question of great importance to our clients: How much exercise is enough?

Many training methods allow us to match specific benefits to the client. Clients' preferences and availability of equipment may also influence our prescriptions. In this chapter, we examine the equipment through which we can achieve our clients' objectives.

Traditional and Emerging Components

We can prescribe exercise programs to produce three potential outcomes: increased overall fitness, performance improvements, and health enhancement.

For years, guidelines for prescribing exercise were based on improvement in athletic ability or physical performance. As overall fitness grew in popularity, led by a surge of interest in aerobics, the guidelines were modified. Intensity levels were reduced, and workouts were structured to include a balance of all fitness components. Exercises were designed to stress the cardiovascular, metabolic, and musculoskeletal systems, thereby creating physiological and structural changes in the components of fitness.

One of the strongest trends in recent history is the adoption of activity as a health-enhancing strategy. Physical fitness and good health are not synonymous, but they are complementary. *Physical fitness* is the ability to carry out daily tasks with vigor and alertness, without undue fatigue, and with ample energy to enjoy leisure pursuits and to meet unforeseen emergencies.

Positive health is not merely the absence of disease—it is a capacity to enjoy life and to withstand challenges. It has social, physical, and psychological dimensions, each characterized on a continuum with positive and negative poles. Health benefits may occur in conjunction with improvements in aerobic power or muscular endurance, or with improvements in physical performance capacity. However, some health benefits appear to be achieved by exercise that normally does not lead to improved physical fitness (IFSM 1990).

Overall Fitness Components

The essential physiological components of physical fitness include cardiovascular endurance, flexibility, strength, muscular endurance, and body composition.

- **Cardiovascular endurance** is the ability to perform physical work involving large muscle groups continuously for an extended period of time. This component depends on the efficiency of the oxygen transport system: In the lungs, oxygen moves across a membrane (diffusion) into the red blood cells; it is transported through the arteries to working muscle cells (diffusion and utilization). End products of cellular metabolism (carbon dioxide and at times lactic acid) are transported back through the veins to the heart and lungs. The heart is the key to the oxygen transport system, since it must continuously pump blood to all bodily systems as well as larger quantities to more active tissues.

- **Flexibility** is the capacity of a joint to move freely through a full range of motion without undue stress. For most joints, the limitation of movement is imposed by the soft tissues, including the muscle and its fascial sheaths; the connective tissue, with tendons, ligaments, and joint capsules; and the skin (Wilmore and Costill 1994).

- **Strength** measures the maximum ability of a muscle or muscle group to exert force against a resistance. For example, a person who can maximally curl a barbell weighing 150 lbs. is twice as strong as the client who can curl only 75 lbs. Lifting as much as possible in one lift is referred to as one repetition maximum (1-RM).

- **Muscular endurance** is the ability of a muscle or muscle group to exert a force repeatedly, or to sustain a contraction for a period of time. A simple measure of muscular endurance involves determining the number of repetitions clients can complete while lifting a fixed percentage of their 1-RM.

- **Body composition** refers to the relative amounts of fat and lean body weight in the body. Exercise often leads to a decrease in total body weight and fat weight, and an increase in fat-free weight (Quinney, Gauvin, and Wall 1994).

Performance-Related and Health-Related Fitness Components

Performance-related fitness components are those necessary for sport performance or optimal work performance. The components include motor skills (e.g., speed, agility, balance, and coordination), cardiovascular endurance, muscular power, strength, endurance, size, body composition, skill acquisition, and motivation.

Health-related fitness components include body composition (e.g., subcutaneous fat distribution, abdominal visceral fat, body mass relative to height), muscle balance (strength, endurance, and flexibility—particularly of postural muscles), cardiovascular functions (e.g., submaximal exercise capacity, blood pressure, lung functions), and metabolic components (e.g., blood lipids, glucose tolerance). Very inactive people benefit most from even low intensity exercise, because the detrimental health-related consequences of extreme inactivity are rapidly reversed.

How Do Client Needs Affect Their Goals and Components?

The need for detail in the exercise prescription varies with the client's goals, desired outcomes, and risks. Skinner (1987) offers a schematic representation of the goals most common for different populations (figure 6.1).

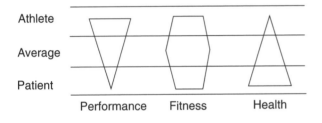

Figure 6.1   Changes in component goals with different clients.

For the athlete, **performance** is the central focus of a physical activity program. Health and fitness are secondary goals. You must be flexible, however—sometimes an athlete will be recovering from an injury (health goal) or building a strong off-season base (fitness goal). Skinner suggests the average client gets involved in activity for **fitness,** with perhaps an added interest in recreational sport performance. Quality of life and reduction of risk factors (health goals) are still in the minds of these clients.

Clients with musculoskeletal injuries or with certain health risk factors obviously are most concerned about improving their **health** and are less oriented toward performance. Clients may have several goals. Consider three hypothetical clients:

- Very active and very fit. This client has progressed with her overall **fitness** goals to a point where she wants to develop a higher level of **performance**.
- Rehabilitation referred, sedentary. In the final stages of rehabilitation for a specific injury or **health** problem, this client will be embarking

on a general **fitness** program to build future resilience.

- The athlete with overuse symptoms. To ensure a **healthy** athlete, you must change the prescription to avoid excessive trauma, regain muscle balance, and reduce inflammation. At the same time, you must help him maintain a competitive level of **performance.**

Clients are increasingly well informed about fitness. Yet the above scenarios show how dynamic their needs can be and how adaptable you must be to serve them well.

Within each component of fitness there are several approaches to the prescription. Look for specific prescription guidelines for each component later in this chapter under "How Much Exercise Is Enough?"

Physical Activity, Fitness, and Health

Much is known about those broad determinants of health that make and keep our clients healthy. We will now investigate how regular physical activity and fitness contribute to health.

Relationships Among Factors Affecting Performance, Fitness, and Health

You must consider more than physiological factors in writing prescriptions. You will benefit from understanding the interrelationships among lifestyle, environment, genetics, occupation, personal attributes, fitness, and health. By helping to orchestrate these factors, you can assist your clients in meeting their prescription objectives. Figure 6.2 presents Bouchard's model that defines these interrelationships.

The model demonstrates how physical activity and fitness influence each other. Just as the most fit tend to be the most active, the most active are frequently the most fit. The components of fitness—particularly health-related fitness—are determined by heredity, diet, and patterns of habitual physical activity. Health status also influences both fitness and physical activity. For example, an injury or illness will limit a client's physical activity and eventually will affect her level of fitness. Wellness is a holistic concept of positive health influenced by social and psychological factors, lifestyle habits (e.g., smoking, stress, diet), the environment, and physical well-being. The model also shows that wellness has a relationship with fitness and physical activity.

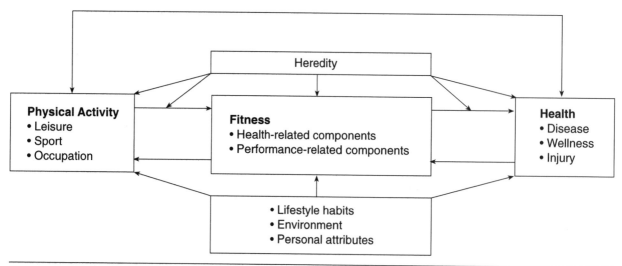

Figure 6.2 Physical activity, fitness, and health model (Bouchard et al., 1993).
Adapted, by permission, from Bouchard, C., 1994, *Toward Active Living, Physical Activity, Fitness, and Health: Overview for the Consensus Symposium.* Human Kinetics, 8.

Implications for Client-Centered Exercise Prescription

A purely physiological approach to exercise prescription would ignore many factors in Bouchard's model. To be client-centered, you must first establish whether your client's main concern is activity, fitness, or health. Then consider how the surrounding factors may directly or indirectly affect him. Carefully spending time with your client in these earlier stages will help both of you develop a clear vision of what he wants to achieve. The relationships in the model will influence how you reach those objectives and how you package the prescription.

For example, you have a client whose health-related fitness **goal** has already been established. The area of **priority** is appearance and a healthy weight. The specific **objectives** include reduction of body fat (especially in the trunk area) and reduction in blood lipids. These objectives are linked to the health-related fitness **components** of metabolism and body composition. The purely physiological approach may provide a very sound aerobic exercise prescription, but this would fail to serve all your client's needs. The model indicates that your client also will benefit from initiatives in the areas of diet, stress management, social environment, occupational activity, and household chores (that provide continuous moderate activity). You will achieve greater success and a more balanced outcome if your prescription for one area is made in light of how that area interacts with the others. This holistic approach is beneficial for athletes, fitness enthusiasts, and health conscious clients.

How Much Exercise Is Enough?

"I've been walking, but I hear that to be fit I should be jogging." "Recently I read that living actively, like taking the stairs and walking the dog, will make me fit." "As a distance runner, should I be doing the same weekly mileage even though I am working in intervals?" These are typical client concerns. How much exercise is enough? Enough for whom? Enough for what goal/objective?

Two Views of How Much Is Enough

The question may not be, "How much is enough?" but rather, "What constitutes an exercise benefit, and how much exercise is required before I see benefits?" Figure 6.3 contrasts two models of the relationship between the acquired benefits of exercise and the amount of exercise performed.

Exercise physiologists traditionally have held that cardiovascular fitness occurs only after a person reaches a threshold of exercise activity. According to this view, there is little or no benefit until the threshold for fitness is exceeded. Benefits continue to accrue as the level of exercise increases beyond this threshold. At an upper limit, the benefits level off (figure 6.3a).

Figure 6.3b shows that some improvements in fitness occur at low levels of exercise, even though the increases are small. At higher exercise levels, benefits accrue at an accelerated rate until an upper limit is reached beyond which the potential for injury and overuse detracts from the positive effects of training. Proponents of the need for some exercise, even at low

a   b

Benefits of
Exercise

Amount of Exercise

Benefits of
Exercise

Amount of Exercise

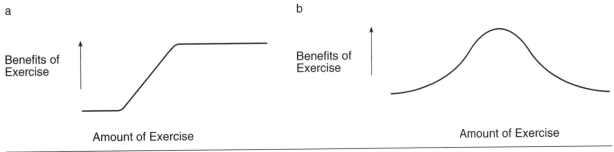

Figure 6.3   Schematic models of the benefits vs. amount of exercise.

levels, believe this gradual increase in benefits is typical of many adaptive responses.

Are the Mechanisms of Change the Same for Health and Fitness?

Improvement in health may be due to biological changes different from those responsible for fitness. For example, endurance training will increase endurance capacity and may help prevent coronary artery disease (CAD). The increase in endurance capacity most likely results from an increase in oxygen transport to and utilization by the skeletal muscles. The reduction in CAD risk may result from alterations in lipoprotein metabolism or blood clotting activity (Haskell 1985).

The accelerated rate of energy production during exercise increases the rate of functioning of other biological systems. With repeated stimulus these systems will increase their capacity or efficiency, providing many of the health-related benefits of exercise (Haskell 1985). This information can be extremely motivating to a client who sees no immediate changes in other measures.

In some circumstances the mechanism for health benefits may relate more to physical or mechanical stress placed on the muscles, connective tissue, or skeleton than to increased energy expenditure. For example, retention of postmenopausal muscle tone and bone calcium through exercise probably results from mechanical stress on muscles and bones from weightbearing activity or resistance exercise (Smith, Reddan, and Smith 1981). Joggers may benefit more from the weightbearing nature of their steps than from elevated heart rates.

Do Health Benefits Build Up or Do They Come and Go?

Although most fitness benefits are somewhat cumulative, this is not always the case with health benefits,

which dissipate quickly and require lifelong regularity of exercise (Haskell 1985).

Numerous biochemical changes occur during or immediately after a workout. Although these changes may be transient, they can favorably alter the progression of a specific disease if they occur often enough. For example, a single bout of endurance exercise will decrease elevated plasma triglycerides. Exercise on consecutive days further lowers the triglyceride concentration for 48 to 72 hours; but if exercise is not performed for several days, the concentration will return to its elevated level (Haskell 1985). Minimum daily exercise may give rise to discernible health benefits for many clients.

How the New Look at Fitness Affects Prescription

Let's examine "How much is enough?" from the perspective of three clients. Client #1 is interested in overall fitness and staying in shape. Client #2 has a number of cardiovascular risk factors and has set a goal of health-related fitness. Client #3 is an athlete interested in performance-related fitness.

Overall Fitness (Client #1)

Your first client wants to be able to perform moderate to vigorous levels of physical activity without undue fatigue and to maintain such ability throughout life (ACSM 1990).

Guidelines for Overall Fitness Prescription

Client #1 wants to see improvements in cardiovascular condition ($\dot{V}O_2max$), body composition, flexibility, and muscular strength and endurance. The ACSM recommendations on page 76 suggest optimal intensity, duration, and frequency for most of the training components. These recommendations are designed for the general population—not for highly trained endurance athletes or persons of poor health.

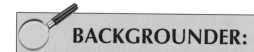

BACKGROUNDER:

ACSM Recommendations for Fitness Training in Healthy Adults

The American College of Sports Medicine (1990) recommends the following for healthy adults:

1. **Frequency** of training: 3-5 days/wk.
2. **Intensity** of training: 60%-90% of maximum heart rate or 50%-85% of maximum oxygen uptake or heart rate reserve.
3. **Duration** of training: 20-60 minutes of continuous aerobic activity. Duration depends on intensity. Lower intensity activity should be done for a longer period of time.
4. **Mode** of activity: Any activity that uses large muscle groups, can be maintained continuously, and is rhythmical and aerobic in nature—e.g., walking-hiking, running-jogging, cycling-bicycling, cross-country skiing, dancing, skipping rope, rowing, stair climbing, swimming, skating, and various endurance game activities.
5. **Resistance** training: Strength training of a moderate intensity, sufficient to develop and maintain fat-free weight (FFW), should be an integral part of an adult fitness program. One set of 8-12 repetitions of 8-10 exercises that condition the major muscle groups at least 2 days/wk. is the recommended minimum.
6. **Initial level of fitness:**

   High = higher workload
   Low = lower workload

Does exercise intensity matter?

The ACSM's minimum intensity recommendations have dropped continually during the past two decades, for two primary reasons: (1) Recent research indicates that some benefits, especially health benefits, are realized with lower intensities (see client #2, page 77); (2) Intensity is an individual factor that depends on a person's current fitness/activity levels. The lower the initial fitness level, the higher the expected change (Wenger and Bell 1986).

Prescribing for Client #1

Intensity is probably the most important variable for improving cardiovascular fitness. Since overall fitness is the primary objective for your client, you must progressively raise the intensity to the recommended level. For instance, if your client is of average capability, the intensity will need to build up to around 70% of his maximum heart rate for substantial cardiovascular improvements.

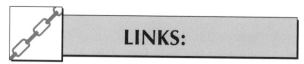

LINKS:

Ten Year Rejuvenation!

Consider an inactive 45-year-old. With his doctor's approval, you design an aerobic program with progressively increased intensity. Over a six-week period, he works up to exercising at 122-125 bpm (70% max. HR) and maintains that intensity regularly for another 16 weeks. The increase in his aerobic capacity is 20%. At his age, on average, 0.5% of his capacity is lost per year—in effect, this client's improvement amounts to a 10-year rejuvenation!

Wenger and Bell (1986) found intensity and duration of training to be interrelated: total caloric expenditure (energy cost) may be the most important factor for cardiovascular and body composition improvements (assuming a minimum intensity of 60% of maximum heart rate). The total energy cost of your client's exercise program, based on a body weight of 70 kg (154 lb.), should be approximately 900 to 1,500 kcal per week or 300 to 500 kcal per exercise session (ACSM 1990).

Even should you not have the resources to measure changes due to training, you can be reasonably sure that if the ACSM guidelines are followed, fitness will improve. The proper combination of intensity, duration, and frequency will improve your client's aerobic capacity 15 to 30% over a period of 4 to 6 months (Wilmore and Costill 1994). Programs of lesser intensity, duration, and frequency, or clients with higher levels of initial fitness, may produce improvements in the 5 to 10% range (Wenger and Bell 1986). If your client stays with the program, he can expect long-term benefits—middle-aged and elderly men who train consistently show less than 5% reduction in aerobic capacity per decade (Wilmore and Costill 1994). Your client may expect slight decreases in his total body weight and in fat weight, and increases in fat-free weight (Hagan 1988). The magnitude of these changes will vary directly with the intensity and duration of the activity and the total caloric expenditure (see chapter 8).

Weight training can increase your client's muscular strength, and cause some changes in body composition, but it will yield only slight improvement in aerobic capacity. Moderate-intensity programs appear superior to high-intensity ones in preventing musculoskeletal injuries and improving adherence to endurance training (Wilmore and Costill 1994).

Exercises for muscle balance (including strength and flexibility) can prevent poor posture, lower back complaints, and osteoporosis. Your client's flexibility will increase with static, dynamic, or PNF (proprioceptive neuromuscular facilitation) techniques of stretching (see chapter 11 for details).

Are strength training benefits difficult to achieve?

Many clients involved in strength training ask, "How much is enough?" Westcott (1991) summarizes a number of recent findings:

- When total work per week (load × sets × reps) was kept constant, there was no significant difference among frequencies of one, two, three, or five sessions per week.

- When two exercises were performed three times a week for 10 weeks, there was no significant difference among groups performing one, two, or three sets of exercise.

- In a study that looked at differences in muscle performance with a given submaximal resistance (75% of maximum), most subjects performed between 8 and 13 repetitions per set.

- A study of adult women following the ACSM guidelines (1 set, 10 reps, 3 days/wk., 8 exercises for 8 weeks) demonstrated 16% increase in leg strength and significant improvements in body composition.

Health-Related Fitness (Client #2)

Physical fitness and health-related fitness, while not synonymous, are complementary. Although your client may experience the health benefits of exercise along with improvements in fitness and performance (Blair et al. 1989), health benefits also may come from frequent performance of low intensity exercise that has no fitness training effect.

Some examples: Strength training may preserve bone mineral content or improve psychological well-being. Resistance training may lead to increased high density lipoproteins, lower diastolic blood pressure, and increased insulin sensitivity (Goldfine et al. 1991). Low intensity dynamic activity ($< 50\%$ $\dot{V}O_2max$) may reduce stress, contribute to weight loss, or improve certain biochemical reactions such as the release of endorphines. Flexibility exercises will improve your client's muscle balance, posture, and musculoskeletal integrity as she ages. It is important that you take a broad perspective when considering what exercise prescription will best improve health-related fitness.

The International Federation of Sports Medicine (1990) reinforces the model in figure 6.2 by describing how physical activity is a valuable component in the therapeutic regimen to control and treat coronary heart disease, hypertension, obesity, musculoskeletal disorders, respiratory diseases, depression, and wellness.

Guidelines for Prescription for Health Benefits

Recent guidelines (ACSM 1995; IFSM 1990; Pate et al. 1995) place less emphasis on vigorous exercise than on moderate intensity exercise (55%-75% max. HR or 40%-60% $\dot{V}O_2max$), particularly for sedentary adults. Moderate aerobic activity performed 30 minutes or more at least three times per week has a significant beneficial effect on blood pressure, lipid metabolism, glucose tolerance, and blood clotting—especially in middle-aged and older persons (Haskell 1995).

Figure 6.4 (Gledhill and Jamnik 1996) illustrates health gains as related to the volume of physical activity. Lower volumes of physical activity (duration × frequency) show more rapid initial improvement in triglycerides and blood pressure. Improvements in several other health-benefit indicators come at higher volumes of participation. Aerobic fitness depends on the intensity of participation, not just its duration and frequency. The other health-benefit indicators, however, depend primarily on duration and frequency of participation. The authors note that figure 6.4 reflects *general* interpretations of the related scientific literature and is meant to show the *collective* improvement in selected health-benefit indicators. The Health-Benefit Zones in figure 6.4 will help your client determine the benefits of his level of activity.

Other metabolic changes, like increases in high-density lipoproteins, appear to respond more to increases in the volume of exercise (amount of time spent) than to intensity. Several studies (Ebisu 1985; De Busk et al. 1990) show that multiple periods of moderate intensity exercise of about 10 minutes each and spread throughout the day can improve metabolism and body

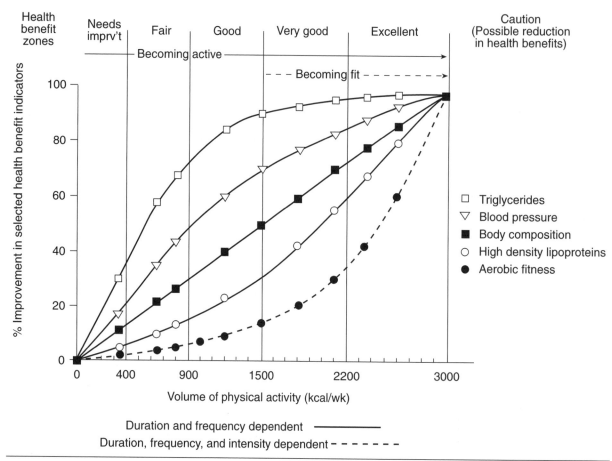

Figure 6.4 Dose-response relationship and health benefit zones for volume of physical activity participation. Reprinted, by permission, from *The Canadian Physical Activity, Fitness and Lifestyle Appraisal: CSEP's Plan for Healthy Active Living*. Published by the Canadian Society for Exercise Physiology, 1996.

composition. Paffenbarger et al. (1986) found that short periods of stair climbing, walking, or light sports proved effective against heart disease.

Prescribing for Client #2

Given equal total energy costs, lower intensity-longer duration exercise will benefit your older or less fit clients as much as higher intensity-shorter duration exercise. Moderate intensity exercise carries lower cardiovascular risk and lower probability of orthopedic injury, and it enjoys higher compliance. If your client is concerned about weight loss, have her exercise at a moderate to low intensity sufficient to burn 300 kcal three days/week, or 200 kcal four days/week (ACSM 1990). Using frequent short bouts of moderate activity, your client may progress up to a target of 1,500 kcal/week (see table 8.1).

In summary, for your client #2, who is pursuing health-related fitness, you should recommend moderate intensity, a minimum of three sessions per week, 20 minutes or longer per session.

Alternatively, have her perform less intense exercise five or six days per week; or 8-10 minute bouts of

moderate intensity exercise several times per day, most days of the week.

For resistance training, have her make extensive use of large muscle mass exercises; use higher volume training (i.e., multiple sets, moderate intensity); and avoid exhaustive sets (Stone, Keith, et al. 1991).

Performance-Related Fitness (Client #3)

For client #3, the serious exerciser or athlete, it is the upper levels of intensity and volume of exercise that are being tested. Optimal training for peak performance can be achieved only with a fine balance between intense training and proper rest. Client-centered prescription for athletes requires individualized training in those components that constitute performance-related fitness: motor skills (e.g., speed, agility, balance, and coordination), cardiovascular endurance, muscular power, strength, endurance, body composition, skill acquisition, and motivation. You can maximize your client's training efficiency only through prudent selection of training methods and by appropriately changing the prescription factors of his program as the need arises.

Since most athletes are highly motivated and tend to overstress themselves, they most frequently err on the side of overtraining rather than undertraining. Both you and your athletic clients must be aware of this problem, since overtraining will deny them their full potentials.

Now consider your third client—the athlete interested in performance-related fitness.

How Much Exercise Is Too Much?

More exercise can be a double-edged sword: it can be helpful or, if poorly directed, it can be harmful. The reinforcement your client receives from her rigorous training regime can easily cross the line to decreased performance and nagging injuries. It is hard to tell such a motivated athlete that she must slow down or change what so far has been a successful prescription. Yet all athletes experience periods when their performance levels off or decreases. This "overtraining" results from failure to tolerate or adapt to the training load.

Guidelines for Prevention of Overtraining

Stone, Fleck, et al. (1991) have observed two types of overtraining: (1) monotonous program overtraining, and (2) chronic overwork overtraining.

1. **Monotonous program overtraining** demonstrates a loss or plateauing of performance due to the consistent, unvarying use of the same type of exercise. It is not due to excessive fatigue. It is akin to a batting slump or a goal-scoring void for athletes, or a feeling of "the blahs," or a lack of energy in the fitness enthusiast. Stone, Fleck, et al. (1991) believe this type of overtraining may be the central nervous system's adaptation to a lack of appropriate stimulation from different movement patterns.

2. **Chronic overwork type overtraining** also can result in a plateauing or loss of performance. It is important to distinguish the differences between chronic and short-term overwork. Decreased performance as a result of a few sessions of high-intensity or high-volume training (short-term) is recovered within a few days. Short-term decreases in performance may also result from changes in training method. For example, a middle distance runner may experience slower times after doing cross-country training for a few weeks. With aerobic exercise, muscles need adequate time to rebuild, restore, and replenish. The recovery period may range from 24 to 72 hours. After an intense bout of weight training, it generally requires 48 hours to repair the microtrauma to the muscles and connective tissue, to remove waste products (e.g., lactic acid), and

to replace energy stores (e.g., muscle glycogen) in the cells (Westcott 1989).

Chronic overwork occurs when the overwork is sustained too long or repeated too frequently and the client no longer responds adaptively to the training. This type of overwork can lead to chronic fatigue, exercise burn-out, and higher rates of injury. Recovery from chronic overwork may take several weeks or months (Kuipers and Keizer 1988).

Prescribing for Client #3

Recognition of overtraining is critically important, yet difficult. Symptoms of monotonous, short-term, and chronic overwork often overlap. By the time they are recognized and differentiated, the client has progressed to a stage where rest is imperative. Prevent overtraining by insisting on (1) adequate short-term recovery, (2) proper variation, and (3) careful monitoring.

1. **Adequate short-term recovery.** If your client performs a 45-minute light aerobic workout with some stretching, she will be able to train harder within 24 hours. If the workout is 90 minutes and is more vigorous and high impact, she may need to wait two or three days before a similar workout.

2. **Proper variation.** Varying volume, intensity, and mechanics of training can reduce the likelihood of overtraining potential. Such variation also encourages a "peaking" at the appropriate time, and helps maintain a high level of performance (Kuipers and Keizer 1988). Adjust the training according to your client's levels of physical or emotional stress. Adjustments often take the form of decreased training volume with normal intensities.

Sudden changes in intensity and volume may create short-term delays in performance gains; but periodic changes in training technique, venue, the use of massage, or stress management techniques can prove rejuvenating.

3. **Careful monitoring.** Keeping a diary or log is essential for the serious performer (see chapter 7). It may include body weight, diet, resting heart rate, sleep patterns, subjective feelings of general health, and ratings of how difficult training felt. You can provide readings of blood pressure and heart rate, both at rest and post exercise. See that infections are treated, with your client gradually returning to normal training levels.

The editor of Runner's World (Burfoot 1995) provides some practical recommendations:

- Run less when you are tired, more when you find that perfect forest trail.

- Run less when you have a cold, more when you feel strong.

- Run more when you are training for a marathon, less when your knee hurts.
- Run less when you are starting a new job, more when your kids head off to college.
- Run more during some weeks, and less during others.

Make running fit into everything else you do. Look at the big picture.

Training Methods: Matching the Client

We are at a point in the prescription journey where a performance, fitness, or health goal has been established for a particular area of priority. The specific objective is linked to one or more fitness components. How to reach those objectives and how to package their prescription is the next stage—that is, matching our client to the training method.

Chapters 7 and 11 describe the many tools at our disposal for designing activity programs. They present the physiological basis and advantages of specific methods of training. Effective exercise prescription depends on our ability to highlight specific benefits for specific clients, using popular methods such as weight, flexibility, aerobic, and anaerobic training.

It is imperative that you integrate the various components of fitness into a balanced workout. To improve or maintain cardiovascular endurance, flexibility, strength, muscular endurance, and body composition, include all the following phases in your client's prescription:

- Warm-up
- Aerobic conditioning
- Flexibility exercises
- Muscular conditioning
- Cooldown

Body composition changes are achieved through a combination of aerobic and muscular conditioning.

There is some room for personal preference in the order of the phases of a workout. Regardless of the order, follow the principle of progressive overload as your client enters the aerobic and the muscular conditioning phases. A gradual increase in intensity will prepare the body for the demands of that phase. The order presented above allows the tissue temperature to be high when your client works on flexibility. It also stretches muscles tightened during the aerobics, in preparation for the resistance training to follow. However, many clients may feel more comfortable doing their flexibility training prior to the aerobic activity.

Both continuous and discontinuous aerobic training can improve cardiovascular fitness (Åstrand and Rodahl 1977). Interval training (discontinuous) consists of a repeated series of exercise bouts with intermittent relief periods. Because interval training permits a variety of activities, it is popular in many sports and has been recommended for symptomatic clients whose primary goal is health (ACSM 1991). Manipulation of the interval prescription factors, such as duration of effort, time of relief, and number of repetitions, can make prescriptions very precise (chapter 7).

You can match strength training programs to your clients' objectives. Almost any form of resistance exercise will stimulate some degree of strength gain, especially if your client is unconditioned. Comfort, convenience, and safety therefore become as important for many clients as results. Again, considering the goals of your clients (performance, fitness, or health) will help you select the appropriate resistance training methods.

Flexibility plays a major role in the maintenance of muscle balance. Your client's objectives will determine how, where, and through what technique you integrate flexibility into the prescription (chapter 11).

Your clients may wish to improve specific aspects of fitness, optimize sport skills, or develop work hardening tasks. For every client, you can match specific benefits provided by weight training, flexibility training, aerobic training, and anaerobic training. Your prescription will take into consideration not only optimal training outcomes, but also your client's preferences and availability of equipment or facilities.

Client-Centered Equipment Selection

As exercise specialists, we must evaluate a variety of resistive, cardiovascular, and home equipment. We should understand the features as well as the design, manufacture, safety, cost, serviceability, etc.

Detailed analysis and client match-ups are discussed in chapter 7 for cardiovascular equipment and in chapter 11 for resistance equipment. Home equipment is examined at the end of this chapter.

Trends in Fitness Equipment and Client Preferences

Who would have predicted five years ago that we would someday be exercising in a virtual reality? Who imagined we could climb a stair machine while seeing and hearing ourselves climb K2, or feel wind and speed changes as we cycle through the French wine country!

The psychological fit of a piece of equipment is as important as its safety and overall workability. Equipment can play a critical role in developing task-specific self-confidence. A person's belief that she *can* stairclimb for 20 minutes, or burn 300 calories on a treadmill, creates strong motivation and adherence. Most modern machines can not only measure variables precisely—they display them throughout the exercise session. For clients who find it difficult to stick to exercise programs, instant readouts of their progress can help focus their efforts.

Computerization may look like a panacea to universal appeal, but looks can be deceiving. Should fitness equipment look like a computer in order to promote greater client satisfaction? Participants over 50 may have minimal computer experience. What appeals to one group may not motivate other groups, especially the inactive. Some personal trainers and consumers have a "back to basics" attitude and shy away from a high tech approach.

Cross training, or the rotation of exercise activities (see chapter 7), is influencing equipment use as well as the variety of equipment a facility must have. A facility's versatility is increasingly important for both aerobic and resistance equipment, as cross training becomes more popular. Most clients rotate through several activities such as stair climbing, cycling, and treadmill usage in a single workout. Strength training shows a similar shift toward using a combination of free weights and machines. People seem less concerned about staying with a single brand name, while they focus more on rotations by function. For example, they may ask for another exercise, using free weights, that is similar to the action on the rowing machine.

LINKS:

Balanced Equipment Inventory

The following offers a proper balance between aerobic equipment, variable resistance equipment, free weights, and some specialized items. It is a functional approach, suggesting a minimum basic selection of equipment to suit general purposes.

Aerobic Equipment

Two types of equipment are needed to allow for the client's ability to bear weight:

- Seated to reduce weight bearing (bicycle ergometers, computerized bikes, recumbent bikes, rowers).

- Upright weight bearing (treadmills, jogging track, stairclimbers, steps).

Variable Resistance Machines

Variable resistance machines alter the effective resistance of a weight stack to match the strength curve of a muscle. Think in terms of a circuit design utilizing selected variable resistance equipment to cover the following areas:

- Chest (e.g., bench press, shoulder press)
- Upper back (e.g., lat pull-down, rowing)
- Shoulders (e.g., lateral arm raises)
- Arms (e.g., curls, extensions)
- Front thigh (e.g., leg press, knee extension)
- Back thigh (e.g., knee curl)
- Calf (e.g., toe raise)

Free Weights

Equipment *should* include the following:

- Dumbbells (with at least a flat and incline bench)—good for isolation and smaller muscle groups.
- Barbells (benches should have spotting racks).
- Olympic bar lifting—for more serious body builders.

Specialty Items

Sometimes rather simple equipment can provide great benefit in return for very low cost:

- Pulley systems (high and low, fixed and swivel base)—allow versatile movements; good for rehab.
- Bands and tubing—similar benefits as pulleys.
- Body weight apparatus (e.g., chin-up bar, dips, stall bars, mats).

People usually do not look for brand names. Rather, they look for types of equipment (e.g., treadmills and bikes) appropriate to their fitness/health goals (Wolkodoff 1995). For example, if a client wants to reduce his risk of heart disease, he will seek a center with treadmills or other cardiovascular training equipment.

Teach your clients how to interpret and use the information provided by displays on their equipment. The readouts can definitely help motivate your clients;

but keep in mind that people prefer displays and controls that are easy to use. The most popular readings show time and calories. People also like machines that permit them to immediately start their workout and then enter personal data later (Robinson & Godbey 1993).

No matter what the equipment choice, educating the client is important to getting the equipment accepted. First become familiar with the machine yourself (equipment suppliers frequently provide product seminars for your own professional development). Try offering orientations to new equipment as soon as it comes in, and to new clients once they have their programs in place.

Model for Equipment Selection

Matching equipment with the needs and priorities of your client depends largely on your asking the right questions and establishing clear objectives. The processes of evaluation and selection are both objective and subjective.

The Model

The model on pages 83-84 provides an effective framework for informed selection of equipment. Optimum equipment selection will increase your clients' compliance and enjoyment, and decrease their frustration and the risk of injury.

Let's look at an example of matching client priorities with the most appropriate machine. A client wants cardiovascular improvement and some upper body toning, but wants something easy and comfortable to use at home that is non-weightbearing. She feels she needs motivation and feedback in your absence. These are all advantages of either a recumbent bike or a rower. The rower has the added benefits that it exercises the upper body, and is relatively affordable for home use. It also can monitor heart rate—a very useful feature that will allow you to chart responses over a period of time and to guide the progressions in work load.

Know your client's needs, and compromise as little as possible on features that are important. It may be better not to buy at all if what your client can afford is not what she truly needs.

Judging Client Needs

Accurately assessing your clients' needs is the most important part of equipment selection. You probably will need to educate and guide your clients in order to show them how certain equipment can contribute to their goals.

LINKS:

The Importance of Client Education

In the preliminary stages of planning an employee fitness center, the CEO of a major sporting goods company was unsure whether to include weights and strength training equipment. An employee survey had rated their interest level high for treadmills and bicycles, their objectives being aerobic fitness and weight control. Despite this message, the CEO obtained *on loan* for three months a multi-gym/stack-weight machine. To assess his decision, the CEO asked me to split the first 30 members into two groups: one that exercised on the aerobic equipment only, and one that spent half their time on aerobic equipment and the other half on both the aerobic equipment and the multi-gym/stack-weight machine. The strength/endurance component of the aerobic program added metabolically active lean tissue that burned calories around the clock. The loss of weight and the cardiovascular improvements in both groups were similar. However, the resistance work brought about changes in measurements and body-sculpting effects that left most of the first group (including the CEO) looking for some cross training! The company purchased the multi-gym.

Equipment should suit the anatomy, interests, and fitness level of your client. For resistance equipment, the client's size and strength are important. Equipment should be adjustable, not just in terms of the resistance but with respect to the seat, position of the pads or straps, position of the moving joint, heights, and range of motion. What feels good to your client is a reasonable indication of suitability.

For aerobic equipment, lack of comfort and boredom are the reasons most often given by dropouts (Dishman 1990). Simplicity and benefits are the major trends in aerobic fitness equipment (Scotti 1985). Most people want simply to get on the machine and start exercising. They want equipment that will not cause overuse injuries, is low impact, provides well-rounded fitness—and most of all, is time efficient.

Home Equipment

The model given on page 83 for equipment selection is appropriate for home equipment—it helps match

EQUIPMENT SELECTION MODEL

1. Circle the * for the most important client priorities.

2. Circle the * for the existing design and safety features (Equipment Profile).

3. Identify match-ups between 1 and 2.

Client priorities

Client Priorities include:

* **Needs**—physiological, structural, and for preventing injury

* **Wants**—areas of interest, expectations, and enjoyment

* **Lifestyle** factors—time, location, availability, partner, motivation, current influences, etc.

* General component (e.g., strength) vs. specific component (e.g., leg power); is your client spending too much time and money on one muscle group, such as thighs or abdomen?)

* Sport-specific outcomes

* Body size/weight (gender)

* Body segment length

* Coordination/skill

* Previous experience

* Biomechanics/ergonomics (safety)

* Fitness level

* Motivation and feedback

* Space/portable (home equipment)

* Partner's priorities

* Current injuries

* Preferred location (e.g., convenient)

* Cross-training

* Economical

* Other: _____

(continued)

EQUIPMENT SELECTION MODEL *(continued)*

Equipment Profile

Equipment: _____

_____

Equipment assessment is based on the design and safety features of a particular piece of equipment.

* Adjustments to suit body size and segment (e.g., check pec-deck on multi-gyms)

* Smoothness and comfort (e.g., can pulley handle heavier weights?)

* Monitoring capabilities

* Ease of use and entry

* Loading capabilities

* User-friendly, quick start-up

* Ability to isolate muscles

* Feel and performance of equipment

* Safety features (e.g., can the limits of ROM be set?)

* Affordable

* Programming capabilities

* Durable

* Pivot locations (active joint alignment) (e.g., leg extensions with no seat adjustment)

* Handles full range of size and fitness levels (e.g., weight stack capacity)

* Stable base of support

* Quality of manufacturing (cables, belts, frames, upholstery, electronics, etc.)

Selecting home equipment

Selecting affordable home equipment presents a unique question: How much should one compromise in quality as compared to equipment in clubs? A good example is with home multi-gyms. The following are some design drawbacks of multi-gyms for home use:

- Assembly time on weight-stack gyms may be half a day.
- Changing resistance may involve rerouting cables around different pulleys.
- Time-consuming setups are required between exercises (no chance for circuit training).
- Cables are too short to go through a full range of motion.
- There is insufficient weight to challenge a majority of clients.
- Equipment is relatively unstable for someone doing leg curls while standing up.
- Exposed bolts or wood can cause chafing.
- It can be difficult to get into starting position.
- Benches are too high, feet do not touch ground, and lower back hyperextends.

specific features of equipment with the needs and priorities of the client. The selection of each piece of home equipment is especially critical, because space and financial limitations demand greater versatility and creativity in its use.

Do Clients Use Home Equipment?

"Muscled aside by time and apathy, home gym equipment is collecting dust and generating guilt in basements and garages across the land" (Turner 1996). This headline in a metropolitan newspaper reflected a genuine problem with home equipment. The explosion of infomercials has been a huge force behind new home equipment sales. Manufacturers romanticize their machines, and the consumer buys a dream.

Is it lack of time, loss of motivation, or poor selection of equipment that finds so many consumers not using their equipment? Because exercise specialists and personal trainers frequently advise clients about suitable equipment for homes or offices, these professionals must be skilled in equipment analysis and selection. Not only must they know product features for various categories of equipment—they must be able to assess their clients' needs, budgets, and space allocations, and determine the genuine value of products for their clients.

What Are the Most Popular "Transportable" Pieces of Home Equipment?

As an exercise specialist, the most effective, versatile, and portable piece of equipment you own is yourself. You are the computer, the feedback display, the variable resistance, the monitor, and the motivation machine. Still, you need some equipment that will enable you to deliver the best possible workout to each client. All exercise equipment need not have blinking lights; not all must be a clone of equipment found in large commercial centers.

Whether advising a client about a purchase or building your own collection, strongly consider adding some affordable and transportable pieces of equipment. Some equipment may be used for cross training; but let's look at suggestions for each of the fitness component areas.

Aerobic Equipment

- **Bench step.** Steps have probably done more to change the face of the industry than most other equipment. Not only have the inexpensive platforms brought more men into the aerobics circle, they've expanded the concept of methods of training. They are effective tools for interval and circuit training, particularly when step training and conditioning exercises are combined (Brooks and Copeland-Brooks 1991). Bench steps are a good alternative for people who would rather not walk/jog or invest large sums of money in aerobic machinery.

- **Slide.** This 8-foot piece of plastic, with angled bumpers and low friction slippers, allows for a reasonably intense lower body and aerobic workout. Various slide techniques and arm movements can increase variety, and can be combined with step or other exercises for an interval or circuit design. Slides can be adapted for sports such as hockey. Clients with ankle or knee instability should be cautious when using slides.

- **Videos.** Commercial fitness videos have expanded to the point where they are targeting specific groups and needs. Whether your client is a senior, an athlete, is overweight, or wants to work her heart, buttocks, or thighs, there is something she can buy! It is critical that you help her screen videos for the appropriate intensity level, style, and degree of safety. Consider videotaping a workout for your client to use during travel, vacation, or when you can't get together.

■ **Recreational/sporting equipment.** Any equipment that helps your client associate fitness with fun will serve you both well. There are many opportunities for one-on-one basketball, in-line skating, throwing Frisbees, even shadow boxing.

■ **Skipping ropes.** A recent survey of personal trainers found that the skipping rope was the least used piece of portable aerobic equipment (Fair 1992). Rope skipping is quite intense, can be high impact, and takes some skill; however, various techniques of lower intensity and lower impact skipping can make it a viable station within a circuit. The rope also can be used as a source of resistance or as a stretching device.

Strength Equipment

■ **Rubberized resistance.** Although rubber for resistance was initially used in rehabilitation and physical therapy clinics, its use has been embellished by the fitness industry. Flat rubber products (e.g., *Dynabands*) and surgical tubing products are equally popular. Four or five levels of resistance are usually available; it is cheaper by the roll. Some products come with built-in handles, pulleys, or door clamps that allow greater comfort and more angles of movement. Tubing with handles looped under a bench step on which the client stands turns an aerobic station into a resistance station. Because the client controls the pull, this source of resistance is one of the most versatile and useful pieces of portable equipment.

■ **Free weights.** Since machines are costly, most men who buy resistance equipment for home use begin with free weights. Women are increasingly buying affordable sets of plastic covered weights (5 to 15 pounds or heavier). Hand or wrist weights are popular add-ons to aerobic activity. Take care to show your clients how to avoid excessive momentum and joint hyperextension.

■ **Weighted bar.** These bars come in 10- to 18-pound sizes and are usually accompanied by an exercise manual. This small addition to the weight of a body segment often provides just the required overload for more rapid gains.

■ **Balls.** Body balls are growing in popularity and are excellent for postural muscle toning and body awareness. They are gaining use in some clinical settings. The old medicine balls have seen a bit of a resurgence with athletic clients, particularly with plyometric training.

Flexibility Equipment

■ **Mats.** A warm, comfortable, padded surface on which to stretch is the most fundamental piece of equipment.

■ **Towels, bars, or tubing.** These items help the client passively stretch a muscle by applying force or leverage. With some thought, these devices could provide a mechanism to perform some PNF (proprioceptive neuromuscular facilitation) stretching (chapter 11).

■ **Sit-and-reach box.** With a little bit of carpentry skill, you can build a box to the specifications of an aerobic bench step test; you also can mark a scale as in a sit-and-reach assessment. Put a handle on it and turn it upside down to carry some smaller items.

■ **Posters.** Posters can provide clear descriptions and good illustrations of the stretches in a client's program. Place the posters on the wall to help the client recall the exercises and develop safe executions.

Support Equipment

■ **Music and cassette players.** Building a client's endurance or time at an activity is a challenge. Music does more than distract from sweat and pain. Studies on perceived exertion have shown that music makes an exercise session feel easier and extends the time required to reach exhaustion (Iknoian 1992). Preparing music for your client is greatly simplified by the availability of commercial speed-adjusted recordings from funky exercise to soft stretch.

■ **Heart rate monitors.** Pulse meters are well suited for clients who want electronic feedback. They allow you or the client to make informed decisions about when to progress or when to cut back. Pedometers measure distance traveled and can also provide motivation—particularly for beginning clients who prefer to be exact.

■ **Water bottles.** Many people work out in hot climates or for long periods of time. Fluid replacement is very important, and educated clients always have water available. Water intake should be at least every 15 minutes during strenuous activity in hot environments.

■ **Shoes.** Incorrect, worn, or poor quality shoes can be a prominent factor in injuries, especially in high impact activities. However, features of some so-called "specialty" shoes are often very similar to those needed in several different activities. For example, court games such as tennis, racquetball, and basketball require similar side-to-side motion and are similar in their requirements for good forefoot and lateral support and for strong heel cups. A mid-cut tennis shoe could certainly be used in an occasional basketball game (Sillery 1996). Similarly, some mid-cut basketball shoes are light enough for other court sports. Encourage your clients to select specialty shoes for any activities they perform more than two or three times a week. Joggers who log more than 10 miles per week should wear running shoes that suit their style of running and their foot mechanics. For example, a "heavy-style" runner should look for running shoes with added cushioning; and a runner who pronates (rolls over on the inside of the foot when bearing weight) should have good arch support and a firm, snug-fitting heel cup. Proper shoes feel more comfortable and leave people less susceptible to injury—and the shoes last longer!

On page 90 is a checklist to use when purchasing home equipment (Turner 1996).

Highlights

- The essential **physiological components** of physical fitness include cardiovascular endurance, flexibility, strength, muscular endurance, and body composition.

- Exercise at the level recommended by the ACSM (1990) leads to beneficial cardiovascular changes.

- When following ACSM prescription guidelines, clients may expect slight decreases in their total body weight, increases in fat-free weight, and decreases in fat weight.

- Significant strength-training benefits can be achieved with minimal workout frequency and time.

- **Performance-related fitness** components are those necessary for sport performance or optimal work performance.

- **Overtraining** results from failure to tolerate or adapt to the training load.

- Prevention of overtraining is largely a result of (1) adequate short-term recovery, (2) proper variation, and (3) careful monitoring.

- **Health-related fitness** is described by Bouchard (1994) as the state of physical and physiological characteristics that decrease the risk of premature development of diseases.

- Lifestyle factors, environment, genetics, occupation, and personal attributes all affect fitness and health. By helping to orchestrate these factors, you can assist clients in meeting their prescription objectives.

- Health benefits of exercise may accompany improvements in fitness and performance capacity (Blair et al. 1989), but some benefits accrue even from exercise that normally does not lead to improved physical fitness.

- Effective exercise prescription highlights, for specific clients, the specific benefits of popular methods of weight training, flexibility training, aerobic training, and anaerobic training. An effective prescription will balance optimal training outcomes with the client's individual preferences.

- People usually look not for brand names but for types of equipment (e.g., treadmills and bikes). As an exercise specialist, you must be able to evaluate the features and benefits of a variety of resistive, cardiovascular, and home equipment.

- You often will need to guide and educate clients to show them how certain exercise equipment can contribute to their goals.

- The selection of each piece of home equipment is critical, because restrictions on space and finances require that home equipment be especially versatile.

- Consider the value of some of the following affordable and transportable pieces of equipment:

  1. **Aerobic Equipment:** bench step, slide, videos, recreational equipment, and skip ropes.

  2. **Strength Equipment:** rubberized resistance, free weights, weighted bar, and balls.

  3. **Flexibility Equipment:** mats, towels, bars, tubing, sit-and-reach boxes, and instructional posters.

  4. **Support Equipment:** music, heart rate monitors, water bottles, and shoes.

CHECKLIST FOR PURCHASE OF HOME EQUIPMENT

_____ **Why do you want the equipment?** Is it to improve a golf game, reduce the risk of heart disease, or help reduce stress? Apply the Equipment Selection Model.

_____ **Take a test drive!** You should be able to obtain a trial visit at a local fitness club or community facility. Take time to try several pieces of equipment, talk to the staff, and determine what the equipment feels like. Choose something you enjoy.

_____ **Compare local retailers.** Prices and product features may differ considerably. A knowledgeable retailer can help you assess equipment design and safety.

_____ **Don't buy on impulse.** If you are unsure, wait and return for another look.

_____ **Beware!** Stay away from items that are touted as no-effort, wonder products. Dramatically cheaper equipment probably is poorly manufactured.

_____ **Be practical.** Make sure the equipment will fit easily into your home. Are assembly time and maintenance reasonable?

_____ **Before making your purchase, check the following:** Is a manual included? What is the warranty? Is it transferable? Where do you go for replacement parts? For service?

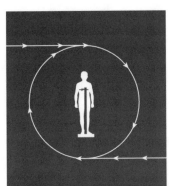

PART III

Selecting Routes: Personalized Prescription for Cardiovascular Conditioning and Weight Management

Clients vary widely in their health and aerobic fitness status, priorities, goals and objectives, occupation, age, motivation, and special needs. It is because of this variety that the client-centered approach to cardiovascular prescription is safer and more effective than the standard approach. Only after we have gathered information about the health, lifestyle, and fitness of our client are we in a position to design, demonstrate, and monitor a personalized exercise prescription. This part of the book details critical steps in the design of a cardiovascular program, including prescription factors, aerobic training methods, and equipment selection. The unique role of exercise in energy balance is the backdrop for discussion of client issues in selecting prescription factors for weight management.

Chapter 7

Personalized Prescription for Cardiovascular Conditioning

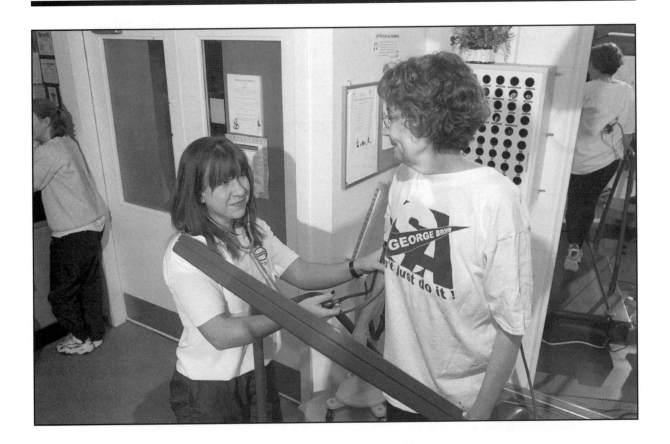

- Cardiovascular Prescription Model
- Client Issues in the Selection of Intensity
- Client Issues in the Selection of Mode/ Training Method
- Client Issues in the Selection of Duration
- Client Issues in the Selection of Frequency
- Client Issues in Selecting the Rate of Progression
- Monitoring
- Warm-Up and Cooldown
- Aerobic Objectives in a Client-Centered Approach
- Matching Aerobic Equipment to the Client

The key to a successful program lies in our ability to help clients maintain the conviction that our prescription will bring about the changes *they* want. Exercise will be a high priority if this personalized connection is maintained. We must provide constant support and reinforcement for this action-benefit relationship. Explaining to a client after four months of aerobic exercise that she can increase her maximum oxygen uptake by 15% may be realistic—but if her goal is to reduce stress, knowing about the oxygen uptake increase will provide scant encouragement.

Although cardiovascular fitness is still the foundation of most exercise prescriptions, the client-centered approach can adjust the outcome to suit more personal goals (e.g., reduction of stress or of CHD risk factors, improved performance). Every personalized goal responds differently to application of the prescription factors: intensity, mode (and training method), duration, frequency, and progression.

Cardiovascular Prescription Model

Below is the Cardiovascular Prescription Model that will serve both as an overview of what is to come and as a useful tool for future review.

Client Issues in the Selection of Intensity

Intensity is probably the most important and complex determinant of the cardiovascular exercise prescription. If it is set too high, our clients will be discouraged and risk injury. If it is set too low, results may be deferred and objectives not met. Before we can prescribe a client's exercise intensity, we must know how to calculate it.

Calculation of Exercise Intensity

The calculation of exercise intensity will depend, in part, on whether a graded exercise assessment was

---

Cardiovascular Prescription Model

Step 1   Consider Assessment Information
- Calculate functional capacity (e.g., maximum oxygen uptake) and normative rating
- Heart rate, blood pressure, and perceived exertion responses (steady states/termination criteria)
- Recovery rate
- Visual signs and symptoms

Note: Although recommended, step 1 may not be possible. A detailed history and subsequent monitoring and follow-up checks are increasingly important.

Step 2   Establish Intensity
- Recommend a training zone
(% $\dot{V}O_2$max, % max METS, % HRmax, % HR reserve, perceived exertion)

Step 3   Establish Mode
- Primary activity and alternate or cross-training activities
- Special needs/problems

Establish Corresponding Workloads
- As related to the training zone (Step 2)

Establish Method of Training
- For example, continuous vs. interval

Step 4   Establish Duration of Work (and Rest)
- Calculate total work/session (kcal/session)

Step 5   Establish Frequency
- Calculate weekly work (kcal/week)

Step 6   Establish Progression
- Stage of progression
- Method of progression
- Monitoring and follow-up checks

Step 7   Design Warm-Up and Cooldown
- Consider the previous steps

Figure 7.1   Cardiovascular prescription model.

done and on the type of test. The most direct way is to use a percentage of the measured functional capacity (e.g., percent of maximum oxygen consumption). If an exercise test was not performed, there are several indirect methods to estimate a training zone. The method selected will also depend on your access to test data, your experience as an exercise specialist, the availability of monitoring equipment, and the client's exercise program and level of fitness.

The following are the primary methods of calculating and prescribing exercise intensity:

- Methods *with* assessment: (1) MET level, (2) graph method, (3) percentage of maximum heart rate.

- Methods *without* assessment: (1) percentage of maximum heart rate (estimated), (2) heart rate reserve (HRR).

Methods With Assessment: MET Level Method

Note: A MET is equal to 3.5 ml/min/kg. Oxygen consumption at any level of exertion can be converted to a MET equivalent by dividing the oxygen consumption by 3.5.

Description

This method uses a percentage of the client's measured $\dot{V}O_2$max (i.e., functional capacity) converted to MET equivalents as described above (1 MET = 3.5 ml/min/kg). Calculate a specified percent max METs (e.g., 50 to 85%). Select activities with similar energy expenditures from table 7.1 (ACSM 1995).

Client Issues

- Useful for clients selecting activities like racquet sports or horseback riding, and who want approximate energy costs.

- Can be quantified for weight loss programs.

- Commonly used measure with referrals.

- Assessment may be difficult and costly.

- Accomodates when test mode is different from training mode.

- Actual energy cost of activity may be affected by environment, weather, clothing, diet, mechanical efficiency, or fatigue.

- When used in conjunction with perceived exertion, "talk test," or heart rate, fine adjustments can be made.

Example:

$$\dot{V}O_2max = 35 \text{ ml/kg} \cdot min$$

$$\text{max METs} = \frac{35 \text{ ml/kg} \cdot min}{3.5 \text{ ml/kg} \cdot min} = 10 \text{ METs}$$

If the intensity prescription is set at 50 to 85% of functional capacity:

$$50\% \text{ of } 10 \text{ METS} = 5 \text{ METs};$$
$$85\% \text{ of } 10 \text{ METS} = 8.5 \text{ METs}$$

Client should use activities that require 5 to 8.5 METs.

Table 7.1 (ACSM 1995) indicates that possible activities include aerobic dance, badminton, conditioning exercise, downhill skiing, hiking, or tennis. Wilmore and Costill (1994) provide a more exhaustive list of physical activities and their respective MET values.

Later in this chapter, we will use MET values to describe total work done in terms of calories (kcal) burned. (The caloric equivalent of 1 MET is 1 kcal/kg · hr. For example, an 80 kg client in average condition, working at 6 METs, would expend 480 kcal/hr or 8 kcal/min.)

Methods With Assessment: Graph Method

Description

Heart rate is linearly related to metabolic load (energy cost), therefore plot it on a graph against oxygen consumption (or MET) equivalents. Do this for each stage of the test, then draw a "best fit" line between the points. Now at any oxygen consumption or MET level, a corresponding heart rate can be read from the graph. Determine the training zone range by taking appropriate percentages of the maximum oxygen consumption and finding the heart rate responses at those points.

Client Issues

- If test mode is same as training mode, the relationship of the prescribed workload and heart rate should be very close.

- Assessment may be difficult and costly, but this method is the most reliable for prescription.

- There may be loss of accuracy if test mode differs from training mode (more monitoring necessary).

Example:

Figure 7.2 shows a functional capacity of 10.5 METs and a training zone of 60% to 80% of max METs.

$$60\% \text{ of } 10.5 \text{ METs} = 6.3 \text{ METs};$$
$$80\% \text{ of } 10.5 \text{ METs} = 8.4 \text{ METs}$$

Table 7.1 Leisure Activities in METs: Sports, Exercise Classes, Games, Dancing

ACTIVITY	MET RANGE	AVERAGE METs	ACTIVITY	MET RANGE	AVERAGE METs
Badminton	4-9+	5.8	Running:		
Basketball	7-12+	8.3	12 min/mile	—	8.7
Canoeing/rowing	3-8	—	10 min/mile	—	10.2
Calisthenics	3-8+	—	8 min/mile	—	12.5
Cross-country skiing	6-12+	—	Skating	5-8	—
Cycling (recreation)	3-8+	—	Skipping: 60-80/min	8-10+	9
Dance (aerobic)	6-9	—	Squash/racquetball	8-12+	9
Downhill skiing	5-8	—	Swimming	4-8+	
Golf (walking)	4-7	5.1	Tennis	4-9+	6.5
Hiking	3-7	—	Volleyball	3-6+	—

Adapted, by permission, from Edward Fox 1979, *Sport physiology* (The McGraw-Hill Companies: New York), 251.

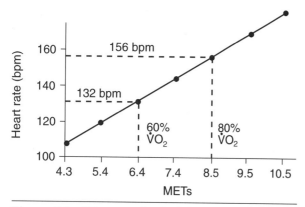

Figure 7.2 Direct method of determining the target heart rate zone.

The graph shows these levels correspond to heart rates of 132 bpm and 156 bpm respectively.

Methods With Assessment: Percentage of Maximum Heart Rate

Description

Percent of maximum HR is linearly related to percent $\dot{V}O_2$max (figure 7.3). Determine maximum heart rate

directly through a maximal functional capacity test using a treadmill or bicycle ergometer and going to a point of fatigue or a limiting symptom. Determine the training zone by taking a percentage of the measured max HR.

Client Issues

- Validated across many populations.
- If test mode is same as training mode, relationship of the prescribed workload and heart rate should be very close.
- Assessment may be difficult and costly, but accurate with use of ECG.
- Discomfort and some risk are possible with the average client.

Example:

ACSM (1995) recommends an exercise intensity of 60% to 90% max HR. If the measured maximum heart rate is 180 bpm, then

60% of 180 = 108 bpm; 90% of 180 = 162 bpm.

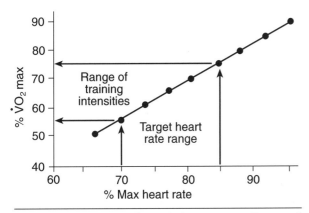

Figure 7.3   Relationship of % Max Heart Rate and % Max Aerobic Power.

Methods Without Assessment: Percentage of Maximum Heart Rate (Indirect Estimate)

Description

Determine maximum heart rate indirectly through age-predicted maximal heart rate tables. Determine the training zone by taking a percentage of the estimated max HR.

Client Issues

■ The formula (max HR = 220 – age) is conservative and variable (± 10-12 bpm).

■ Adding 15% to the training heart rate is suggested (Pollock and Wilmore 1990).

■ Important: If not added, threshold for cardiovascular (CV) improvement may be underestimated.

Example:

Heart Rate Training Zone = [(220 – age) × Training Zone %] × 1.15

For a 30-year-old client training between 70%-85% max HR,

[(220 – 30) × 70%] × 1.15 = 133 × 1.15
= 153 bpm

[(220 – 30) × 85%] × 1.15 = 161 × 1.15
= 185 bpm

Methods With Assessment: Heart Rate Reserve (HRR)

Description

Heart Rate Reserve is the difference between the maximum heart rate and the resting heart rate. Deter-

mine at what intensity you want the client to exercise. Take that percentage of the "reserve" and add it on to the resting HR to determine the heart rate training zone. The percentage of HRR is approximately equal to the percentage of $\dot{V}O_2$max (figure 7.4).

Client Issues

■ Very popular.

■ True resting HR not always available, but this does not seem to introduce a serious error.

■ Max HR estimates may be inaccurate.

■ Physiologically represents reserve of the heart for increasing cardiac output.

Example:

Heart Rate Training Zone = [(max HR – rest HR) × (50 to 85%) + rest HR (ACSM 1995).

For a 40-year-old client with a resting heart rate of 70 bpm at an intensity of 60%,

[(180 – 70) × 60%] + 70 = 66 + 70 = 136 bpm.

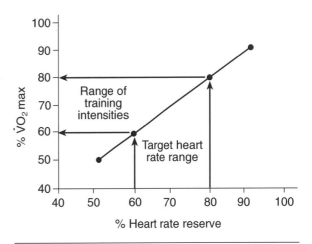

Figure 7.4   Relationship of % Heart Rate Reserve and % Maximal Aerobic Power.

General Guidelines for Selecting Intensity

You can vary the prescribed intensity level for your clients, depending on their fitness level, exercise history, objectives, and risk factors. Chapter 6 discussed health gains possible at lower levels of intensity (Haskell 1995). Intensities that provide adequate cardiovascular improvement for most of the population are in the following ranges (Howley and Franks 1997):

- 60% to 80% of $\dot{V}O_2$max (max METs)
- 60% to 80% of HRR
- 70% to 85% of max HR

[Note: These ranges are narrower than but still within the ACSM guidelines (1995)]

Intensity guidelines based on client descriptions in table 7.2 provide a greater degree of client specificity.

Ratings of Perceived Exertion (RPE) is a subjective measure of exercise intensity that takes into account the client's feelings of exercise fatigue, including musculoskeletal, psychological, and environmental factors. The Borg Scale of PE assigns a numerical value between 6 and 20 (table 7.3). You can use RPEs from a graded exercise test independently or in combination with heart rate to prescribe exercise training intensities.

Pollock and Wilmore (1990) show the relationship of perceived exertion and relative intensity (table 7.4).

Client-Centered Tips for Setting Cardiovascular Intensity

Here are some practical considerations to help you set the correct intensity for a client. Following these principles will put you well on the way to successful prescription.

1. **Consider the information gained from the cardiovascular assessment.** Graded exercise tests provide general categorizations of fitness status, to help you select the training zone. For example, table 7.2 shows an intensity of 50%-65% HRR for a client in a low fitness category and 65%-80% for an average fitness category.

The following "flags" identify the point just *above* which you should set the intensity:

- A sudden jump in heart rate, blood pressure, or physical effort during a test (or supervised change in workload if a test was not done)
- Systolic blood pressure rising significantly or rapidly

- A long time to steady state
- A slow recovery

Often it is helpful to start at a lower intensity and increase the volume of work gradually. Also consider using intervals to encourage adaptation in smaller increments. Set relief times based on recovery heart rates. The final cooldown should be gradual.

2. **Consider the relationship of intensity to the other prescription factors.** Duration, frequency, and mode interact with intensity in terms of total work and the stage of progression. Duration and frequency are often chosen to accommodate the selected intensity: intensity may be dangerously high if selected to accommodate low duration or low frequency. Duration of the work (or the work interval) provides the safest initial progression. Wider intensity ranges may be appropriate for some interval training programs. For example, you may prescribe an upper heart rate limit slightly beyond the standard aerobic training zone because the work interval is short; or you may prescribe a lower heart rate limit below the standard zone because it represents an interval recovery rate (see Interval Training later in this chapter). The aerobic warm-up intensity at the beginning of a workout should approach the lower end of the heart rate training zone.

3. **Consider the personal goals of your clients.** What your clients want must be balanced against your physiological objectives. Although the most rapid improvements usually occur when intensity is increased, the type of improvement your clients want (e.g., sport specific) should influence intensity selection. High intensity intervals will produce aerobic and anaerobic benefits; moderate, steady intensities improve stamina and aerobic endurance. Listen to your clients and their perceptions of the intensity. The Borg Scale is an excellent tool for tracking your clients' accommodations to their workloads, whether you are present or the ratings are logged.

Table 7.2 Client-Centered Intensity Prescription

CLIENT DESCRIPTION	INTENSITY (% $\dot{V}O_2$MAX/% HRR)
Low fitness status/inactive/several risk factors/wants lower intensity, longer duration	50%-65%
Average fitness status/normal activity/few risk factors	65%-80%
Excellent fitness status/very active/low risk/an athlete/intervals	80%-90%

Table 7.3   Borg's Ratings of Perceived Exertion Scale

6	No exertion at all
7	
8	Extremely light
9	Very light
10	
11	Light
12	
13	Somewhat hard
14	
15	Hard (heavy)
16	
17	Very hard
18	
19	Extremely hard
20	Maximal exertion

Note: From *An Introduction to Borg's RPE-Scale* by G. Borg, 1985, Ithaca, NY: Movement Publications. Copyright 1985 by Gunnar Borg. Reprinted by permission.

Table 7.4   Methods of Classification of Exercise Intensity

% MAX HR	% $\dot{V}O_2$MAX/% HRR	RPE (BORG SCALE)	CLASS OF INTENSITY
<35%	<30%	<10	Very light
35-59%	30-49%	10-11	Light
60-79%	50-74%	12-13	Moderate (somewhat hard)
80-89%	75-84%	14-16	Heavy
>90%	>85%	>16	Very heavy

Client Issues in the Selection of Mode/Training Method

In the past, many exercise specialists treated all clients alike. Even when they knew better, they often didn't know what factors were important in personalizing their prescriptions. The following discussion will help you target what is and is not important.

Selection Criteria

Select an exercise mode based on the client's

- stated preferences/interests,
- goals and objectives,
- availability and convenience (facility/equipment/time),
- skills and/or background,
- suitability (e.g., level of fitness/high risk), and
- other desired benefits (e.g., anaerobic, skill, social, etc.).

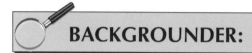

BACKGROUNDER:

Cardiovascular Endurance Activities—Grouping by Intensity

Any activity that uses large muscle groups, can be maintained, and is rhythmical and aerobic in nature can increase cardiovascular endurance. The American College of Sports Medicine (1995) classifies cardiovascular endurance activities into three groups:

Group 1: Physical activities in which exercise intensity is easily sustained with little variability in heart rate response: walking, aerobic dancing, swimming, jogging, running, and cycling.

Group 2: Physical activities in which energy expenditure is related to skill but for a given individual can provide a constant intensity: figure skating, swimming, highly choreographed dance exercise, cross-country skiing, and skating.

Group 3: Physical activities that are quite variable in intensity and skill: soccer, basketball, racquetball, etc.

Group 1 activities are most appropriate for beginning clients who need to carefully control intensity.

Group 2 activities are often outside of the "gym," providing an enjoyable venue. Combining a group

1 and 2 activity can reduce boredom and attrition and improve skill levels.

Group 3 activities may be the most fun and provide variety and cross-training opportunities. They are often group-oriented, adding a social element. The sporadic changes in intensity demand caution: People should spend time in a group 1 activity (e.g., preseason conditioning) before entering into a group 3 activity.

Aerobic Training Methods: Continuous or Interval

The two broad categories of aerobic methods are continuous and interval training. Research indicates that both are effective in improving cardiovascular fitness (Åstrand and Rodhal 1977; MacDougall and Sale 1981). The methods differ in their physiological bases, types of demand, and benefits. You must select the method and the training factors that match the needs of your client.

Continuous Training

Continuous training (CT) involves exercise (walking, jogging, in-line skating, cycling, stairclimbing, swimming, etc.) at a moderate intensity with no rest intervals. Runners often call this LSD or long, slow distance training.

Determining the Appropriate Level

Depending on the client and the desired outcome, the optimal prescription can vary considerably based on the following guidelines:

- **Athletes and well-conditioned.** Continuous exercise involving large muscle groups at 75% of client's aerobic capacity or $\dot{V}O_2$max (around 85% max. heart rate) optimally train the central oxygen transport system (MacDougall and Sale 1981).
- **Average client.** Training gains for the average client initiating a program may start at 50 to 70% $\dot{V}O_2$max or 65 to 80% MHR (Heyward 1998).
- **Sedentary client.** Health benefits may be seen at as low as 40% of $\dot{V}O_2$max (60% MHR) (ACSM 1995).

When the intensity level causes a sharp increase in lactic acid production and in fatigue, your client has reached the *anaerobic threshold*. The duration of the training session will be shortened dramatically if she exercises above this intensity level. The greatest benefits without early fatigue are provided with intensities just below the anaerobic threshold. Anaerobic threshold can be measured accurately in a laboratory. With some guidance, however, your client can learn to recognize the abrupt increase in ventilation and RPE that occurs when she exceeds her threshold.

If you have not determined an anaerobic threshold through aerobic assessment or a submaximal test, you can calculate a crude but generally effective target heart rate from the equation THR = RHR + 75%(MHR – RHR). THR = the target heart rate; RHR = the resting heart rate; and MHR = the maximum heart rate (estimated as 220 – age). The percentage is based on the guidelines described previously. Use the target heart rate initially as an approximate guide. Then by trial and error adjust the intensity to stay just below the anaerobic threshold. Your client can maintain or adjust the intensity level for continuous training by monitoring her peak training heart rate and her perceived exertion level.

Advantages and Client Suitability of CT

- Low to moderate intensities (e.g., 40%-70% $\dot{V}O_2$max or 60%-80% MHR) are safe, comfortable, and able to produce health and cardiovascular benefits for less fit individuals.

- CT is generally well-suited for clients initiating an aerobic exercise program.

- Dropout rates for adults may be half those for high-intensity interval programs (Pollock et al. 1977).

- A prescribed exercise intensity is easily maintained in an evenly paced workout.

- More easily than with interval training, your client can maintain a training effect simply by reducing the training load (Brynteson and Sinning 1973).

- It is generally less taxing physiologically and psychologically and therefore requires minimal motivation.

- Daily workouts are possible, since glycogen is not sufficiently depleted that it cannot be replenished within 24 hours (MacDougall et al. 1977).

- Continuous submaximal training is appropriate for athletes during off-season, and during the competitive season as a light day alternating with heavier interval days.

- Benefits to the oxygen transport system from continuous training are more easily transferred from one mode of training to another or to a specific sport. This provides a variety of training activities and is well-suited to incorporation of cross-training techniques.

- Fewer injuries are reported in CT than in interval training (Pollock et al. 1977).

Interval Training

In interval training (IT), periods of low-intensity exercise (which use the body's aerobic energy system) are alternated with periods of higher-intensity exercise (which use anaerobic energy systems). Kosich (1991) refers to interval training as a high-intensity effort designed to enhance performance, usually in a competitive sport. Because one energy system can recover while the other is being used, your client is able to exercise for long periods of time with a greater total amount of work performed.

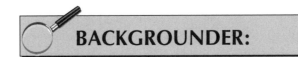

BACKGROUNDER:

Energy Systems Used by the Body

1. ATP (adenosine triphosphate) is the immediately usable form of chemical energy stored in muscle cells and used for muscular activity. The **ATP-PC system** is an anaerobic energy system that resynthesizes ATP from energy released when phosphocreatine (PC) is broken down. It is a very rapid but limited source of ATP that is used predominantly during high-power, short-duration activities. It is restored for reuse during each relief interval (50% in 30 seconds, 75% in 60 seconds, 95% in 2 minutes), thereby reducing reliance on the lactic acid system.

2. The **lactic acid (LA) system**, also anaerobic, resynthesizes ATP from energy released during the breakdown of glycogen (sugar) to lactic acid. Accumulation of the latter causes muscular fatigue. This sytem is used mainly during activities that require between one and three minutes of maximum effort.

3. The **oxygen (O_2) system** utilizes both glycogen and fats as fuels for ATP resynthesis. By a series of reactions that take place in the mitochondria of the cells, the system yields large amounts of ATP but no fatiguing by-products. The aerobic system is used predominantly during endurance tasks or low power output activities (Fox 1979).

Advantages of Interval Training

Interval training (IT) improves the body's ability to adapt and recover. Like continuous training, it improves cardiorespiratory fitness (Heyward 1998). It provides paced training that athletes can monitor and modify to suit their training phase and purpose. These and other advantages make interval training attractive for more than just the athlete.

When you know which energy systems you want to emphasize, interval training allows for great variations. You can regulate it to develop mainly aerobic, anaerobic, or muscular systems. You can target specific energy systems' improvements.

Interval training often stimulates the aerobic system without producing the high levels of lactic acid that occur with continuous higher-intensity exercise. The repeated bouts of high-intensity work nevertheless increase stroke volume and myocardial strength (Wilmore and Costill 1994).

Programming Advantages and Client Suitability of IT

- Achieves the greatest amount of work possible with the least fatigue (although longer workout times are usually necessary).

- By examining the requirements of a particular event and the energy systems used, you can design an IT program that accentuates the specificity of training.

- If used late pre-season and selectively during the season, IT can peak an athlete's performance.

- For clients in poor condition who have trouble maintaining their training intensity, the work-relief intervals will allow them to complete more total work.

- The ACSM (1995) recommends IT for symptomatic individuals who can tolerate only low-intensity exercise for short periods of time (1 to 2 minutes).

- The frequent breaks in activity facilitate monitoring of your client and making appropriate adjustments.

- The possibility of greater variety is a motivating factor.

Interval Training Prescription Terms

In prescribing interval training, you generally will use the following terms (Fox 1979):

- **Work Interval:** That portion of the interval training program consisting of the work effort (e.g., a 220-yard run performed within a prescribed time).

- **Relief Interval:** The time between work intervals in a set. The relief interval may consist of light activity such as walking (rest-relief) or mild to moderate exercise such as jogging (work-relief).

- **Work-Relief Ratio:** The ratio of the work and relief intervals. A work-relief ratio of 1:2 means that the work interval is half as long as the relief interval.

- **Set:** A group of work and relief intervals (e.g., six 220-yard runs, each performed within a prescribed time, separated by designated relief intervals).

- **Repetition:** The number of work intervals per set. Six 220-yard runs would constitute six repetitions.

- **Training Time:** The rate of work during the work interval (e.g., each 220-yard run might be performed in 28 seconds).

- **Training Distance:** Distance of the work interval (e.g., 220 yards).

- **ITP Prescription:** The specifications for the routines to be performed in an interval training workout. For several sample prescriptions, see page 103, "Sample Interval Training Prescriptions."

Writing an Interval Training Prescription

Table 7.5 shows which energy system athletes should develop, according to their sport (Fox 1979). For example, because a basketball player relies heavily on anaerobic systems for ATP energy, it is on anaerobic systems that his IT program should focus.

Match your interval training prescription to the reality of your client's outside activities. For a specific sport, for example, find out the typical length of time during which your client puts in continuous, strenuous effort. Consider ice hockey, which typically has players on the ice for about a 45-90 second shift. Use tables 7.5 and 7.6 together. According to table 7.5, ice hockey predominantly uses the ATP-PC-LA energy system. Therefore your hockey-playing client's prescription should emphasize this same system. Now go to table 7.6, find ATP-PC-LA in the left column, and note the training time that is closest to the range of a hockey shift (i.e., 1:00-1:10 min.). According to table 7.6, the prescription for your client should include five repetitions and three sets, with a work-relief ratio of 1:3 or perhaps 1:2. The relief interval should be of the work-relief type.

Table 7.5 Various Sports and Their Predominant Energy System

SPORT OR ACTIVITY	% EMPHASIS OF ENERGY SYSTEM:		
	ATP-PC AND LA	LA AND O_2	O_2
Basketball	85	15	—
Ice hockey	80	20	—
Recreational sports	—	5	95
Skiing—downhill	80	20	—
Skiing—cross-country	—	5	95
Swimming—100 m	80	15	5
Swimming—1500 m	10	20	70
Tennis	70	20	10

Adapted, by permission, from E. Fox and D. Mathews, 1974, *Interval Training* (All rights reserved to author: Ohio State University), 60.

To review, here are the steps for constructing the ITP prescription:

1. Using table 7.5, determine which energy system is to be improved.
2. Select the type of exercise to be used during the work interval (e.g., running, cycling, stairclimbing, a sport).
3. From table 7.6, select the training times (per work interval), the number of repetitions and sets, the work-relief ratio, and the type of relief interval.

These IT prescription factors may need fine tuning if

- the work is not difficult or is too difficult,
- your client is in poor or very good condition,
- your client is fresh or near the end of the workout, or
- the training signs (e.g., recovery heart rates) do not seem appropriate.

Two of the most important considerations with an IT prescription are sufficient work rate and sufficient relief/recovery. For short, highly intensive performance, the relief interval may be three times as long as the work interval. For longer, less intensive work periods, the relief interval may be equal to or less than the work interval. When the work interval has produced lactic acid, the most rapid removal rate occurs during continuous aerobic activity.

The intermittent nature of interval training allows you to monitor the heart rate at the end of work intervals and relief intervals (Fox 1979). Table 7.7 provides some guidelines for this monitoring.

Other Aerobic Training Methods

Although continuous and interval training are two of the most popular training methods, it may be more suitable for your clients to use circuit training, cross training, fartlek training, or simply active living.

Circuit Training

Circuit training usually consists of 10-15 different exercise stations with the circuit repeated two or three times.

Principles of Circuit Training

The stations are either calisthenics (such as stride jumps, stepping, sit-ups, high knee hops, push-ups, pull-ups, skipping, etc.); resistance equipment (such as machines, free weights, bands, etc.); or a combination. Stations are near one another to facilitate efficient movement. The exercises are selected to avoid repeated use of the same muscle group and early fatigue.

Table 7.6 Guidelines for Writing Interval Training Prescriptions

MAJOR ENERGY SYSTEM	TRAINING TIME (in min:sec)	REPS PER WORKOUT	SETS PER WORKOUT	REPS PER SET	WORK-RELIEF RATIO	TYPE OF RELIEF INTERVAL
ATP-PC	0:10 0:15 0:20 0:20	50 45 40 32	5 5 4 4	10 9 10 8	1:3	Rest-relief (e.g., walking, stretching)
ATP-PC-LA	0:30 0:40-0:50 1:00-1:10	25 20 15	5 4 3	5 5 5	1:3	Work-relief (e.g., light exercise, jogging)
LA-O_2	1:30-2:00 2:10-2:40 2:50-3:00	8 6 4	2 1 1	4 6 4	1:2 1:1	Work-relief Rest-relief
O_2	3:00-4:00 4:00-5:00	4 3	1 1	4 3	1:1 1:1/2	Rest-relief

Adapted, by permission, from E. Fox, 1979, *Sports physiology* (The McGraw-Hill Companies: New York), 205.

Table 7.7 Monitoring IT Prescription Target Heart Rates (Men and Women)

AGE (YEARS)	WORK HR (BPM)	RELIEF HR (BETWEEN REPS)	RELIEF HR (BETWEEN SETS)
Under 20	190	150	125
20-29	180	140	120
30-39	170	130	110
40-49	160	120	105
50-59	150	115	100
60-69	140	105	90

Adapted, by permission, from E. Fox and D. Mathews, 1974, *Interval Training*, W.B. Saunders, 60.

When you prescribe weights, select a moderate intensity (40%-60% of maximum capacity) with either a repetition limit such as 15 reps or a timed limit of around 30 seconds. The relief periods between the stations are an important part of the design. For example, with lighter intensity exercises (or lighter weights), rest periods between stations need be only 15 seconds—or about the time to move to and get set up at the next station. Circuit weight training typically has an exercise-to-rest ratio of 1:1 (Baechle 1994). Greater aerobic gains are achieved when relief times involve aerobic activities such as jogging or use of aerobic machines (space and facilities permitting). A client training in the basement can use the stairs, a skipping rope, an aerobic video, or any number of aerobic calisthenics such as stride jumps, high knee hops, or leg exchange lunges between the weight stations.

Circuit weight training is a compromise between muscular conditioning and aerobic conditioning. Monitoring the maintenance of a target heart rate is important. The metabolic requirements of circuit weight training usually meet minimum requirements for the development of aerobic capacity with an aerobic cost of 40%-60% $\dot{V}O_2$max or 60%-75% MHR (ACSM 1995). Gettman and Pollock (1981) reported that circuit weight training produced a 5%-11% increase in aerobic capacity, as compared to a 15%-20% increase with other methods of aerobic training.

LINKS:

Sample Interval Training Prescriptions

1. A moderately fit 34-year-old wants to follow her favorite aerobic video while interval training for cardiovascular condition. The prescription is as follows:

> 4 × 4:30 (4:00) where
>
> 4 = number of repetitions
>
> 4:30 = training time in minutes and seconds
>
> (4:00) = time of relief interval in minutes and seconds

Each work interval consists of following the video for 4 1/2 minutes followed by a relief interval of walking on the spot and stretching while the video is on pause for 4 minutes. Four repetitions of this sequence constitute a set. The prescription works the oxygen system, with a work to rest-relief interval of 1:1. For most moderately fit clients, exercise intensities should fall within the range of 70 to 85% of $\dot{V}O_2$max (80% to 90% of MRH), starting at the lower end of this range. Create the initial overload by progressively increasing the length of the work period; later, you can decrease the length of the rest-relief interval.

2. A competitive squash player complains of fatiguing too early. The ATP-PC and LA systems are predominant (table 7.5). It is pre-season, so you decide to start by working his LA-O$_2$ system. You design a series of carefully timed, on-the-court drills:

> ***Set 1:*** 6 × 2:30 (3:45) where

each of six drills last 2 1/2 minutes (high intensity) with a 3-minute, 45-second light exercise (jogging, or using a nearby bike or treadmill).

> ***Set 2:*** 8 × 1:30 (3:00)

These drills are slightly shorter but use the same format, intensity, and energy system. Because the recovery intervals will be incomplete, the client will increase his tolerance to lactic acid as well as his anaerobic capacity—important for a squash player. As the season approaches, you progress to a more intense work-out of his ATP-PC-LA system. According to the guidelines in table 7.5, this progression will mean shorter (more intense) training intervals and more repetitions per workout—so you will need to prescribe a slightly longer work-relief ratio.

Advantages and Client Suitability of Circuit Training

- Efficient use of time for the benefits obtained.
- Moderate gains in aerobic fitness, muscular strength, and endurance.
- Adaptable for beginners or athletes.
- Keeps a focus and a challenge to the training.
- Can maintain fitness levels when client is recovering from an injury.

Cross-Training

Cross-training involves a variety of fitness activities. It provides the flexibility of mixing activities, allowing joints and soft tissues to rest without stopping workouts. Appropriate for the beginner as well as the athlete, cross-training can expand the training benefits of a single-sport exerciser.

Yacenda (1995) explains how runners can use aerobics and swimming to shorten the duration of fatigue in their legs. Runners typically have a high incidence of lower leg overuse problems, but missing workouts means losing an acquired level of aerobic conditioning. Their chronic knee and shin problems may also be mediated with complementary cycling or circuit weight training workouts. Swimmers can gain endurance and joint stability from low-impact aerobic classes. The contrasting stresses are a positive challenge. Cross-training is often selected at a time of injury recovery, since most aerobic training gains are maintained if another mode of activity is substituted for several

LINKS:

Sample Calisthenic Training Circuit

Circuit training does not need weights or machinery. A circuit of 8-10 aerobic calisthenics will elevate and maintain a heart rate more effectively than weights. For this sample circuit, a 4 to 6 foot piece of surgical tubing or Dynaband can provide added resistance but is not necessary. The compact versatility of this circuit is a major advantage for clients working in their home with little space or equipment.

In the first or second workout, and then about every tenth workout, you should perform an assessment of each exercise. Establish the client's starting level by noting, with ample time for recovery between each exercise test, the maximum number of perfectly executed exercises done at each station during 30 seconds. Watch for excessive momentum, incomplete ranges of motion, and poor alignment. Allot your client one minute at each station to do the number of repetitions performed on the assessment. With fifteen seconds between each station, one full circuit should take 10 minutes. After the first circuit trial, you can fine tune the number of reps. Start with two sets or circuits per session and progress by adding reps to selected stations; you can also progress by including the Dynaband, or by adding a third circuit. The following calisthenics involve large muscle groups, including most of the major groups, and should minimize local muscle fatigue.

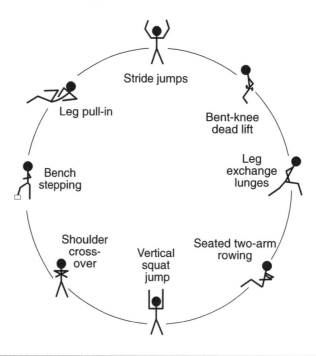

weeks while an injury is allowed to heal. If your client maintains the cross-training after the injury recovery, it will serve as a preventative measure against other single-activity overuse injuries.

The four primary prescription factors for cardiovascular fitness (FITT: Frequency, Intensity, Time, Type) can be approximately duplicated regardless of the activity selected. Table 7.8 will help you select aerobic activities based on intensity levels. You can calculate the intensity of exercise as a percentage of your client's maximum MET value (chapter 4). If you don't know the appropriate MET training level, start by identifying the activity level that your client can consistently maintain and move across the row to the workload. Any other activity in this column should be close to what your client can perform. Kosich (1991) and the ACSM (1995) have published extensive lists of activity energy expenditures.

Table 7.8   Intensity Levels of Aerobic Activity

ACTIVITY		3-4	4-5	5-6	6-7	7-8	8-9	10+
	METs	3-4	4-5	5-6	6-7	7-8	8-9	10+
	kcal/min	4-5	5-6	6-7	7-8	8-10	10-11	11+
Walking	mph	3.0	3.5	4.0	5			
	min/mile	20	17	15	12			
Jogging	mph					5	5.5	6 7 8
	min/mile					12	11	10 8½ 7½
Stationary bicycle	130 lb	½	1	1¼	1¾	2	2¼	3+
(tension Kp)	175 lb	¾	1¼	1¾	2¼	2¾	3¼	4+
Outdoor	mph	6	8	10	11	12	13	15
cycling	min/mile	10	7:30	6	5:30	5	4:40	4
Swimming	mph		0.85	1.0	1.25	1.5	1.7	2.0
	sec/25 yd		60	50	43	35	30	25
Bench stepping [70 kg/154 lbs]		8" × 12/min	8" × 18/min	8" × 24/min 11" × 18/min	11" × 24/min 12-6" × 18/min	8" × 30/min 12-6" × 24/min	11" × 30/min 15-8" × 24/min	(11 mets) 15" × 30/min
Recreational sports		Bowling Golf (pulling a cart) Light calisthenics Light games	Table tennis Volleyball Golf (carry clubs) Tennis doubles Badminton doubles Most calisthenics	Ice/roller skating Badminton singles Moderate dancing Jog-on-spot (60-70/min)	Tennis singles Water-skiing Group aerobic exercise class Jog-on-spot (90-100/min)	Downhill skiing Paddleball Basketball Fast & hard dancing Jog-on-spot (120/min)	Squash Handball Cross-country skiing Rope skipping (<75 rpm)	Most competitive sports, if continuous activity Rope skipping (>75 rpm)
Other activities		Cleaning windows Mopping floors Light gardening Painting Active child care/play	Scrubbing floors Mowing lawns Chopping wood	Shoveling Manual labour Hand sawing				

Fartlek Training

Fartlek (translation of Swedish term that means "speed play") is a form of training developed in Sweden. It combines elements of continuous training with interval training. Although timed and formalized by athletes as a serious mode of training, you can adapt it as an interesting change to a fitness program that can be a lot of fun alone or in a small group.

Principles of Fartlek Training

Fun is the main goal, and distance and time are secondary. People are relatively free to run whatever course and speed they prefer, although the speed should periodically reach high intensity levels. Fartlek involves fast-paced accelerations interspersed with endurance running. The accelerations vary in distance, and the "form" may be a sport-specific action, straight running, or simply playful in nature. Fartlek training is often performed in the countryside where there are a variety of hills and terrain. Warm-up is important for this type of training. More than 10 minutes of jogging and long static stretches of the running muscles are necessary. Runs may last for forty minutes or longer.

Many city parks have fitness trails with exercise stations spread along the pathway. Whereas the true cross country speed play of a fartlek may prove to be too intense for many exercisers, a customized park fitness trail is well-suited for many clients.

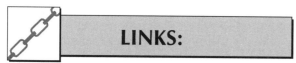

LINKS:

A Sample Fartlek Prescription

To simulate a **_Swedish fartlek_**, you may start in the country by a lake. After a walk-jog warm-up and some lower body static stretching, begin with a moderately paced kilometer run on flat paths. Coming upon a hill, attack it at near top speed, walking back down the hill, and repeating this four or five times. Follow this with a level run at about 75% speed for 3-4 minutes, and repeat this sequence two or three times. A few short sprints over local obstacles and an easy jog will bring you back to the lake. Follow with a social sauna, fluid replacement, some stretching, and a plunge in the lake!

Advantages of Fartlek Training:

- The break in monotony from changing speeds and scenery make it psychologically stimulating.

- It improves both anaerobic and aerobic capacity.

- It is an enjoyable means of achieving cardiovascular fitness, and to a lesser extent other health-related aspects of fitness.

- It is a good training break for a small group of athletes and a welcomed addition to a serious training program.

- If your client has a cottage, the match is a natural one.

Active Living

Gord Stewart (1995) describes active living as an enhancement of the simple activities in a daily routine, like walking to the corner store instead of taking the car, or climbing stairs instead of riding the elevator. At first sight, this may not seem like a method of training; but for a majority of adults the leap into an aerobic class, weight room, or running track is too large a step (see "Stages of Change" in chapter 1).

Advantages of Active Living

Recent research has shown that regular moderately intense activity can provide impressive health benefits (Blair et al.1989; Haskell 1985). Active living is particularly well-suited for a previously sedentary or older client concerned about blood pressure, blood lipids, heart health, and preventive medicine. It can relieve stress, improve energy, inject enjoyment, and provide feelings of well-being.

In a recent study with adolescents, Horswill, Kien, and Zipf (1995) demonstrated how the choice of a leisure activity such as playing a musical instrument rather than watching television can increase energy expenditure by 41%. Even these small changes in lifestyle habits can have a substantial, cumulative effect on long-term energy balance and weight management. For your older clients, the benefits of being an "active liver" translate to greater independence and the prevention of disabilities.

Suggested Active Living Prescription

If your client is inactive, initially prescribe an expenditure of 1000 calories a week, striving eventually for 2000. Any one of the following will burn about 1000 calories:

- 5 hours of housework
- 5 hours of active child care/play
- 3.5 hours of gardening or yard work
- 3 hours of dancing
- 3 hours of walking
- 2.5 hours of ice-skating
- 2.5 hours of manual labour
- 2 hours of tennis

The variety is limited only by your ingenuity. Help your clients see their opportunities: stationary cycling while watching television, alternatives to the car for transportation, more manual tools for daily chores, playing with the kids, an active vacation, cartless golf, or a walk at lunch.

Active living extends beyond the physical and has the potential of becoming a way of life. Your clients may need some initial guidance, but active living is about their making choices—it is truly client centered.

Client-Centered Tips for Setting Cardiovascular Mode or Training Method

Whenever possible, the test mode should be specific to the training mode—if your client will be training on a bicycle, test her on a bicycle. Monitor your clients to verify that the workload you prescribed is eliciting the desired heart rate. This is especially important if no assessment was done or if the training mode is different from the assessment mode.

If the total work (intensity × duration × frequency) and initial fitness status are similar, the mode of activity does not significantly influence the cardiovascular training effect. However, there are some local or specific muscle benefits from each activity. Therefore consider selecting a mode that will enhance other objectives such as isolating a body area or pursuing cross-training benefits for a sport.

Consider the possibility of overuse or acute injury when selecting the mode. For athletes, this may mean selecting a fitness mode that provides some rest for overused joints. You can use metabolic calculations and charts (table 7.8) to match activities with energy costs, but you will need to monitor and fine-tune the results (see Metabolic Calculations, below).

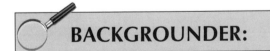

BACKGROUNDER:

Metabolic Calculations

You can use ACSM equations (1995) to calculate the speed or workloads corresponding to a specific MET intensity for walking, jogging, running, cycling, and bench stepping activities.

Example 1: How fast should a client jog on a level route to be exercising at an intensity of 8 METs?

$\dot{V}O_2$ = 8 METs × (3.5 ml/kg · min)

$\dot{V}O_2$ = 28 ml/kg · min

ACSM running equation:

ml/kg · min = [speed (m/min) × 0.2 ml/kg · min] + 3.5 ml/kg · min

28 ml/kg · min – 3.5 ml/kg · min = speed (m/min) × 0.2 ml/kg · min

24.5 ml/kg · min = speed (m/min) × 0.2

122.5 m/min = speed

If 1 mph = 26.8 m/min, 122.5 m/min ÷ 26.8 m/min = 4.57 mph.

If Pace = 60 min/hr ÷ mph; Pace = 60 min/hr ÷ 4.57 mph; Pace = 13.1 minutes per mile.

Example 2: What workload should be set for an 80 kg (BW) client on a bicycle ergometer, exercising at an intensity of 4.3 METs?

VO_2 = 4.3 METs × (3.5 ml/kg · min)

VO_2 = 15 ml/kg · min

VO_2 (ml/min) = 15 ml/kg · min × 80 kg

VO_2 (ml/min) = 1200 ml/min

ACSM leg ergometer equation:

VO_2 (ml/min) = work rate in 2 kgm/min + 3.5 ml/kg · min × kgBW

1200 ml/min = 2 kgm/min + 280 ml/min

Work rate = 460 kgm/min

Client Issues in the Selection of Duration

The optimal duration of an exercise session depends on the prescribed intensity. Generally, the higher the intensity, the shorter the duration. We must know our clients well enough to prescribe an appropriate mix of intensity and duration to challenge their cardiovascular systems without overexertion.

Total Work Done

The most important variable for cardiovascular gains is the total work done. Although other health gains are possible at quite low intensities, cardiovascular improvements appear to require a minimum threshold for the total work done in an exercise session.

Total work may be expressed in terms of the caloric cost of an activity. The caloric equivalent of 1 MET is 1 kcal/kg · hr. For example, if an 80-kg client in average condition works at 6 METs, he expends 480 kcal/hr (6 METs × 80 kg) or 8 kcal/min (480 kcal/hr/60 min).

In the previous example, the client working at an intensity of 6 METs and a recommended total work/session of 200 kcal would have an initial workout of 25 minutes (200 kcal/workout ÷ 8 kcal/min). If the duration gradually increased to 40 minutes at the same intensity, the total work/session would be 320 kcal. Figure 7.5 shows that improvements in oxygen uptake increase with the duration of the exercise session. The body responds well to workouts lasting 20-30 minutes, with benefits leveling off after this time. Figure 7.5 also shows that, with moderate intensity, workouts much longer than 40 minutes increase the risk of orthopedic injury.

RECOMMENDATIONS:

Low fitness	10-20 min.	100-200 kcal/workout
Average fitness	15-40 min.	200-400 kcal/workout
High fitness	30-60 min.	> 400 kcal/workout

Client-Centered Tips for Setting Cardiovascular Duration

If your client's objective is cardiovascular improvement, "duration" should refer to the time within the training zone. Activity below the training zone still may positively affect body composition or decrease risk factors. Longer durations can help your client

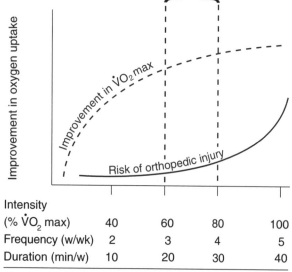

Figure 7.5 The effects of intensity, duration, and frequency on cardiovascular improvements.

tolerate submaximal challenges, but they are less effective in changing maximum oxygen uptake.

Determine the duration of higher intensity "spurts" of activity in those sports that demand cardiovascular endurance; then design interval training programs with similar durations.

Duration is an important prescription factor for clients who have intensity restrictions (symptoms that limit their level of intensity). Because such people have less chance of intensity-related injury, you can progressively increase the duration of their activities. Note: if recovery is incomplete within one hour, or heart rate is still more than 20 bpm above the pre-exercise level after 10 minutes of recovery, then either total work or duration may be too high.

Client Issues in the Selection of Frequency

The frequency of exercise depends on the duration and intensity of the session. If the intensity is kept low and duration is short, plan more sessions per week.

Being Realistic

Frequency—or the number of times your clients are motivated and able to workout—may be the most difficult factor within the fitness formula. The number of sessions/week depends on many limitations imposed by your clients' lifestyles. Perhaps this is one reason why the personal training phenomenon has been so successful. Selection of frequency can influence clients' priorities and personal objectives. The American College of Sports Medicine (1995) recommends 3-5 days a week for most aerobic programs.

RECOMMENDATIONS:

Very low fitness	1-2 day (if intensity and duration low)
Low fitness	3/week
Average fitness	3-5/week
Maintenance	2-4/week

Figure 7.5 shows that improvements in oxygen uptake (cardiovascular endurance) increase with the frequency of the exercise sessions. These benefits begin to level off after four days/week. In fact, if a client has been previously sedentary, exercising more

than four days per week seems to be too much and the incidence of injuries and dropouts rises (Powers and Howley 1990). If sessions are shorter and less intense, frequency can safely increase.

Client-Centered Tips for Setting Cardiovascular Frequency

Frequency is a key prescription factor in building a habit. Daily walking routines appear to have lower attrition than less frequent programs. It becomes part of your clients' lifestyles. Daily doses of lower-intensity activity for those with a lower functional capacity will minimize fatigue and help build muscular endurance.

The work-a-day then rest-a-day routine will improve cardiovascular health, lower the incidence of injury, and achieve weight-loss goals (ACSM 1995). If aerobic improvement is a primary objective, there should be no more than two days between workouts.

Although exercising only twice a week may cause some CV improvements, the higher intensity necessary to bring about the improvements can be hazardous. If your client is just beginning a weightbearing activity such as jogging or aerobic classes, suggest 36-48 hours of relative rest between aerobic workouts to prevent overuse injuries. The rest is even more important for overweight people or those who have lower leg alignment problems. No restrictions on stretching!

Client Issues in Selecting the Rate of Progression

The rate of improvement depends on an individual's age, functional capacity, health status, and objectives. Clients who are more fit or closer to their genetic potential and some older individuals will not improve as much as those less fit (Heyward 1998). The fastest rate of progression is during the first 6-8 weeks, when physiological changes enable clients to significantly increase the total work performed. Sharkey (1984) claims that aerobic endurance may improve as much as 3% a week during the first month, 2% a week during the second month, and 1% a week or less thereafter. Your clients can achieve safety and comfort by building a level of endurance before initiating higher intensity workouts or engaging in competitions.

Stages of Progression

The three stages of progression for cardiovascular exercise programs are

- initial conditioning,
- improvement conditioning, and
- maintenance conditioning (ACSM 1995).

The **initial conditioning stage** usually lasts four to six weeks and is characterized by longer warm-ups and cooldowns, intensities of 40% to 60% of HRR, durations of 12 to 15 minutes progressing up to 20 minutes, and frequencies of three times per week on nonconsecutive days. Active clients with better than average fitness may skip this stage.

The **improvement conditioning stage** usually lasts 16 to 20 weeks and is characterized by more rapid progressions, intensities moving from 50% to 85% of HRR, durations increasing every two to three weeks up to 30 continuous minutes, and frequencies of three to five times per week.

The **maintenance conditioning stage** usually begins after six months of training. It is characterized by maintenance of an energy cost comparable to that of the conditioning stage, but altered to include some cross-training activities, more Group 2 or 3 activities (see Cardiovascular Endurance Activities, page 98) involving skill and variety, a change of training method for some of the workouts, or a change of goals.

Client-Centered Tips for Setting Cardiovascular Progression

Table 7.9 will help you establish prescription factors appropriate to your clients' stages of cardiovascular progression. During the first few weeks, move your clients through gradual increases in duration, holding intensity nearly constant until they have achieved 20-30 minutes of endurance in the training zone. Building frequency and duration will increase workout volume, with resulting beneficial changes in body composition, reduction of risk factors such as blood lipids, and physiological changes at the submaximal levels (McArdle, Katch, and Katch 1991). With an interval training program, you can maintain the total duration of the workout, but prescribe progression by changing the ratio of work time and relief time. Base your progressions on data from regular monitoring. For example, monitoring of resting (morning) heart rate over a 4-5 week period of aerobic endurance training should reveal a drop of about 5 to 10 bpm. An increase in resting heart rate over several days, however, may indicate physical or mental fatigue. Suspect overtraining or possible illness in such a case, and adjust the workouts accordingly. The cardiovascular prescription summary (page 116) provides a concise reference to a client's prescription factors.

Monitoring

Follow-up and monitoring provide

- information that allows clients to receive regular feedback,

Table 7.9   Cardiovascular Progressions

STAGE	WEEK	FREQUENCY (WORKOUTS/WK)	INTENSITY (%HR RESERVE)	DURATION (MIN)
Initial stage	1 2-5	3 3	40-50 50-70	12 15-20
Improvement stage	6-10 11-24	3-4 3-5	70-80 70-80	20 20-30
Maintenance stage	25+	3	70-85	30-45

- a basis to judge the effectiveness of our prescriptions, and
- trends that are invaluable for planning changes or progressions.

Recording Data

Some data, such as heart rates, times, perceived exertions, training loads, and other fitness measures, are best collected during the workout on a monitoring form or program card. It may be as simple as recording weekly mileage or keeping a multipurpose exercise diary. The charts on pages 111 and 112 may be copied for your clients' use.

Monitoring Heart Rate

Heart rate has long been a key physiological parameter. It is reliably used to estimate the relative intensity of an exercise and to quantify training loads. Note the following guidelines when you use heart rate to monitor the cardiovascular part of a prescription:

- Determine training intensities on a individual basis. Time spent at a specific heart rate can vary considerably among clients exercising at the same workload.

- Establish training zones from the results of graded exercise tests (see chapter 4). The tests should use the same modes of exercise as you will be prescribing for the clients.

- At a given submaximal workload, heart rate will tend to be higher in children and females than in adult males (on whose data most heart rate norms are based!).

- Because of dehydration and increased core temperature, heart rate tends to be higher toward the end of a prolonged exercise even though the intensity remains constant (Marion, Kenny, and Thoden 1994).

- Overdressing or protective equipment (e.g., while hiking or engaging in sports such as lacrosse) will cause higher heart rates at submaximal exercise and recovery.

- Day-to-day variations can account for up to ± 5 bpm for the same individual at identical sub-maximal workloads (Åstrand and Rodhal 1986).

- During interval training, a pulse rate check at the end of the relief period can verify if the client is ready to repeat the work interval.

- Your client's heart rate can tell you when it is time to apply the progressive overload principle. Record the heart rate at the end of a standardized workload on a daily basis. As the heart rate decreases (figure 7.6), increase the intensity of the workout.

Unfortunately, many adults—particularly those just starting an exercise program—find it difficult or inconvenient to monitor their heart rate. In this case, you can use ratings of perceived exertion (RPE) to monitor exercise intensity (table 7.3). This approach is very client-centered; it sensitizes people to judge local cues (such as muscular discomfort) as well as central cues (such as breathing and heart rates).

Table 7.10 uses heart rate and RPE to provide guidelines for either the adjustment of an exercise session or the progression of the prescription after a training effect has taken place.

WEEKLY MILEAGE

Week	Weekly mileage total	Total to date
1		
2		
3		
4		
5		
6		
7		
8		
9		
10		
11		
12		
13		

EXERCISE DIARY—MULTIPURPOSE

Date	Type of exercise	Distance (miles)	Duration (minutes)	Pulse before Pulse after	Observations/ comments

From *Client-Centered Exercise Prescription* by John C. Griffin, 1998, Champaign, IL: Human Kinetics. Copyright 1998 by John C. Griffin.

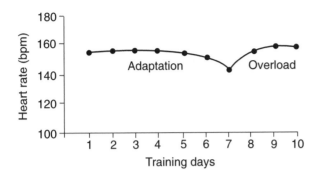

Figure 7.6 Progression based on heart rate adaptation.

Warm-Up and Cooldown

The cardiovascular prescription model (figure 7.1) suggests that the design of the warm-up and cooldown should occur as a final step. These components must be prescription-specific and client-centered. It is important to understand the purpose as well as the methods of both warming up and cooling down.

The Warm-Up

The warm-up should increase heart rate, blood pressure, and oxygen consumption; dilate the blood vessels; and increase elasticity of muscle and connective tissue in a gradual fashion. As seen in table 7.11, range of motion exercises, stretches, and gradual low-level aerobic exercise are essential for safety, delay of fatigue, and economy of movement.

Your client's warm-up activities should provide a graduated level of activity mechanically similar to that within the aerobic segment. This will improve mechanical efficiency and facilitate the transmission of neural impulses that augment coordination and power (Nieman 1990). For example:

- participants in racquet sports should begin with a light jog or brisk walk, followed by a gradually increased tempo of volleying;

- swimmers should begin with a slow crawl (perhaps in intervals) and gradually increase stroke pace;

Table 7.10 Interpretation of Intensity Monitoring

| INTENSITY MONITORING METHOD | | EXERCISE PRESCRIPTION |
%HRR*	RPE**	
>85%	>16	Decrease intensity, duration, or both. Continue to monitor at the reduced intensity.
80-85%	15-16	Caution. Monitor heart rate. Make sure client is working at the prescribed workoad. Appropriate for an athlete or a client with good fitness status.
60-80%	12-15	Appropriate for clients with average fitness status and few risk factors. Increase duration when RPE remains lower for consecutive workouts. Increase intensity instead of duration every 3rd and 4th progression.
<60%	<12	If low fitness status and/or several risk factors, this may be appropriate. Progress with longer durations. Usually means intensity or duration need to increase.

*HRR = Heart Rate Reserve (see chapter 4)

**RPE = Rating of Perceived Exertion (table 7.3).

Table 7.11   Warm-Up (Preparation) Segment Design

PRESCRIPTION	DESIGN ISSUES
Range of motion (major joints are moved through their ROM)	• increases joint lubrication and synovial fluid (protect) • client's first check on how body feels before work • some flexibility gains (stage 1)
Circulatory warm-up (light aerobic; same mode as CV work)	• increases tissue temperature and synovial fluid in preparation for stretching • gradual preparation for heart and circulatory system • simulates joint mechanics with low trauma
Stretch (emphasis on static stretching)	• flexibility gains (stage 2) • target muscles used, especially if used eccentrically • dynamic stretches for sport preparation
Transition (ease into next segment)	• warm-up continues with a light overload in the activity to follow (start of progressive overload) • look for opportunities to do a mini-warm-up and skill practice (especially in intermittent sports such as baseball)

■ outdoor cyclists should begin on flat terrain in lower gears;

■ stationary cyclists should begin at half the intended work setting and a slower speed;

■ joggers should warm up with a walk-jog interval or a slower-paced jog.

Duration of the warm-up should be longer if the intensity of the aerobic segment is high or the level of fitness of your client is low.

The Cooldown

The cooldown should gradually decrease the cardiac work and metabolism with low-level aerobic activity similar to the preceding aerobic segment. For clients with higher cardiovascular risk, the cooldown is crucial. Lower extremity blood pooling and high concentrations of exercise hormones can significantly strain the heart. Table 7.12 shows that circulatory cooldown should be followed by stretching—particularly of the active muscles.

The length of the cooldown segment is proportional to the intensity, mode, and duration of the aerobic activity and to your client's level of fitness. After a moderate intensity workout, most people should allot for their cooldown a period equal to about 15% of the time they spent exercising.

Aerobic Objectives in a Client-Centered Approach

Small alterations to the prescription factors (intensity, mode, duration, frequency, and progression) can favor different aerobic objectives in different clients. Table 7.13 (page 117) illustrates how you can manipulate the prescription factors to highlight the potential gains for specific aerobic objectives.

Matching Aerobic Equipment to the Client

The wide variety of available training methods allows us to match our clients with the specific benefits

Table 7.12 Cool-Down Segment Design

PRESCRIPTION	DESIGN ISSUES
Circulatory cool-down/transition	• CV indicators (e.g., heart rate, depth of breathing, blood pressure) should be well down • muscles should feel worked but not sore or tight • any "hot spots" or minor injuries?—if so, ice them • tier-down gradually; avoid final sprints or sudden stops (better CV adaptations permitted)
Stretch (emphasis on static stretching)	• greatest flexibility gains—tissue is warm • hold for up to 30 seconds • target muscles used, especially if used eccentrically • consider PNF if flexibility is a priority

provided by different training methods. Our prescriptions will account for our clients' preferences as well as the availability of equipment. See chapter 6 for general guidelines and a model for the selection of exercise equipment.

Types of Aerobic Equipment

Your clients generally will be most satisfied with modes of exercise that allow them to sustain intensity with little variability and with ease of monitoring. These modes include walking, jogging, running, swimming, cycling, cross-country skiing, ice skating, in-line skating, stepping, skipping, rowing, etc. Cardiovascular improvements are comparable for most modes of aerobic exercise as long as intensity, frequency, and duration of exercise are prescribed in accordance with sound scientific principles (Heyward 1998). Most aerobic fitness equipment simulates one of the aerobic modes of exercise. Most commercial clubs, many corporate fitness centers, and an increasing number of home gyms include treadmills, stationary bicycles, rowing machines, stair-climbing simulators, and cross-country ski simulators.

Product Features That Match the Client

Although comfort, appearance, durability, and cost are important factors in exercise machines, the mechanism of providing the resistance and the mechanics of the movement are the most critical features to scrutinize.

The following sections will apply the Equipment Selection Model (chapter 6) to some of the aerobic

equipment listed above. We will examine the design and safety features of the machines and then identify the type of client for which these features are most beneficial (tables 7.14 to 7.17).

Treadmills (Table 7.14)

In 1994, 16.2 million Americans walked for fitness at least twice a week; nearly half that number jogged or ran (Sillery 1996). This adds up to the largest identifiable group of exercisers. It is not surprising that treadmills have become so popular. Treadmills burn more calories than any other simulator at heart rates of 65%, 75%, and 85% of age-adjusted maximum (Allen and Goldberg 1986).

Stationary Bicycles (Table 7.15)

The choices here include

- electronic, in which the pedaling effort is controlled electronically; and
- nonelectronic, in which the resistance mechanism is a belt circling a heavy flywheel.

Your clients may choose either an upright or a recumbent style bike. The upright bike is the most common piece of equipment in most centers.

Rowing Machines (Table 7.16)

Rowers have come a long way since the squeaky spring-loaded models tucked away in attics and garages. Except for a few designs like the hydraulic-resistance rowers, most provide a realistic feel to the rowing action. Most nonelectronic machines utilize a flywheel for resistance; many people like the feel of the air machines more than the more expensive electronic models (Wolfe and Richie 1991).

CARDIOVASCULAR PRESCRIPTION SUMMARY

Prescription factors essential to systematic, individualized exercise prescriptions include appropriate intensity (workload), mode (method of training), duration, frequency, and progression of physical activity. The Cardiovascular Prescription Summary provides a quick, concise reference to this information.

Client name _____

Functional capacity _____ ml/kg · min _____ METs

Assessment comments _____

Initial training level _____ % of [   ] bpm; WL _____

Upper training limit _____ % of [   ] bpm; WL _____

Mode _____ Method of training _____

Duration: _____ work/session _____ kcal/session _____ Frequency: ____/wk ____ kcal/wk

Progression _____

Table 7.13   Prescription Factors for Specific Aerobic Objectives

AEROBIC OBJECTIVE	PRESCRIPTION FACTOR SELECTION
1. Ability to do prolonged work (>30 minutes)	• alternate increasing intensity then duration • apply these progressions regularly (approximately every 2 weeks during improvement stage) • will develop aerobic capacity and a tolerance to lactic acid • encourage supplemental activity and cross training
2. Ability to resist fatigue and maintain high levels of work	• interval training is well-suited (e.g., upper to lower training zone) • gradually decrease time of relief • relief should remain reasonably active
3. Ability to rapidly recover from higher rates of work	• work very hard for short intervals (<2 minutes) • allow quite a lengthy and yet active recovery • good for sport preparation
4. Ability to adapt to psychological stress and gain a feeling of well-being	• low to moderate intensity of a longer, continuous nature (no fatigue) • lengthy, gradual recovery • mood and climate around the exercise is important
5. Weight loss	• avoid lactic acid buildup by staying below the anaerobic threshold • non-fatiguing, longer activity will better mobilize fats and continue to burn calories

That rowing machines provide an upper body workout is an attractive added benefit for many clients. Because these machines permit such great freedom of technique, however, clients risk doing themselves harm. Remember to show them how to use their legs to push off, not their backs, and to maintain a smooth pull with the arms in and just below chest level.

Stair-Climbing Simulators (Table 7.17)

An attractive feature of these machines is that, in addition to excellent aerobic benefits, they provide muscular conditioning to the lower body. Many people should begin with a short range of motion and a slow stepping rate. To reduce stress on the knees, clients should not lean into the machine or move their knees forward over their toes during stepping. Leaning forward also increases strain on the lower back.

Highlights

- The seven steps of the Cardiovascular Prescription Model are as follows:

  1. Consider assessment information.

  2. Establish intensity.

  3. Establish mode, corresponding workloads, and method of training.

  4. Establish duration of work (and rest).

  5. Establish frequency.

  6. Establish progression.

  7. Design warm-up and cooldown.

- The **intensity** that provides adequate cardiovascular improvement for most people is 60% to 80% of $\dot{V}O_2$max (max METs), 60% to 80% of HRR, or 70% to 85% of max HR.

Table 7.14 Treadmill-Client Match-Up

DESIGN/SAFETY FEATURE	CLIENT MATCH-UP
• Alternative to the hazards of outdoor running/walking	• Clients in inclement weather locations (e.g., too hot/cold/stormy) or unsafe times/locations/health conditions
• Precise measurement	• Useful for stress testing, rehabilitation, and medical assessments (prescription is more accurate if the treadmill was also used for the assessment)
• Fingertip control of speed and elevation	• Personalized, fine-tuning
• Course and pace set for stature and condition	• Prescription can be fed into the electronic circuitry to control workout
• Ease of use and learning	• Can feel awkward to mount and control the panel while using the machine
• Reduced impact vs. outdoors for runners	• Clients with lower extremity or back irritation or overweight
• Monitoring features	• Helpful for higher risk client or for feedback and motivation
• Pre-programming capabilities	• Encourages proper warm-ups and cooldowns because they are part of the program; interval/continuous options

- **Continuous aerobic training** is safe and well-suited for many clients and different types of activities. Dropout rates are lower than with interval training. Daily workouts are possible with fewer injuries reported.

- By adjusting the duration of high-intensity exercise and the alternate relief periods, **interval training** (IT) is effective in working any energy system.

- To design an IT program: (1) determine the energy system; (2) select the type of exercise; and (3) select work interval, number of reps and sets, work-relief ratio, and type of relief.

- Interval training achieves the greatest amount of work with the least fatigue. It can be tailored to suit a specific demand (e.g., a sport), yet it is also adaptable for clients in poor condition.

- **Circuit training**, with or without weights, can provide gains in aerobic fitness, muscular strength, and endurance to fulfill a variety of client needs.

- **Cross training** allows a mixing of activities and causes a minimum of strain from repetitive forces.

- **Fartlek training** allows a freedom of choice of speed and terrain that is stimulating and that provides both aerobic and anaerobic benefits.

- **Active living,** well-suited as a first step in exercise, encourages everyone to take advantage of lifestyle opportunities for increased activity.

- The optimal **duration** of an exercise session depends on the prescribed intensity and total work done.

- The **frequency** of exercise depends on its duration and intensity.

- The **rate of improvement** depends on an individual's age, functional capacity, health status, and individual objectives.

Table 7.15 Bicycle-Client Match-Up

DESIGN/SAFETY FEATURE	CLIENT MATCH-UP
• Non-electronic are long-lasting, heavy-duty, affordable	• Suitable for home programs • Space-efficient and portable
• Electronic often have exciting computer graphics	• Immediate feedback increases motivation (e.g., simulated hills)
• Pedaling effort may be controlled by heart-rate response to the ride	• Optimizes training level and is a safety feature
• Precise measurement	• Useful for stress testing, rehabilitation, and medical assessments (prescription is more accurate if the bike was also used for the assessment)
• Pre-programming capabilities on most electronic models	• Encourages proper warm-ups and cooldowns; interval/continuous options
• Recumbent bikes offer greater comfort	• Suited to clients with back problems; greater loading for gluteals and hamstrings • Reduced lower leg weightbearing

Table 7.16 Rower-Client Match-Up

DESIGN/SAFETY FEATURE	CLIENT MATCH-UP
• Low impact, esp. lower body	• Good aerobic alternative if weight bearing is a problem
• Air and flywheel provide quality simulation	• Affordable for home use and comfortable to use
• Works muscles of the legs, shoulders, back, and arms	• Overall muscular endurance benefits for large muscle groups of the body
• Some compression and shearing forces in the lower back	• Not suitable for clients with low-back pain
• Some home models are smaller	• Space-efficient and portable
• Some electronic models have color TV, audio, and modulation of workout variables (e.g., competition, time, speed)	• Immediate feedback increases motivation; interval/continuous options

Table 7.17   Stair-Climber–Client Match-Up

DESIGN/SAFETY FEATURE	CLIENT MATCH-UP
• Foot platforms must hinge to remain parallel to the floor	• Clients with ankle or knee problems will have added stress if platforms don't hinge (e.g., knee hyperextension)
• Independent-step allows both steps to go up or down while dependent-step has one go up when the other comes down	• Dependent takes a little more practice to learn but offers more control and often less weight shifting
• Electronic models offer programming and monitoring displays	• Tracking of floors climbed, floors/minute, calories, elapsed time, etc., increases interest and motivation
• Motor skill and balance are an issue with some models	• May be inappropriate for some seniors or clients with a balance/coordination problem • Weightbearing with arms may cause elbow overuse injuries
• Some models have an aerobic self-test option	• Care should be taken not to place too much confidence in the self-test results

- The three **stages of progression** for cardiovascular exercise programs are the initial (4-6 weeks), improvement (16-20 weeks), and maintenance conditioning stages.

- During the **warm-up**, range of motion exercises, stretches, and gradual low-level aerobic exercise are essential for safety, delay of fatigue, and economy of movement.

- The circulatory **cooldown** should be followed by stretching, particularly of the active muscles.

- Exercise specialists can manipulate prescription factors to highlight the potential gains for specific aerobic objectives.

- The most effective machines to prescribe are those that simulate traditional modes of aerobic exercise, that allow intensity to be sustained with little variability, and that provide ease of monitoring. The traditional modes include walking, jogging, running, swimming, cycling, cross-country skiing, ice skating, skating, stepping, skipping, rowing, etc.

Chapter 8

Personalized Prescription for Weight Management

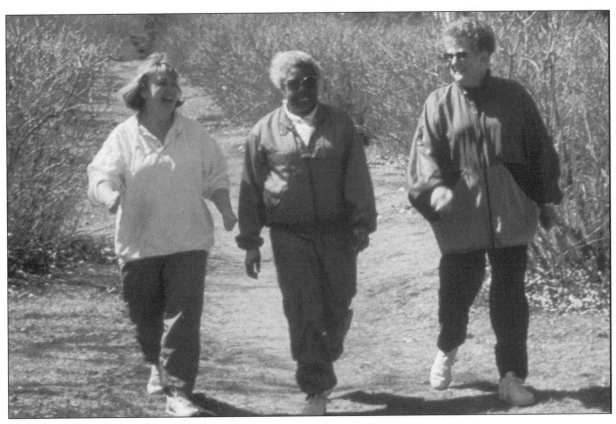

© CLEO Photography

- Focusing on Client Factors That Affect Weight Management
- Reframing the Positive: Energy Balance
- The Unique Role of Exercise in Weight Management
- Client Issues in the Selection of Prescription Factors

Penny was a 35-year-old working mother with a long-standing weight problem. Her story followed the classic stages of change (chapter 1) as she attempted to modify her behavior. This chapter examines personalized prescription for weight management by following Penny's journey. Struggling through the contemplation stage, Penny wondered if anything new would help. As she began to reframe her situation in a more positive light, her intentions moved to a preparation stage.

Understanding the unique role of exercise in the management of her weight provided enough focus and motivation to shift into an action stage. This journey took us over three weeks of regular sessions, the highlights of which are presented here.

Focusing on Client Factors That Affect Weight Management

In our first session, Penny asked, "Why do I put on weight when my food intake appears to be the same as my friends' and they are thinner?" I assured her that the problem with losing weight is much more than willpower. Weight gain usually involves a long period in which energy intake exceeds energy expenditure. In order to personalize my approach to Penny, I sought to learn more about her. Specifically, I wanted to look at three issues that could affect her weight management: heredity, levels of energy expenditure, and the relative importance of overeating and diet.

Heredity

Penny's genetic risk of weight gain left her more prone to putting on weight than others. I explained that studies of twins and adopted children have led to clear recognition of a genetic contribution to obesity (Nieman 1990). These genetic factors relate to the number and size of fat cells. Most fat cell proliferation occurs during specific periods: before birth and during adolescence. However, adults can increase cell number when existing cells reach their maximum capacity.

I described a theory of weight regulation called set point theory, which claims that each person has a biologically determined point at which the body regulates weight and fat. In spite of any changes of weight above or below this set point, the body eventually will tend to return to this point (Brownell and Steen 1987). High fat foods and inactivity may raise the set point, and exercise may lower it, but people generally have a genetically predetermined setting.

Clearly, Penny had some genetic limitations. I had to keep in mind what was realistic yet positive for Penny. The next session, I brought in some popular magazines that showed how she could feel good about her body and positive about her self-image.

Levels of Energy Expenditure

Penny was pleasantly surprised that there are several ways to expend energy: resting energy expenditure, metabolizing food (thermic effect of food), and physical activity.

Resting Energy Expenditure

Resting energy expenditure (REE) represents the energy expended to maintain normal body functions if we are simply lying in bed. It is usually the primary source of energy expenditure (60%-75%) and would be about 1600 kcal/day for Penny at 154 pounds—the equivalent of jogging 16 miles!

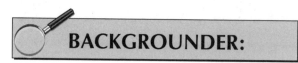

BACKGROUNDER:

The World Health Organization (1985)

The World Health Organization (1985) provides equations to estimate resting energy expenditure:

Male (30-60 years): $11.6 \times$ body weight* (in kg) + 879 kcal/day

Female (30-60) years: $8.7 \times$ body weight* (in kg) + 829 kcal/day

*In lb divide by 2.2.

Obese people have daily REEs approximately 500 kcal higher than nonobese people. Penny said this seemed like good news. However, when an obese person loses excess weight, the REE may drop to 15%-20% *below* that of a normal-weight person of similar height and weight (Nieman 1990). This makes it even more difficult to lose weight at the same levels of energy expenditure than before the dieting. This was very disheartening—Penny's dramatic dieting had caused her to lose lean body tissue, so that her "internal furnace" had slowed down!

Penny would feed her children in the morning and pack them a lunch, but she would not eat until dinner. By this time, her furnace was on low (reduced resting energy expenditure) and much less efficient at burning fuel. Sometimes after dinner or in place of dinner she would binge eat, which resulted in the calories being more easily stored as fat. My message: *"Spread your calories throughout the day."*

Thermic Effect of Food (TEF)

The thermic effect of food is the increase in energy expenditure above the REE that can be measured for several hours after a meal. The average client's TEF is 7%-10% of the total ingested calories and may last over three hours. I explained to Penny that it is important to realize that the TEF is higher after carbohydrate and protein meals than after fat meals (Miller 1991). With appropriate adjustments in her meal plans, she could eat more and still lose weight!

Physical Activity

All physical activity, all muscular movement, expends calories. During periods when Penny is sedentary, she may expend energy at the rate of only 300-800 kcal/day. The amount of time watching television significantly correlates to development of obesity. Klesges et al. (1993) indicated that the resting energy expenditure (REE) decreases while watching television in approximately inverse proportion to the temptation to consume high-calorie snacks.

Looking for a positive spin, we talked about the potential for living actively (chapter 7). A full-blown exercise program at this stage seemed a bit much. Instead I suggested that every daily routine she performed *without* work-saving devices would add to her total caloric expenditure. The tally at the end of the week could be quite substantial, even without a formal workout.

Once clients like Penny have become committed to active living, we can encourage them to exercise even more for added benefit. The thermic effect of exercise includes additional calories burned after exercise as a result of an increased metabolic rate. Athletes and clients who exercise regularly and vigorously obviously burn a large number of calories, but the thermic effect of their exercise is also quite significant in increasing their energy expenditure. Present this bonus to your clients as their physical condition improves and their enjoyment of activity increases.

Overeating and Diet Composition

We had established for Penny a less than ideal heredity profile and low levels of energy expenditure. I knew overeating could be a sensitive topic. It is unfair, and for the most part unproven, to suggest that all people with weight problems overeat. I maintained an unconditional trust of Penny and her food records of what she had eaten.

Although further information may emerge later, we must build our relationships on trust. Even if the cause of increased fat deposit is not overeating, treatment for overweight clients usually involves a reduction in daily energy intake. Yet dieting can reduce the resting metabolic rate, shift the energy balance back in the direction of energy storage, and counteract the caloric reduction (Williams 1995). Penny's repeated diets may have decreased her ability to lose weight and increased her ability to gain weight (Blackburn et al.

1989). With the questionable usefulness of traditional restrictive diets, I wanted to examine other factors, such as low-fat diets, and their relationship to body fatness.

The average American consumes nearly 40% of calories from fat (25% to 30% is recommended). This amount of dietary fat can itself be a cause of obesity. It has been shown that naturally lean people have a difficult time gaining weight on a low-fat diet but gain easily on high-fat diets (Tremblay et al. 1989).

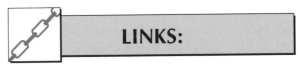

LINKS:

Fast Food Fat

I told Penny about a friend who often found himself on the road at meal time. He usually picked up a cinnamon bun with butter in the late afternoon, to hold him till dinner. His wife prepared wonderful nutritious dinners such as chicken breast, baked potato, salad and juice. What changed his habit was his shock in learning that the afternoon snack had more calories than his dinner! He was also surprised that not all hamburgers are created equal. For example, McDonald's *Big Mac* has almost 600 calories with its high fat sauce, while a regular hamburger contains only 150 calories (from carbohydrate, fat, and protein).

Fast food snacks may be high fat meals—*choose carefully*.

Eating a high-fat diet promotes body fat formation. The body uses one-fourth to one-third less energy to process dietary fat than it does to convert protein or carbohydrate to body fat (Dattilio 1995). In other words, a given caloric quantity of excess dietary fat is more fattening than a calorically similar quantity of excess carbohydrate. To Penny this meant that what she ate (diet composition) may be as important as total calories in the promotion of obesity.

Miller (1991) demonstrated that middle-aged obesity is characterized by reduced carbohydrate intake. His data suggested that consumption of natural or complex carbohydrates (such as whole grains) assists in weight loss, whereas obesity correlates with excess consumption of "added" or refined sugars. He also found that a high fiber intake assists in weight loss because of the increased consumption of natural carbohydrates (vegetables, fruits, grains).

Penny was becoming very interested in nutrition, recognizing things she had done in the past that had contributed to her problem. She relayed a story to me from a few years earlier when she and a girlfriend had joined a fitness center together and planned to help each other get ready for the summer. Their activity interests and fitness levels were similar, and they ended up doing the step class and power walking together three or four times a week. She said they were diligent about keeping track of the calories in their food and often selected "lite" or "low-calorie" labels. They both consumed a similar total calories/day. Yet Penny's friend lost weight and she did not! I knew we were making progress when Penny asked if the difference may have been that her diet had a higher level of dietary fat. She had believed that the pasta, potatoes, and bread made her fat—not recognizing that the high fat sauce, sour cream, and margarine used with them were the real culprits. I added that once her ratio of dietary fat was changed by substituting more complex carbohydrates or even protein, she would find that she was less hungry and had fewer glucose fluctuations.

The principle is nearly universal: *Try to choose food items that get less than 25%-30% of their calories from fat.*

Reframing the Positive: Energy Balance

By our second session, Penny was showing clear signs that she was moving into the preparation stage. She was starting to see how changes in her behavior could bring about personal benefits, and was intending to take some action. It was time for me to focus on the "pros," provide some resources, and encourage some small changes.

Is Calorie Counting Valid?

The first question Penny asked in our second session was, "Should I be counting calories?" I explained that every calorie we eat must be expended or conserved in the body. Dietary fat is stored as body fat more efficiently than other sources of calories; but if you routinely consume more calories than you expend, you will gain weight regardless of the composition of your diet. I explained that protein and carbohydrate contain only 4 calories per gram, fat contains 9 calories per gram, and water contains no calories (McArdle, Katch, and Katch 1991).

Since the body comprises different components (water, fat, fat-free mass), changes in these components may bring about weight fluctuations that appear to contradict the caloric balance concept. For instance, early weight loss may be primarily loss of water. Also, exercise increases the fat-free mass (which is heavier, though more compact than fat) while it is decreasing fat, so weight loss on the scales may be slower than might be expected (figure 8.1). I told Penny that perhaps the question should be "Is calorie counting

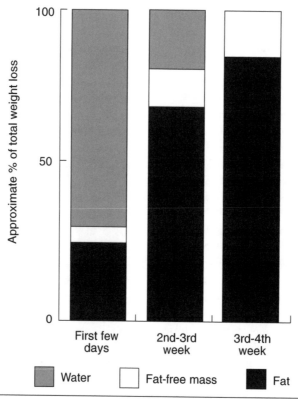

Figure 8.1   Percent composition of weight loss.

LINKS:

Counting Calories for the Blue Jeans

Gwen entered our employee fitness program weighing 150 pounds and set realistic goals of losing 10 pounds and fitting into her blue jeans. She had been maintaining her weight for the last year and felt that she could achieve a daily 500 calorie deficit (3,500 calories per week) by reducing her diet by 250 calories and increasing her activity by 250 calories, on average. Gwen joined our noon aerobics class three days a week (3×300 calories) and started walking to work five days a week (5×150). A weekend golf game or tennis match burned an extra 500 calories. At the end of each day, Gwen recorded food deficit calories and the caloric worth of her activities. Each day did not add up to 500 calories, but the week's total gave her a 3,500 calorie deficit. After a greater than one pound loss in the first two weeks (probably water loss), it looked like things were starting to plateau. However, by the end of 10 weeks, she had lost the 10 pounds. More importantly for Gwen, she arrived at work that Friday casually dressed in blue jeans.

---

valuable?" rather than "Is it valid?" I told her about my client Gwen, who benefited from counting calories.

Which Is More Effective: Diet or Exercise?

In the latter part of our session, Penny began to show some interest in the benefits of exercise. I explained that there are pros and cons to using exercise alone or dieting alone, but that either can be effective in reducing weight. One challenge I faced was in matching Penny to an appropriate treatment strategy. Overweight clients are somewhat less likely to stay with an exercise program. Inactivity may be the cause of the problem, or it may be the result of the excess weight. Penny felt that she should exercise; but if she didn't, and only followed a calorie-restricted diet, she risked losing lean body tissue. Walberg (1989) has shown that diet-only programs lead to decreased resting energy expenditure and ongoing weight management difficulties. The slower metabolism helps conserve a dwindling energy reserve from lack of food. But the restrictive dieting also makes it progressively harder to lose weight. It may be only a matter of time before the

weight is gained back and another crash diet starts a "yo-yo" effect. Penny had already tried diet restriction alone for some time, and thus far had been one of the 95% of all people who lose weight only to gain it back within two years.

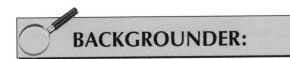

BACKGROUNDER:

Compared to exercise alone, dieting can produce more rapid weight reduction early in a program. Although exercise may provide slower results, it can help maintain lean body mass and prevent any decrease in resting energy expenditure. Weight lost by dieting is about 75% fat and 25% protein. Combining exercise and diet can reduce that protein loss to only 5% (Garfinkel and Coscina 1990). Exercise counterbalances the disadvantages of dieting; and once excess body fat has been lost, continued exercise is important to maintaining a stable, healthy body weight. Marks et al. (1995) have shown that aerobic cycle exercise and resistance training are equally effective in maintaining fat-free mass while encouraging weight loss.

The Unique Role of Exercise in Weight Management

Dieting was familiar ground for Penny. But to convince her to undertake a new behavior—exercise—I would have to present compelling arguments. Knowledge of the effect exercise has on fat metabolism and metabolic rate, if presented convincingly, could help move Penny from a preparation stage to one of action.

What Effect Does Exercise Have on Fat Metabolism?

The two major sources of energy during exercise are fats (in the form of fatty acids) and carbohydrates (in the form of muscle glycogen).

A mixture of fats and carbohydrates is usually used during exercise, the ratio depending on the intensity and duration of the exercise and on the diet and physical condition of the individual.

Fat cells are specialized for the synthesis and storage of triglycerides. Prior to energy release from fat, triglycerides are broken down into free fatty acids (FFAs). Although some fat is stored in all cells (some in the muscle cells and a small amount in the blood), the most active sources of FFAs are the fat cells within adipose tissue. Once FFAs diffuse into the blood stream, they are delivered to active tissues where they can be utilized for energy (figure 8.2a). As blood flow increases with exercise, more FFAs are removed from fat cells and delivered to active muscle (figure 8.2b). During exercise, the muscle cells first use fatty acids from the blood and from the muscles' own stores of triglycerides. As exercise continues or increases in intensity, the blood FFAs begin to be in short supply and must be replenished by the vast stores of triglycerides in the adipose tissue.

During rest, the body metabolizes only about 30% of the FFAs that are released from adipose tissue. The other 70% are converted back into fat (i.e., triglycerides) (figure 8.2a). During exercise, only about 25% of these FFAs are reconverted into triglycerides, providing much more FAA to the muscle cells (figure 8.2 b).

During light exercise (25% to 50% of $\dot{V}O_2$max), about 30% to 50% of the total energy cost is derived from carbohydrate while the other 50% to 70% comes from FFAs. As the exercise intensity increases toward 60% to 65% $\dot{V}O_2$max, the muscle triglycerides become

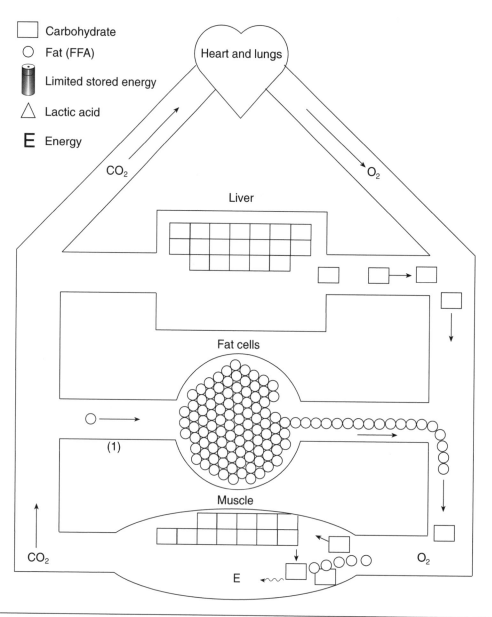

Figure 8.2a Schematic of energy production during rest.

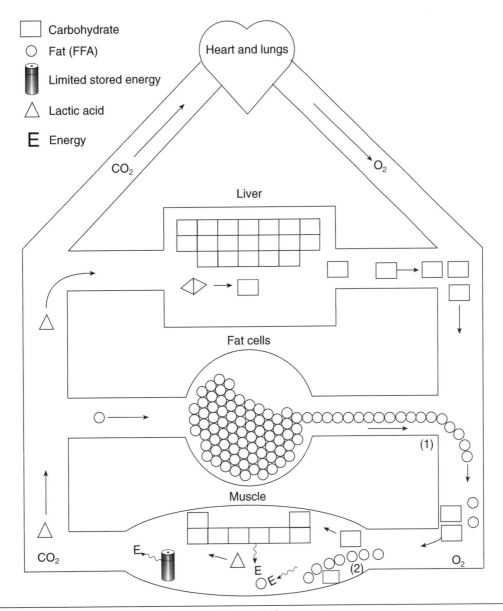

Figure 8.2b Schematic of energy production during light exercise.

increasingly important as the source of fatty acids (Romijn et al. 1993) (figure 8.2c).

Carbohydrate is the preferred energy source during high intensity exercise, such as 65% to 70% of $\dot{V}O_2$max and above (figure 8.2c). FFAs alone cannot sustain exercise at this intensity, and their contribution diminishes. Hodgetts et al. (1991) suggest that an increase in blood lactic acid levels may block release of FFAs from the adipose tissue (figure 8.2c).

Although carbohydrate becomes more important as an energy source during high-intensity exercise, trained endurance athletes may be able to use fats more efficiently at higher exercise intensities.

What convinced Penny was the fact that even lower-intensity exercise is effective for weight loss. I said that, once she had been successful at a "beginner's"

level, we could talk about even more effective ways of burning fat!

How Does Exercise Affect Metabolic Rate?

The baseline rate of metabolism at rest is the resting energy expenditure (REE). Any physical activity will raise the REE. The energy expended for physical activity is the thermic effect of exercise (TEE). The most significant factor affecting this TEE is the intensity of the exercise. For example, a briskly walking average-sized adult male may expend 5 calories per minute (compared to 1 calorie per minute in a lying rest). The same man jogging easily may burn 10 calories per minute. And if the intensity is up to a level

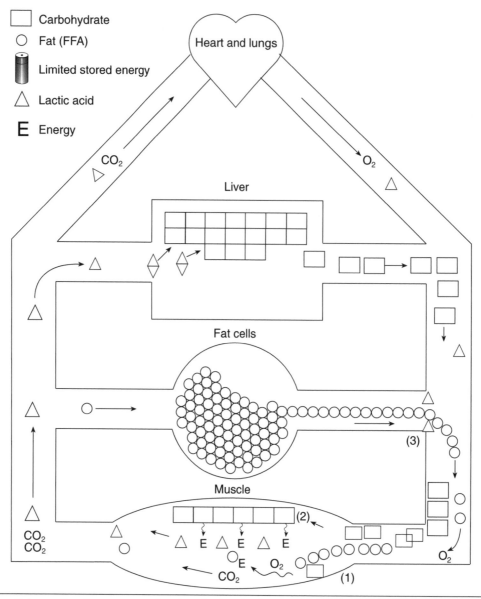

Figure 8.2c Schematic of energy production during high-intensity exercise.

barely sustainable by the best athletes for a full workout (10-12 mph), the rate of caloric expenditure may be over 20 calories per minute (Williams 1995).

Energy expenditure is affected not only by the intensity but also by the efficiency of movement. A more awkward swimmer or runner will burn more calories going the same distance at the same speed as an expert swimmer. Heavier people also burn more calories for any given amount of work, because it takes more energy to move a heavier load.

Penny thought this was wonderful: her extra weight and poorer motor skills were actually an advantage to burn more calories! I explained that any awkwardness she may have while walking briskly could help her burn more calories than a jogger moving at a similar speed.

Exercise may also facilitate weight loss by causing an increase in post exercise REE (Brehm 1996). Cy-

cling at 70% $\dot{V}O_2$max for 20 to 80 minutes is reported to produce a 5% to 14% elevation in REE for 12 hours after exercise.

What Role Does Exercise Play in Weight Management?

The human body is a remarkable machine. It can consume nearly a ton of food in a year and not change its weight. We constantly harness and expend energy through the intricacies of our metabolism in order to maintain energy balance. Nevertheless, creeping obesity is a major problem today and a personal concern for the estimated 40% of the American population who are overweight. About one-third of men and women in Canada also consider themselves to be beyond the "generally acceptable" range (Health and Welfare Canada 1988).

The late Jean Mayer, an international authority on weight control, reported that no single factor is more frequently responsible for obesity than lack of physical activity. If inactivity is not a major cause for obesity, it is the consequence of obesity and plays a definite role in maintaining it. My challenge was to find for Penny a prescription that provided a comfort level that would keep her exercising.

If at rest the average-sized adult burns 60-70 kcal per hour, with even light activity this can be tripled. As conditioning increases to allow a moderate level of activity such as tennis, walking briskly, or low-impact aerobics, the furnace can be stoked to about eight times its normal burning capacity.

Many resources (including table 7.8) list the energy costs of a wide variety of physical activities and sports (Dusek 1989; Heyward 1998). When using these lists, remember that

- they refer only to the time that your client is actually moving, which may be only 35-40 minutes of an hour-long basketball game;
- actual energy expenditure may vary because of skill level, air resistance, terrain, etc.; and body weight and gender can affect the data.

Penny's final argument against exercise as a means of weight loss was that it expended so few calories: "One piece of cake and I've blown my whole aerobics class!" In the short term this is true. But I compared mild exercise with the return we expect when we invest money at interest. The immediate payback usually is not large; but if we are patient and stay with the investment, it will grow substantially over time. Similarly, I knew I must help Penny look at the long haul for weight control. If she walked briskly for about two miles a day, it would expend enough calories in a month to six weeks to account for a loss of nearly 2 pounds.

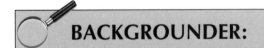

BACKGROUNDER:

Aerobic Training Results

Heyward (1998) describes four changes relating to fat loss and the conservation of lean body tissues that results from aerobic training:

- A larger percentage of the energy used during submaximal exercise is derived from the metabolism of FFA than the percentage used during rest or intense exercise.
- Endurance training raises the point at which lactic acid levels sharply increase (called the

anaerobic threshold). Since lactic acid inhibits fatty acid metabolism, conditioned people burn more fat during exercise than do unconditioned people.

- Resting energy expenditure (REE) may not decrease during calorie-restricted diets if regular exercise is maintained.
- Increased levels of epinephrine and norepinephrine released during exercise stimulate the mobilization of fat from storage and active the enzyme lipose, which breaks down triglycerides into free fatty acids.

Client Issues in the Selection of Prescription Factors

Penny and I were in our second week by now—a seemingly long time, but it is important not to skip stages when attempting behavioral change. She was now ready to take some action.

Is High or Low Intensity Best for Burning Fat?

People have been told for years that they must exercise at a threshold stimulus for a minimum intensity to produce significant CV effects. This belief is incorrect. I told Penny she could expect improvements at low levels of exercise, even with her calorie-burning furnace set on low. She could progress in duration and frequency even with lower intensities, and still produce some significant middle- to long-term results.

A second myth is the feeling that the optimal exercise intensity for burning fat is low intensity, comparable to walking. At very low intensities, our bodies rely predominantly on fat stores. At higher intensities, carbohydrates are the predominant energy source. This has led some people to conclude that to burn fat, low intensity exercise is preferable. The fact is that higher intensity exercise burns more calories. Even though the *proportion* of fat calories is smaller, the *total number* of fat calories used in high intensity exercise greatly exceeds those used in low intensity workouts of equal duration.

Penny could expend more fat calories jogging than walking (Brehm 1996):

Walking, 30 min:
240 kcal @ 41% fat calories = 96 kcal

Jogging, 30 min:
450 kcal. @ 24% fat calories = 108 kcal

Other physiological factors also support higher intensity activity. First, the REE can stay elevated for hours after a bout of intense exercise. Second, the cardiovascular training effect created by higher intensity training increases the activity of certain muscle enzymes involved in burning fat. These enzymes favor the burning of fat rather than glycogen (Bean 1996).

Penny was surprised to hear that lower intensity exercise may not be the fastest way to burn fat even if she is burning a higher percentage of fat calories. However, there are many health benefits to regular lower intensity exercise that may normalize metabolic disorders common in obese clients (chapter 6). We must always turn back to our clients in making prescriptive decisions—in many cases, as with Penny, lower intensity (longer duration and frequent) exercise may be most suitable. Showing obese clients how to live more actively on a daily basis may prove more successful than regimented programs (see table 8.1). Many overweight clients have orthopedic limitations, and they will sustain fewer injuries with a lower intensity. Weight-supported activities such as swimming are excellent choices, especially for deconditioned or restricted clients. If previously inactive clients can get into the habit of exercise, their fitness may gradually improve to the point that we can prescribe higher-intensity levels of activity without driving them away.

How Should the FITT Principle Be Applied?

Recent American and European surveys (Williams 1995; Simopoulos 1992) have shown that approximately 35% to 40% of adult women and from 25% to 30% of adult men are currently attempting to lose weight. Any exercise prescription must be suited both to the goals of weight control and to the individual client. Knowing how to apply the FITT principle (Frequency, Intensity, Time [or duration], and Type [or mode] of exercise) is an important skill.

Type or Mode of Exercise

Aerobic exercise is the best type of program for losing body fat. It also provides significant other health and cardiovascular benefits (see chapters 6 and 7). Aerobic exercise involves large muscle groups, so you can look beyond walking, jogging, stairclimbing, and bicycling to activities that also incorporate shoulder and trunk muscles (e.g., cross-country skiing, swimming, skipping, rowing, aerobic dance, holding weights while walking); or you can combine these activities with some cross training or a circuit (chapter 7). Other activities such as tennis, squash, basketball, baseball,

hockey, and so on have an aerobic component to them. Remember that the action should be continuous, maintaining the energy expenditure level.

Even with all these choices, there remains a single mode of exercise that consistently maintains adherence, suits the overweight client, and has a proven track record for weight management. I refer to walking or its progressive extensions, walk-jog-run. Penny had been doing some walking, but it was too leisurely to provide effective stimulus. I urged her to walk more briskly, with more vigorous arm action, a slightly longer stride length, and an increased step rate. For hypertensive clients, carrying weights in the hands tends to increase blood pressure more than weights strapped to the wrist. With hand weights, energy expenditure may increase 5%-10% (nearly 1 kcal/min); for Penny, however, simply walking faster or longer without weights provided similar results (Williams 1995).

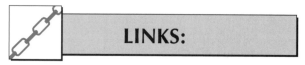

LINKS:

The Zen of Walking

My 63-year-old neighbor was approaching retirement and knew he wanted to play golf everyday. His weight and blood pressure had been creeping up, and he was concerned about his future quality of life. He bought a Walkman and set aside his "walking time" after work each day. Gradually building loops to his walking route to progressively extend his time, my neighbor had lost almost a pound a week in the first three months. The walking time became a cherished time of sanctuary and rejuvenation. It would never replace golf, he told me, but it has become more than just a means of losing weight. Surely there is a Zen of walking.

Commonly advertised weight-reduction programs like "fat-burner," "slimnastics," or "trimfit" seemed both attractive and confusing to Penny: weight loss was linked to sophisticated weight training equipment, weight loss clothing, and special vibrating machines. I suggested that she assess each claim against the principles I had taught her, such as the need for continuous large muscle activity for a minimum of 15-20 minutes. Our bottom line, of course, is to help clients select activities that are convenient and enjoyable, since adherence is the most important factor in any program.

Intensity

The merits of high or low intensity of exercise have been discussed. Every client has an optimal intensity, depending on her condition and the length of the exercise. The intensity must be adapted to the duration of the exercise.

Duration

If losing weight is a priority of your client, your prescription should stress duration or total energy expenditure (intensity × duration). One of your initial challenges is to bring your clients to a point of sufficient aerobic fitness that they can sustain moderate intensity for enough time to burn a lot of calories. If a client is jogging at a 7-minute-mile pace and fatigues after three miles, she has burned approximately 325 kcal (21 min × 15.5 kcal/min). If she reduces her speed to an 8-minute-mile pace, she can complete four miles and burn 448 kcal (32 × 14 kcal/min). Duration and total distance are more important than speed (intensity) alone. The slower pace also avoids the inhibiting effect of lactic acid on fat mobilization.

Similarly a jogger, because her activity is continuous, uses considerably more calories in an hour than a tennis player who may be moving for only 40% of the game. Be aware of this principle if you base your prescription on a chart of caloric expenditures per minute for various activities.

The benefits of avoiding labor-saving devices—taking the stairs, walking to work, and generally living more actively—accumulate during the day, and effectively extend the daily energy expenditure. This was the approach I initially took with Penny. It suited her lifestyle and level of commitment and firmly implanted her in the action stage of change. Penny could use frequent short bouts of moderate day-to-day activities to burn the equivalent of 2 lb of body fat per month (table 8.1).

Frequency

It is quite evident that the more a person exercises, the greater his weekly caloric expenditure. Exercise frequency complements duration and intensity. A daily program is most likely to establish a behavioral habit and promote adherence. Four sessions per week are satisfactory, provided duration and intensity are adequate. An active living lifestyle, like Penny's, can effectively complement a more formal exercise prescription and make a significant difference in the speed of weight loss or the ease of weight maintenance. Active living (chapter 7) may not produce profound

Table 8.1 Health-Related Fitness Prescription

DAY	ACTIVITY (150 LB PERSON)	KCAL
Monday	30 minutes at fitness club—aerobic	250-300
Tuesday	brisk walk to work—30 minutes stairs—5 minutes	200-250
Wednesday	30 minutes at fitness club—aerobic	250-300
Thursday	brisk walk to work—30 minutes stairs—5 minutes	200-250
Friday	brisk walk to work—30 minutes stairs—5 minutes wash & wax car—30 minutes	300-350
Saturday	gardening—30 minutes housecleaning—30 minutes	300
Sunday	mow lawn—30 minutes rake & yard work—30 minutes	400-450
	TOTAL	1900-2200

cardiovascular benefits; but for energy expenditure, "every little bit counts." Every time Penny thought she was about to relapse from her exercise program, I reminded her that washing the car, mowing the lawn, vacuuming the carpet, gardening, or doing house repairs were bonus calorie-burners rather than work, and every bit as valid as a trip to the gym.

Is Resistance Training for Weight Loss or Weight Gain?

Most clients want resistance training programs to build muscle strength, endurance, power, or size. However, resistance training can also be a valuable adjunct to a weight management prescription.

A weight reduction program can cause loss of protein tissue (primarily muscle) along with body fat. Weight training can prevent significant loss of lean body mass, while also preventing decreases in resting energy expenditure. It keeps the furnace fire stoked! In fact, each additional pound of muscle tissue can raise the REE by 35 kcal per day (Campbell et al. 1994). I told Penny that if she *adds* two pounds of muscle tissue as the result of resistance training, it could raise her REE by 70 kcal/day (35 × 2), which equals 25,550 kcal/year (70 × 365), or the equivalent of 7.3 pounds of fat (25,550/3,500).

Although resistance training does burn calories, the effect is relatively small compared to that of aerobic exercise. Lifting lighter weights for more repetitions (e.g., 15-25) and one or two sets can maintain muscle endurance and tone with little chance of significantly altering muscle size. Many clients need to be reminded that it is physiologically impossible for muscle cells to turn into fat in the future. The optimal prescription for Penny, once she was ready for a more formal program, was a combination of aerobic exercise and light resistance training.

How Do You Counsel Clients Who Want to Change Their Appearance?

Our eyes see what our brains tell them to see. Body image is the mental image we have of our own physical appearance. Penny was one of more than 50% of adult women who are dissatisfied with their weight. Her concern with weight started in high school, and she has felt handicapped ever since in terms of personal and professional fulfillment.

The image in Penny's mind of her appearance at her "ideal" weight was distorted. An acceptable and realistic standard may be a "tolerable" weight that is within a healthy standard (chapter 4).

Fitness professionals often take a physiological approach, examining weight and health in terms of metabolic normality, body composition (leanness and fat), and functional capacity. This approach tends to focus on health enhancement, on an acceptable standard, on performance, or on aesthetics. Such a focus, however, may not connect with your client's needs.

You must always consider the psychological and social pressures your clients face. Once Penny realized that I didn't simply see her weight as a risk factor, the doors were open to talk about her weight in relation to well-being, body image, and social acceptance. I de-emphasized any absolute measure of weight or body composition in our counseling, and encouraged Penny to find her own desirable and healthy weight. I had her ask herself if she was happy with her weight. To really enjoy a high quality of life, it is important to be happy with yourself. Then I had her ask herself if she wanted to change enough to implement exercise and dietary changes. These simple questions helped establish a degree of commitment to define a "tolerable" weight for her.

For clients with a body image goal, I like to use a "mirror" analogy: I challenge them to change the reflection they see. It becomes an attitude challenge. Our goal is to promote a personal acceptance of a large range of healthy weights and variations in body size. I had Penny search through magazines to find appropriate images of body shape. Less frequent use of her scales and a few new pieces of clothing also helped toward a more positive self-attitude. Penny was realistic about her "reflection," but recognized the continuing benefits of appropriate eating and physical activity habits.

Highlights

- Each of the following affects weight management: heredity, levels of energy expenditure, and the relative importance of overeating and diet composition.

- There are several ways to expend energy: resting energy expenditure, metabolizing food (thermic effect of food), and physical activity.

- Remember: "Try to spread your calories throughout the day"; "Fast food *snacks* may be high fat *meals*—choose carefully"; "Try to choose food items that get less than 25%-30% of their calories from fat."

- With diet only, there is often an accompanying decrease in resting energy expenditure that contributes to ongoing weight management difficulties.

- During light exercise about 30% to 50% of the total energy cost is derived from carbohydrate, while the other 50% to 70% comes from FFA. As exercise intensity increases, muscle triglycerides become increasingly important as the supplier of fatty acids. Carbohydrate is the preferred energy source during high intensity exercise, such as 65% to 70% of $\dot{V}O_2$max and above.

- Higher intensity exercise burns more calories than low intensity exercise; and even though the proportion of fat calories is less, the total number of fat calories by the end of equal-length bouts of exercise will be higher for the high intensity client.

- Walking is the mode of exercise that best seems to maintain adherence, suit the overweight client, and lead to good weight management. Brisk walking is at a faster-than-normal pace involving more vigorous arm action, a slightly longer stride length, and an increased step rate.

- Prescriptions should stress duration or total energy expenditure (intensity × duration) for a given workout. The benefits of avoiding labor-saving devices, taking the stairs, walking to work, and generally living more actively can accumulate during the day and increase the daily energy expenditure.

- Weight training can prevent significant losses of lean body mass and decreases in resting energy expenditure. The optimal prescription is a combination of aerobic exercise and light resistance training.

- Our goal is to help clients accept a large range of healthy weights and variations in body size, and recognize the continuing benefits of appropriate eating and physical activity.

Chapter 9

Cardiovascular and Weight Control Case Studies

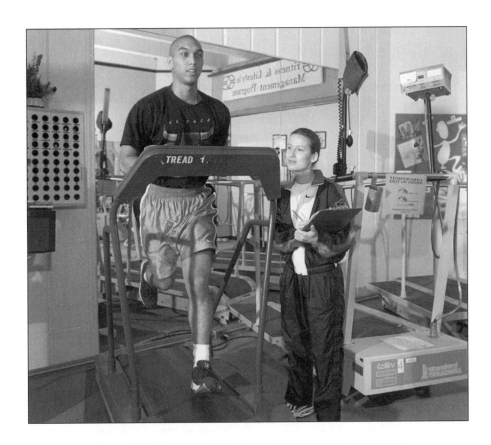

- Case Study #1: Well-Conditioned Woman
- Case Study #2: Prescribing Without Cardiovascular Assessment
- Case Study #3: Twenty-Three-Year-Old Male Sprinter
- Case Study #4: Male With Creeping Obesity
- Case Study #5: Thirty-Five-Year-Old Working Mother

Chapters 7 and 8 dealt with personal prescription for cardiovascular conditioning and weight management. The following case studies deal with specific client situations and demonstrate the application of many of the prescription tools.

Case study #1 has a cardiovascular concern and involves a 37-year-old woman in good condition interested in cycling. The second case is a 27-year-old male for whom no fitness assessment was administered. The third client is a sprint athlete interested in a longer-term plan. The fourth case study involves a middle-aged executive with a progressing weight problem that is starting to affect his health. For the final case, I refer you back to chapter 8 where Penny, the 35-year-old working mother, struggles through a long standing battle with weight management.

Case Study #1: Well-Conditioned Woman

Ingrid was a 37-year-old woman in good condition, interested in cycling. She was at a maintenance stage but interested in a progressive prescription that would get her over her fitness plateau.

Assessment

I assessed Ingrid on a bicycle ergometer using a multistage graded exercise protocol. Her blood pressure, perceived exertion, and other signs were within normal

ASSESSMENT	DATA
Age	37 years
Sex	Female
Weight	70 kg [154 lb]
Resting heart rate	72 bpm
Maximum heart rate (estimated)	183 bpm
Maximum heart rate (during assessment)	180 bpm
$\dot{V}O_2$max	37 ml/kg · min × 70 kg = 2590 ml/min Since 1 MET = 3.5 ml/kg · min, 37/3.5 = 10.6 METs
Assessment mode	Bicycle ergometer
Fitness classification	Good

ranges. The following is a summary of the assessment data:

Figure 7.2 plots heart rate against MET levels. Ingrid's final heart rate was 180 bpm. The point on the horizontal axis that corresponds to 180 bpm, according to the plotted curve, is 10.6 METs.

Assessment Discussion and Action

Given Ingrid's "good" rating (Howley and Franks 1997), I selected a training zone of 60% to 80% of max METs (60% to 80% of 10.6 METs = 6.4-8.5 METs).

The graph in figure 7.2 shows that these levels correspond to heart rates of 132 bpm and 156 bpm, respectively.

At an initial intensity of 60% of the functional capacity:

$$\dot{V}O_2 = 6.4 \text{ METs} \times (3.5 \text{ ml/kg·min})$$
$$\dot{V}O_2 = 22.4 \text{ ml/kg·min}$$
$$\dot{V}O_2 \text{ (ml/min)} = 22.4 \text{ ml/kg·min} \times 70 \text{ kg}$$
$$\dot{V}O_2 \text{ (ml/min)} = 1568 \text{ ml/min}$$

The American College of Sports Medicine (1995) provides an equation for calculating work rate on the bicycle ergometer.

$$\dot{V}O_2 \text{ (in ml/min)} = 2 \times \text{Work Rate} + 3.5 \text{ [body weight (in kg)]}$$
where Work Rate is in kg·m/min

Substituting the measurements for Ingrid:

$$1568 = 2WR + 3.5(70)$$
$$2WR = 1568 - 245$$
$$WR = 661.5 \text{ kg · m/min}$$

It is most practical to assign a 525 kgm/min workload (i.e., 1 3/4 kg @ 50 rev/min). Although Ingrid is not primarily concerned with burning calories, it may be useful to remember that the caloric equivalent of 1 MET is 1 kcal/kg { hr. For example, if our 70 kg client worked at 6.4 METs, she would expend 6.4 3 70 = 448 kcal/hr, or 7.5 kcal/min.

Prescription

The general prescription is summarized below, with Ingrid starting at the lower levels for each of the prescription factors.

The essential segments of a cardiovascular exercise program include warm-up and cooldown; aerobic segment prescription factors (intensity, mode and train-

FACTOR	PRESCRIPTION
Mode	Stationary cycling (ergometer)
Intensity	60%-80% $\dot{V}O_2$max or 60%-80% max METs (i.e., 6.4-8.5 METs)
Training zone heart rates	132 bpm (minimum) 156 bpm (maximum)
Duration	20-45 minutes
Frequency	3-5 days per week

ing method, duration, frequency); and a progression plan.

The warm-up I prescribed was standard: range of motion (lower body joints moved through their ROM); circulatory (light aerobic activity, such as stationary cycling, walking, or calisthenics); stretch (emphasis on static stretching legs and trunk); and transition (easing into the aerobic segment with easy cycling).

The prescribed cooldown also was rather standard: circulatory cooldown (light cycling); transition (reverse of warm-up parts); and stretch (emphasis on static stretching of the legs added a good opportunity to work on whole body flexibility).

During the initial stage of the exercise program, I assigned Ingrid a workload corresponding to 60% of $\dot{V}O_2$max (6.4 METs or 525 kgm/min) for 3 weeks. The workload is calculated using the ACSM formula for leg ergometry (see page 136). Her heart rate was near or slightly above 132 bpm; duration was 20 minutes; and frequency was three times per week.

Results

After a few weeks, Ingrid's heart rates were regularly below 132 bpm even with slight increases in duration. I increased the workload about 10% in the fourth week. With gradual increases in duration during this initial stage, her energy expenditure progressed from 150 to

Aerobic Segment: Summary of Progressions

PHASE (WEEKS)	INTENSITY (% $\dot{V}O_2$MAX)	INTENSITY (METS)	WORKLOAD (KG · M/MIN)	DURATION (MIN)	FREQUENCY
Initial					
1	60	6.4	525	20	3
2	60	6.4	525	25	3
3	60	6.4	525	30	3
4	60-65	6.4-7.0	525-600	30	3
Improvement					
5-6	65-70	7.0-7.5	600-660	30	3
7-8	70-75	7.5-8.0	660-720	30	3
9-10	70-75	7.5-8.0	660-720	35	4
11-12	75-80	8.0-8.5	720-800	35	4
13-14	75-80	8.0-8.5	720-800	40	5
15-16	80	8.5	800	40	5
Maintenance					
17+	80	8.5	800	40-45	3
	80-85	8.5-9.0	squash	40-50	1
	80-85	8.5-9.0	aerobics	40-50	1

250 kcal per workout (7.5 kcal/min), excluding warm-up and cooldown.

As the summary of progressions chart indicates, I progressively increased intensity, duration, and frequency during the "improvement" stage. Although I varied the prescription factors to suit Ingrid's schedule, the total work per week remained the same. In this stage, the caloric expenditures ranged from 250 to 400 kcal per workout. Within 8-10 weeks, she reached her objective of progressing beyond her earlier fitness plateau. In order to add variety and keep Ingrid's interest high in the "maintenance" stage, after about four months I had her supplement the cycling with squash and aerobic dancing.

Case Study #2: Prescribing Without Cardiovascular Assessment

I met Josh while working with a fitness center that does not offer cardiovascular fitness assessments, claiming they were too expensive—an unfortunate but not uncommon situation. When hard data are in short supply, we have to be creative in obtaining information that will guide us in our prescription designs.

Counseling Assessment

Josh wanted to significantly improve his cardiovascular fitness. More extensive questioning during the counseling stage revealed that

- this 27-year-old had been active in several aerobic sports, but in the last four months had only been using a home exercise bicycle once or twice a week;
- he did not mind the cycling but found it hard to motivate himself;
- after only 10-12 minutes on his bike, his legs were tired—and he felt it took him a long time to recover;
- on the rare occasions when he did a warm-up, it consisted of two or three stretches that were completed in less than a minute; there was never a cooldown;
- he was interested in improving his squash game and in beginning to compete;
- he had no injuries or other health problems, and his weight was controlled;
- most days he had an hour to work out and was confident he could get out four times per week.

Assessment Discussion and Action

I had to use an indirect method to estimate a training zone. Heart Rate Reserve (HRR) physiologically represents the reserve of the heart for increasing cardiac output (see chapter 7). I had Josh monitor his resting heart rate on three consecutive days before he got up in the morning, and found a consistent 62 bpm.

Josh was young, healthy, and was still somewhat active. Some of his early fatigue appeared to be caused by an inappropriate intensity (workload setting) and the lack of proper warm-ups or cooldowns. His history of involvement in multiple sports suggested that he would enjoy the squash competition, and I considered the intensity level and interval nature of squash in the program design.

Prescription

Calculation of exercise intensity:

$$max \ HR = (220 - age) = (220 - 27) = 193 \ bpm$$

Using the Heart Rate Reserve (HRR) method and a moderate to high training zone of 70%-80% HRR:

$$
\begin{aligned}
Heart \ Rate \ Reserve &= [(max \ HR - rest \ HR) \times \\
&\quad \%Training \ Zone] + rest \\
&\quad HR \\
&= [(193 - 62) \times 70 \ to \ 80\%] \\
&\quad + 62 \\
&= [(131) \times 70 \ to \ 80\%] + 62 \\
&= [92 \ to \ 105] + 62 \\
&= 154 \ to \ 167 \ bpm
\end{aligned}
$$

One of the difficulties of prescription without assessment is allocation of a workload. Sometimes Josh used his home exercise bicycle, sometimes the bicycle ergometer at the fitness center. At home I had him cycle at a load and speed about half of what he had been using, then check his heart rate after three minutes of steady cycling. If it was less than 154 bpm, he increased the workload for another three minutes and monitored heart rate again. He continued this process until the heart rate was between 154 and 167 bpm, at which point he recorded the tension setting and speed for the next session. The ergometer at the center gave a more precise measure of work. Remember that perceived exertion should be "somewhat hard" (about 13-14 on the Borg scale).

Josh's warm-up included light cycling for five minutes followed by static stretches for his quadriceps, hamstrings, calves, shins, and lower back. The first three minutes of the cycling were at half to two-thirds of the training zone. For the cooldown, he tapered the cycling for the final three to five minutes and redid the warm-up stretches—holding them longer, since tissue temperature was high, for added flexibility gains.

Results

Once Josh began to tolerate intensity levels closer to his upper limit for 25-30 minutes, I introduced him on alternate days to some interval training. He started with three-minute periods of cycling at his upper limit load but at a faster speed, then three minutes cycling at his warm-up level. He repeated this cycle six to eight times. Squash eventually became his primary focus, and I adjusted the intervals accordingly (see chapter 7).

Case Study #3: Twenty-Three-Year-Old Male Sprinter

A serious 23-year-old male sprinter, Rory specialized in the 200-meter event. He wanted to train all year long and was looking for a safe, progressive program.

Assessment

I used the treadmill for Rory's aerobic assessment because I want him to achieve his highest measurable oxygen uptake, because he was familiar with the device, and because he wanted a prescription for running. Not surprisingly, his results were in the excellent category. And when the assessment was redone in three months, we had a benchmark for comparison. Perhaps most valuable for a client-centered prescription was Rory's personal best in the 200 meters at 24 seconds.

Discussion and Action

Rory's program spanned three phases: preparation, competition, and transition.

Preparation Phase

The early portion of Rory's preseason effort emphasized aerobic training, flexibility and strength balance, and muscular endurance. The volume of training was high and the intensity low. As the preseason progressed, however, I had him ease up on volume and increase intensity. The technical skill preparation involved drilling fundamental techniques such as running the turn. The progression was from simple to complex skills as the preseason advanced. For example, he practiced with basic acceleration form before preceding to block form.

Competition Phase

Rory's next phase included high intensity and a decline in volume. The training was specific, concentrating on fitness and motor components that simulated sprinting. Adequate recovery from workouts was important. As is true in many sports at this stage, Rory needed increased emphasis on speed of movement, reactive training (e.g. plyometrics), and technique work.

Transition Phase

The off-season provided an opportunity for Rory to recover physiologically and psychologically, through a period of active rest that involved lower-intensity activities that required motor skills similar to those needed for sprinting.

Prescription

Now for more details on Rory's daily workout prescriptions during these phases. Refer to chapter 7 to review training methods.

In the early preseason, the preparation was general: continuous runs, fartleks, or cross-country runs. I prescribed specific times, not distances, such as starting with 20 minutes and building up to 45 minutes. In the late preseason, the volume or total work was double that of the competitive phase. For Rory, this was a mixture of continuous and interval work. A 400 meter runner typically may be given a volume of 2400 m (4 × 600 m). Since Rory ran 200 meters, I gave him a volume of 1200 m (6 × 200 m or 4 × 300 m). The intensity at the start was 60% of his personal best of 200 m/24 sec, or 24 sec × (100/60) = 40 seconds for 200 m. He worked up to 70% (34-35 sec) in five to six weeks. After this time, I increased the intensity by 5% and decreased the volume by 10% (20 m for every 200 m) every two to four weeks.

In the competitive phase, interval training was at a 1:3 or 1:4 work to relief ratio. The volume was about half that of the late preseason, or about 3 to 4 times the racing distance. For example, I prescribed a volume of 600 m (3 × 200 m) at 90% intensity. Since his personal best in the 200 meters was 24 seconds, 24 × (100/90) = 26.6 seconds was the workout time. Therefore, the prescription was 3 × 200 m @ 26.6 sec with a walking recovery lasting 1 1/2 to 2 minute or until his heart rate returned to 120-130 bpm.

Results

Initially, Rory needed a longer recovery time near the end of a workout than I expected. As the volume dropped and his condition improved, he no longer needed to extend his recoveries. In the competitive season, Rory ran better than his personal best in all but one competition. He never sustained a serious injury the whole year and his personal best dropped to 22.6 seconds.

In the off-season, Rory jogs at his family's cottage and plays some recreational soccer.

Case Study #4: Male With Creeping Obesity

A 42-year-old insurance broker, Fred was a prime example of creeping obesity. He had coached basketball for 17 years, but had done nothing for the last five years. He claimed that a busy insurance practice and a new cottage had left him little time for regular exercise. He had noticed the weight problem, but it was his last medical checkup (elevated cholesterol and borderline hypertension) that motivated him to come in for help with an exercise program.

Our first task was to focus on his priorities—to determine what *he* wanted to achieve, not just what his doctor wanted. His objectives were to

- lose 12 pounds in the first six months and a total of 20 pounds in the first year,
- reduce his elevated cholesterol level to a normal range, and
- reduce the fat around his waist (if possible) and strengthen that area.

Assessment

The assessment provided me with the following data:

BODY COMPOSITION

Weight	185 lb
Height	5'8"
BMI	28 (grade 1 obesity, overweight)

Body fat	24.5% (moderately high trunk measure)
Abdominal girth	38" (4" less than chest)

CARDIOVASCULAR

Resting heart rate	80 bpm
Resting blood pressure	135/88 (high normal)
Oxygen uptake	Below average, with early leg fatigue and slow recovery

MUSCLE BALANCE

Flexibility	Tight hamstrings, hip flexors, and spinal extensors
Strength	Weak abdominals, but average upper body strength on push-ups
Posture	Lumbar lordosis and rounded shoulders

Discussion and Action

After I explained the assessment results and the implications of his doctors' findings, Fred was committed to making some immediate changes. He decided to walk the twenty minutes to work each day and to set aside three twenty-minute sessions in his office each week to do muscle balance exercises. There was a basketball team that he decided to coach, with plans to be physically active in their 1 1/2 hour practice once a week. We discussed the possibilities for cross-country skiing at his cottage during the winter. After Fred's wife attended the follow-up session, she eliminated high cholesterol/fat snacks at night and reduced between-meal "junk" eating. The rest of their menu appeared reasonable except for the number of times they ate at fast food outlets.

PRESCRIPTION

Brisk walk to work (10 trips × 20 min each) @ 8 kcal/min	1600 kcal/wk
Basketball practice (approx. 40 min active) @ 10 kcal/min (Substitute cross-country skiing at the cottage as suits schedule)	400 kcal/wk
Diet modification (reduce snacks and fast food)	1500 kcal/wk
Deficit:	3500 kcal/wk
Strength/endurance work on abdominals:	3 abdominal exercises for various muscles, 2 sets of 10-15 each (progress with 3rd set)
Strength/endurance work on upper back:	3 tubing exercises (attached to office door) for posterior shoulder joint and shoulder girdle muscles; cross-country skiing at the cottage for 30 to 45 minutes as conditions permit.
Flexibility:	1 exercise each for hamstrings, one-joint hip flexors, two-joint flexors, spinal extensors, calves, and chest; best done after walk to work (warm), hold each for 15-20 seconds then try to increase range of motion and hold for another 10 seconds.

Results

For the first month of the program, Fred followed the program very closely and lost 4 pounds (3500 kcal/wk). He set up a corner of his office with a mat, the tubing, some music, and a monitoring chart. His wife continued to be a good support; and besides a few meal celebrations, by the sixth month both had significantly modified their eating habits. Weather and work pressures permitted Fred to walk to work an average of three days per week for the remainder of the six months. By this time the weight loss was almost 15 pounds, his waist girth was down 2 inches, his blood pressure was consistently 130/84, and the basketball was a lot of fun! Although the cardiovascular results showed no significant improvement (perhaps the intensity was too low), he felt less fatigue and generally more energized. He certainly "carried" himself better and avoided any injuries in the six months. His physician was pleased with the lowered weight and blood pressure, and was confident that his blood cholesterol would soon follow.

Case Study #5: Thirty-Five-Year-Old Working Mother

Like so many, Penny had a long-standing battle with weight management. Chapter 8 follows Penny extensively, describing a number of counseling strategies as they were applied to her stages of change (chapter 1). The study follows Penny for three weeks to the point where she made definite progress toward more positive self-esteem and recognized the continuing benefits of correct eating and active living.

Highlights

- We have given detailed accounts of four individuals who sought the help of a fitness professional.

- We have seen how, by listening carefully to clients and learning details of their values and their lifestyles, it is possible to prescribe creative fitness programs that are effective and that make **adherence** easy and attractive.

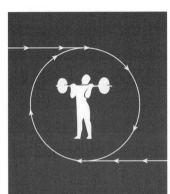

PART IV

Selecting Routes: Personalized Prescription for Musculoskeletal Conditioning

One of our first challenges was to get a very clear picture of what and how our client wanted to change. Client-centered counseling techniques determined individual needs, wants, and lifestyle. Next, we gathered more detailed information from selected assessments which allowed us to fine-tune goals, making them measurable and progressive. In making the transition between counseling and the program design, we select appropriate elements of the exercise prescription that suit the client and the client's goals in the areas of musculoskeletal fitness.

In order to prescribe exercises in the area of musculoskeletal fitness, we must be able to analyze various exercises, sport skills, and work tasks. This analysis allows us to tailor an exercise to suit our client's specific needs.

Chapter 10

Exercise Analysis and Exercise Design

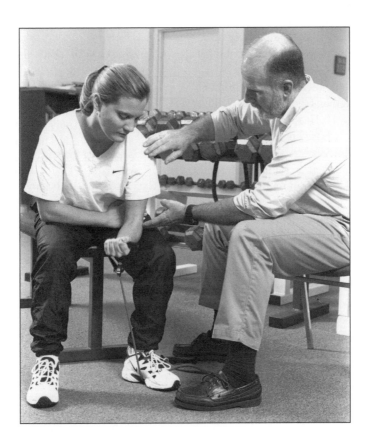

- Anatomical Analysis of Exercise
- Biomechanical Analysis of Exercise
- Anatomical and Biomechanical Analysis of a Weight Training Exercise
- Exercise Design
- Five-Step Approach to Exercise Design
- JAM (Joint-Action-Muscle) Charts

Exercise design is optimized when each exercise is client-centered. There are three broad criteria that form the anchor points for client-centered exercise design:

1. Meeting the client's needs
2. Achieving the purpose for which it was designed effectively and safely
3. Being accepted by the client as something he wants to do

Information from analysis of an exercise allows us to select or modify that exercise. The exercise selection approach to prescription involves a judgment based on the analysis—if it meets the above criteria, the exercise will be part of the prescription.

The process of client personalization comes a step closer with the "selection + modification" approach. Modification is a tuning process that molds an exercise to meet exact specifications—for example, to simulate a movement pattern used in a work task or sport skill. Figure 10.1a shows a resisted horizontal adduction of the shoulder joint that strengthens the pectoralis major and anterior deltoid. Figure 10.1b shows a modification suitable for an athlete whose sport includes the skill of throwing. The modified exercise involves the same muscles, but works them at a slightly different angle and includes a medial rotation (subscapularis) and some trunk rotation.

We must meet the needs of our clients with appropriate modifications. We change designs based on answers to a number of questions: Does it work the targeted muscle? Does the joint action(s) suit the purpose? Is the difficulty level appropriate? Does this exercise maintain a balance with the rest of the prescription? Does the client need unique modifications? Is the starting position and range of motion safe and effective? If equipment is used, is it the right piece; is

it needed at all? Will the client enjoy or value the exercise? What is the effectiveness vs. risk ratio? Do monitoring techniques need to be integrated? Our system of exercise design must be simple to employ but sensitive enough to deal with these issues.

The skills in this chapter involve *breaking down* exercises to determine their purpose (i.e., **analysis**) and *building* exercises from the concept of a need (i.e., **design**). We can use exercise analysis skills in three situations:

1. **Exercise analysis:** To aid in selection or modification of an exercise to be added to a program design
2. **Sport skill analysis:** To aid in selection of exercises that simulate the movements and muscular patterns of a skill
3. **Work task analysis:** To aid in design of exercises that may build the required muscular strength/endurance, or to balance the overuse effects of repetitive or prolonged tasks

Exercise specialists should be able to anatomically analyze the joint movements, muscles used, and types of contraction for exercises and activities common to fitness programming. Understanding the anatomy of the targeted area, recognizing the degree of risk, knowing how to deal with alignment issues, and being able to provide modifications and alternatives are required skills for exercise analysis and design.

This chapter outlines two types of exercise analysis: anatomical and biomechanical. Numerous examples of popular exercises are used, and their suitability to

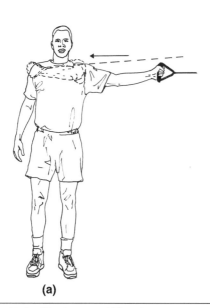

(a)

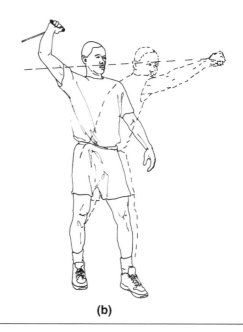

(b)

Figure 10.1   Design modifications.

client needs are determined. A pivotal point in the prescription model is presented at the end of the chapter in the five-step approach to client-centered exercise design.

Anatomical Analysis of Exercise

It is critical that we differentiate the muscular focus of an exercise and know if that focus is appropriate for our client. To the untrained eye, identifying the muscles responsible for various exercises can be very confusing. The following should help you judge your current skills of anatomical analysis.

Imagine you are with a client at the local fitness center and he asks what the difference is between exercises being done by the people in figure 10.2.

Since the movements of the arm look very similar, one might assume the same muscles are responsible for each exercise. In each case, rubber tubing is providing the resistance in a muscular conditioning exercise for the upper body. However, this is where the similarities end.

In figure 10.2, the muscles working are as follows:

Exercise #1. Middle and posterior deltoid, middle and upper trapezius, and rhomboids

Exercise #2. Pectoralis major, anterior deltoid, serratus anterior, and pectoralis minor

Exercise #3. Infraspinatus and teres minor

Even the seasoned exercise specialist must scrutinize an exercise very carefully. Watch the exercise several times and perhaps repeat it yourself slowly. Notice which body parts are moving and which are stabilizing without movement. Are joints bending or straightening through a full range of motion, or to the end of their range of motion? Are the muscles being stretched or are they contracting; and if so, how? The following anatomical analysis section shows how to determine the targeted muscle group for each exercise.

Four-Step Approach to Exercise (Anatomical) Analysis

You should systematically analyze every exercise you prescribe. Apply your system when critiquing an existing program (written or demonstrated), observing a class or workshop, reading a fitness journal or book, receiving a program from a rehabilitation referral, seeing exercise equipment promotions, or trying new things yourself. With practice, the following simple four-step approach to anatomical analysis will become second nature to you: (1) analyze phases; (2) analyze joints and movements; (3) analyze types of contractions; (4) analyze which muscles are being used.

Step #1: Analyze Phases

Break the exercise into phases. Most exercises have two discernible phases: up and down; in and out; push and pull; or left and right. For example, exercise #1 in figure 10.2 has "out" and "back" phases. The phases are not technical terms but are chosen as brief and descriptive. New phases generally are determined by

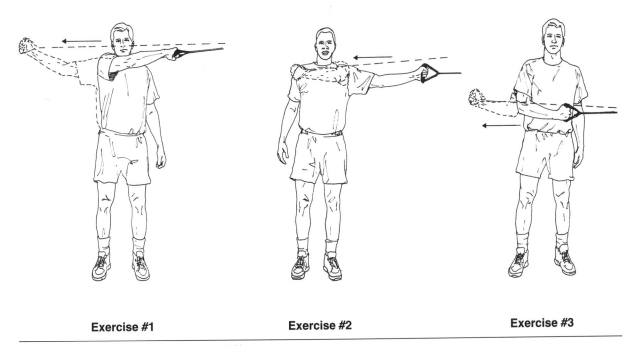

Exercise #1   Exercise #2   Exercise #3

Figure 10.2 Determining exercise differences.

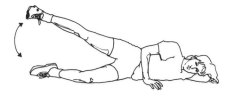

Figure 10.3 Side leg raise with up and down phases.

the point when a joint movement stops and a new movement begins. In muscular conditioning exercises such as with free weights or calisthenics, the phases are usually "up" and "down" to take advantage of gravity's opposition on the up phase. In figure 10.3, the side-lying position optimizes the force of gravity in the up and down phases of the exercise.

Some complex sports skills have several phases. The *power phase* is illustrated in the batter example (figure 10.4). The power phase is the time of the greatest force generation and is often the part of the movement just preceding contact (e.g., in batting) or release (e.g., in throwing). The *preparatory phase*, or wind-up, precedes the power phase it is usually in the opposite direction, and serves two functions: to increase the range of motion through which the force can be applied in the power phase and, if done quickly, to pre-stretch the muscles responsible for the power phase and thereby increase their force.

After the power phase is the *follow-through* phase. This phase has no effect on the amount of force transferred from the body (or bat). These three phases are typical of many sport skills. As a trainer, you will focus your analysis on the power phase—for this is where the client will need the greatest strength or power.

Step #2: Analyze Joints and Movements

Within specific segments of exercise phases, determine which joints are involved and what movements they are performing. Joints move when muscles crossing those joints contract. During concentric (shortening) contractions, the insertion of the muscle moves toward the origin. To be more effective in exercise analysis, you should review your knowledge of anatomy so that you can accurately describe major joint movements (see figure 10.5).

Definitions of Movements Performed at Several Joints

The following are definitions of the major movements at joints throughout the body (Batman and Van Capelle 1992). All movements are from the anatomical position. The *anatomical position* involves the body standing at an erect position, arms and legs straight, head

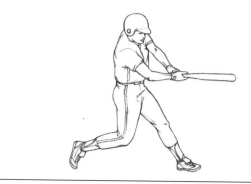

Figure 10.4 The power phase of batting.

facing forward, with palms and toes also facing forward.

- **Flexion:** Bending; bringing the bones together; reducing the angle at a joint. The exception is flexion at the shoulder joint which occurs when the humerus is moved forward.
- **Extension:** Straightening; moving bones apart; increasing the angle at a joint. The exception is extension at the shoulder joint where the humerus is brought back toward the body.
- **Abduction:** Movement away from the midline of the body—for example, moving the arms and legs away from the trunk in a sideways motion.
- **Adduction:** Movement toward the midline of the body—for example, moving the arms or legs toward the trunk in sideways motion.
- **Medial rotation:** Rotation of a limb toward the midline of the body—for example, rotating the arms or legs towards the trunk.
- **Lateral rotation:** Rotation of a limb away from the midline of the body—for example, rotating the arms or legs away from the trunk.
- **Supination:** Lateral rotation movement at the radioulnar joint (below elbow) or a roll to the outside of the heel at the subtalar joint (below the ankle).
- **Pronation:** Medial rotation movement at the radioulnar joint (below elbow) or a roll to the inside of the heel at the subtalar joint (below the ankle).
- **Horizontal abduction:** Movement of a limb away from the midline of the body in a horizontal plane—for example, moving the arm from a front horizontal position to a side horizontal position.
- **Horizontal adduction:** Movement of a limb toward the midline of the body in a horizontal plane—for example, moving the arm from a

side horizontal position to a front horizontal position.

- **Circumduction:** Circular movements at a joint; combines many other movements—for example, occurs at shoulder joint, hip joint, and spinal joint.

Definitions of Movements Unique to Specific Joints

Some movements occur only at one pair of joints.

The Shoulder Girdle. The shoulder girdle is a combination of three joints that work together. The movements are often difficult to see. The following actions describe movements of the shoulder girdle, which comprises the scapula and clavicle.

- **Elevation:** Movement of the scapula upward.
- **Depression:** Movement of the scapula downward.
- **Abduction:** Movement of the scapula away from the spinal column.
- **Adduction:** Movement of the scapula toward the spinal column.

- **Upward rotation:** Rotation of the scapula upward. The inferior angle (bottom) moves outward and upward.
- **Downward rotation:** Rotation of the scapula downward. Inferior angle moves down and in.

Although its joints can move independently, the shoulder girdle functions mainly to support and assist movements of the shoulder joint. The shoulder girdle moves in a series of actions to allow the arm (humerus) to move through a wide range of motion. When you analyze shoulder joint and shoulder girdle movements, it might be helpful to use table 10.1 to identify the action at the shoulder joint and then look across to the corresponding shoulder girdle action.

The Pelvic Girdle. The following actions are specifically related to the pelvic girdle.

- **Forward tilt:** Movement of the pelvic girdle forward.
- **Backward tilt:** Movement of the pelvic girdle backward.
- **Lateral tilt:** Movement of the pelvic girdle such that one side drops.

Table 10.1 Combined Shoulder Girdle and Shoulder Joint Actions

SHOULDER JOINT ACTION	SHOULDER GIRDLE ACTION
Abduction	Upward rotation Abduction
Adduction	Downward rotation Adduction
Flexion	Upward rotation Abduction
Extension	Downward rotation Adduction
Medial rotation	Abduction
Lateral rotation	Adduction
Horizontal abduction	Adduction
Horizontal adduction	Abduction

The Foot. The following actions are specifically related to the ankle and foot.

- **Dorsiflexion:** Same as flexion only at the ankle joint.
- **Plantar flexion:** Same as extension only at the ankle joint; pointing the foot.
- **Eversion:** Turning the sole of the foot outwards where the weight is taken on the inside of the foot. Occurs at the subtalar joint.
- **Inversion:** Turning the sole of the foot inwards

where the weight is taken on the outside of the foot. Occurs at the subtalar joint.

Actions at Specific Joints

Figure 10.5 shows actions performed by specific joints. Some of those listed before as unique to certain joints are not listed.

Practicing Steps 1 and 2

At this point, you are able to divide the exercise into phases, identify all joints that are involved for each

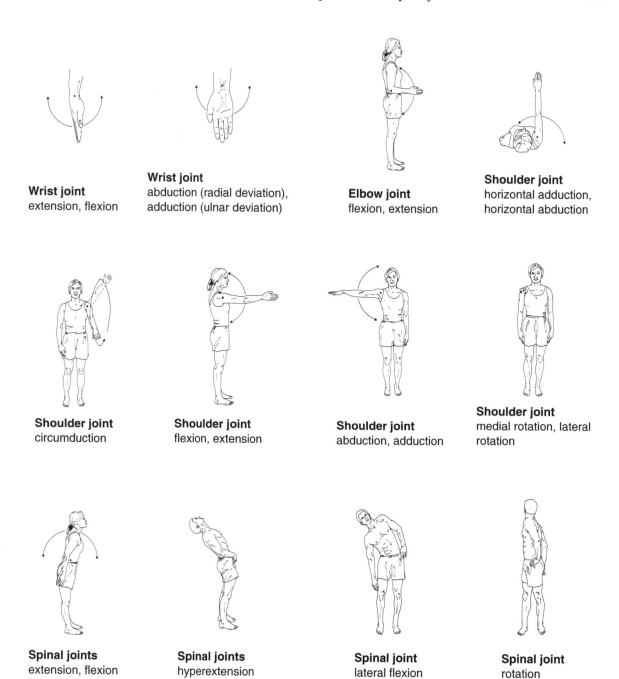

Wrist joint
extension, flexion

Wrist joint
abduction (radial deviation),
adduction (ulnar deviation)

Elbow joint
flexion, extension

Shoulder joint
horizontal adduction,
horizontal abduction

Shoulder joint
circumduction

Shoulder joint
flexion, extension

Shoulder joint
abduction, adduction

Shoulder joint
medial rotation, lateral
rotation

Spinal joints
extension, flexion

Spinal joints
hyperextension

Spinal joint
lateral flexion

Spinal joint
rotation

(continued)

Figure 10.5 Action at specific joints.

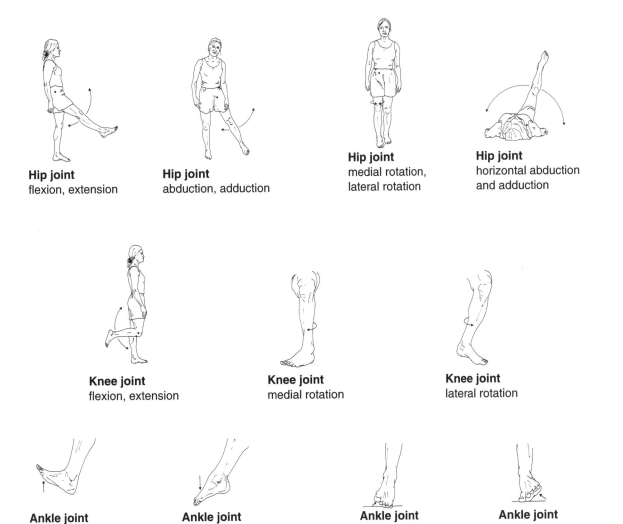

Hip joint
flexion, extension

Hip joint
abduction, adduction

Hip joint
medial rotation,
lateral rotation

Hip joint
horizontal abduction
and adduction

Knee joint
flexion, extension

Knee joint
medial rotation

Knee joint
lateral rotation

Ankle joint
dorsi flexion

Ankle joint
plantar flexion

Ankle joint
inversion

Ankle joint
eversion

Figure 10.5   *(continued)*

phase, and determine the movement or movements for each joint.

You should practice these skills. In the following exercises, determine the phases, the joints involved, and the movement(s) taking place at those joints.

First, do an anatomical analysis of a curl-up, and determine which muscles it targets.

Exercise: curl-up (raise head and shoulders from floor, tilt pelvis backward to flatten back)

Phases: up and down

Joint(s): spine (lumbar)

Movements: flexion (up); extension (down)

To facilitate the analysis, use the following table.

Table 10.2 Exercise: Curl-Up

PHASE	JOINT	MOVEMENT
Up	Spine (lumbar)	Flexion
Down	Spine (lumbar)	Extension

:
Here are some other examples:

Table 10.3 Exercise: Resisted Toe Points
(With tubing around foot, press foot down.)

PHASE	JOINT	MOVEMENT
Out	Ankle	Plantarflexion
In	Ankle	Dorsiflexion

Table 10.4 Exercise: Prone Scapular Retraction
(Pinch shoulder blades together with arms out from sides and elbows bent.)

PHASE	JOINT	MOVEMENT
Up	Shoulder joint	Horizontal abduction
Up	Shoulder girdle	Adduction
Down	Shoulder joint	Horizontal adduction
Down	Shoulder girdle	Abduction

Step #3: Analyze Types of Contractions

To cause a movement, a muscle must produce tension and contract. While under tension, the muscle may shorten during the contraction, lengthen, or stay the same length

With a *concentric contraction*, the muscle develops tension great enough to overcome a resistance and produces an action by shortening. The "up" phase of calisthenics, free weights, sports skills, and many resistance machines involves concentric contraction of the muscles producing joint movements in that direction. For example, in the up phase of a biceps curl, the biceps shorten under tension (concentric contraction) to produce the action of flexion at the elbow. The biceps are creating enough tension to overcome the resistance of gravity, the weight of the arm, and the external weight.

With an *eccentric contraction*, the tension generated by the muscle is less than the resistance and the muscle will lengthen. Eccentric contractions occur when

- muscles attempt to counter the force of gravity, such as when the body or a limb is lowered, or
- muscles attempt to counter the force of momentum by slowing down the action (for example, the ballistic action of the follow-through of a batter).

Eccentric contractions do not increase flexibility, because the muscle is producing tension while it is lengthening. In fact, eccentric contraction can generate more tension than a shortening contraction (Wilmore and Costill 1994). The "down" phase of calisthenics, free weights, sports skills, and many resistance machines involves eccentric contraction of the muscles that produce joint movements in that direction. Remember, the force of gravity produces significant acceleration if an object or limb is allowed to fall freely. In most exercises, the down phase involves eccentric contractions of the muscles that initiated the up movement. We control the speed of the descent with eccentric contractions. For example, the biceps lower the weight in the biceps curl at a rate slower than gravity, thus controlling the free fall.

It is sometimes a difficult concept that the same muscle groups are responsible for both the up and down phases of an exercise. They shorten on the way up with a concentric contraction and lengthen on the way down with an eccentric contraction. Eccentric contractions are a big part of everyday life—e.g., the landing phase of each step of a jog; or lowering yourself to sit, walking down the stairs, lowering a fork from your mouth, and bending down.

Eccentric contractions also occur when we slow down something that is moving quickly or that has significant momentum (momentum = mass × velocity). We are still attempting to control a movement. When a person throws a ball, for example, the anterior shoulder muscles contract concentrically to produce the movement (power phase); but after the ball has been released (follow-through phase), the arm must be slowed down to prevent injury. This control comes from tension in the muscles on the posterior shoulder. The momentum of the arm keeps it moving forward, but the lengthening contraction slows the movement. Many high-power sports and ballistic exercises (such as arm actions with hand weights) involve rapid eccentric contractions. The greatest muscular forces are generated with rapid eccentric contractions; and more strain is placed on connective tissue when it is elongated under tension.

Proper execution of an exercise or skill may involve the stabilization of a joint. If a muscle develops tension but there is no visible movement of the joint, it is called an *isometric contraction*. Although the information is not included on our analysis chart, you will do well to identify the major muscles involved in any isometric contraction where stabilization is a critical part of your client's activity. For example, most upper body exercises involving barbells or dumbbells require the shoulder girdle to be stabilized. An isometric contraction of the shoulder girdle elevators and adductors will form a strong base for shoulder joint movements.

It is useful, then, to expand the analysis chart to include the type of contraction (T of C).

Table 10.5 Exercise: Lateral Arm Raises
(Raise arms out from the body)

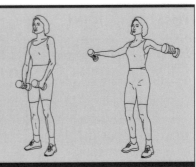

PHASE	JOINT	MOVEMENT	CONTRACTION TYPE
Up	Shoulder joint	Abduction	Concentric
Up	Shoulder girdle	Upward rotation Abduction	Concentric
Down	Shoulder joint	Adduction	Eccentric
Down	Shoulder girdle	Downward rotation Adduction	Eccentric

Note:

- There is no movement in the elbows and wrists, which are stabilized (isometric contractions) during both phases of the exercise.

- In the first 60 degrees of shoulder joint abduction, there is little or no movement of the shoulder girdle. Shoulder girdle adductor muscles contract isometrically to stabilize.

Step #4: Analyze Which Muscles Are Being Used

Here are two helpful visualizations for exercise analysis: (1) Muscles affect movement of the joints that they cross. An obvious example is the biceps at the elbow. Flexion of the elbow is the primary movement; but the biceps also crosses the radioulnar joint and the shoulder joint, and can be recruited to cause movements at these joints. (2) If alignment of the muscle-tendon unit is in the direction of the movement, the influence of that muscle will be optimal (see biomechanical analysis).

Once you have determined the joint action and type of contraction, your final and most important step is to identify the active muscles. Determining individual muscles responsible for a movement can be simplified by following this principle: *The muscle group causing the action is named by that joint and action (if the contraction is concentric).* For example, in the up phase of a biceps curl, the elbow flexes—and the muscle group is the elbow flexors. In lateral arm raises, the shoulder joint abducts in the up phase—therefore the shoulder joint abductors are responsible.

Table 10.6 Exercise: Bench Press
(Press bar up; lower bar near chest.)

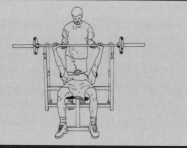

PHASE	JOINT	MOVEMENT	CONTRACTION TYPE	MUSCLES
Up	Shoulder joint	Horizontal adduction	Concentric	Pectoralis major Anterior deltoid (Shoulder joint horizontal adductors)
Up	Shoulder girdle	Abduction	Concentric	Serratus anterior Pectoralis minor (Shoulder girdle abductors)
Up	Elbow	Extension	Concentric	Triceps (Elbow extensors)
Down	Shoulder joint	Horizontal abduction	Eccentric	Pectoralis major Anterior deltoid
Down	Shoulder girdle	Adduction	Eccentric	Serratus anterior Pectoralis minor
Down	Elbow	Flexion	Eccentric	Triceps

For a more detailed analysis, we will look at a bench press.

The analysis chart concisely presents the active joints, their movements, the primary muscles, and how they are contracting during the phases of the exercise. The most challenging part of the anatomical analysis is recalling the specific muscles responsible for the joint actions (Shier, Butler, and Lewis 1996). To facilitate this step, the end of the chapter presents **JAM** charts: quick references indicating **J**oint, **A**ctions, and **M**uscles (tables 10.11-10.17).

Let's apply the JAM charts for anatomical analysis of a partial squat designed to strengthen the lower body—particularly the quadriceps. The exercise is effective in producing gains but does carry some risk. The patellar-femoral pressure increases dramatically as the angle of the knee approaches 90 degrees. Use a light weight and restricted range of motion to begin.

Remember the principle: The muscle group causing the action is named by that joint and action (if the contraction is concentric). This directs us to the JAM chart column for: (1) Hip extensors (table 10.14); (2) Knee extensors (table 10.15); and, (3) Ankle plantarflexors (table 10.16). Reading down each column, select the prime movers (PM) and insert them in the analysis chart. Remember, the down phase is the

Table 10.7 Exercise: Partial Squat
(Keeping back straight and head up, lower the bar by flexing the knees to 90 degrees. Return.)

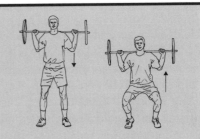

PHASE	JOINT	MOVEMENT	CONTRACTION TYPE	MUSCLES
Up	Hip	Extension	Concentric	Gluteus maximus Semitendinosus Semimembranosus Biceps femoris
Up	Knee	Extension	Concentric	Rectus femoris Vastus lateralis Vastus intermedius Vastus medialis
Up	Ankle	Plantar flexion	Concentric	Gastrocnemius Soleus
Down	Hip	Flexion	Eccentric	Gluteus maximus Semitendinosus Semimembranosus Biceps femoris
Down	Knee	Flexion	Eccentric	Rectus femoris Vastus lateralis Vastus intermedius Vastus medialis
Down	Ankle	Dorsiflexion	Eccentric	Gastrocnemius Soleus

opposite movement but the same muscles are contracting eccentrically. Notice the advantage in always analyzing the "up" phase first.

Purpose, Effectiveness, and Risk

Having completed the anatomical analysis of an exercise, you know what muscles it will work. Is this what you want for your client? With the client-centered counseling approach, you have established her priorities by considering her needs, wants, and lifestyle. It is time now to evaluate the effectiveness of the exercise, how well it fills its purpose, and the degree of personal risk it carries with it.

Purpose

Establish the general purpose of the exercise, that is, which primary fitness component is being challenged. The purpose of the exercise must coincide with the component and body area identified by the client as an area of priority. Discussion in this chapter will focus primarily on the components of flexibility and muscular conditioning. It is sometimes difficult to differentiate between a flexibility and a strengthening exercise. To assist, try these three simple checks.

CHECKS	STRETCH	STRENGTH
Attachment points (i.e., origin and insertion)	Pulled further apart	Come closer together (concentric contraction)
Muscle tension	Slight	Moderate to high
Gradual feeling	Relief and relaxation	Hardness; fatigue

Define the purpose more specifically by referring to the area(s) of the body targeted by the exercise. For example, the purpose of an exercise may be "to stretch the calves," or "to strengthen the abdominal area," or "to develop power needed for a vertical jump."

Effectiveness

Effectiveness refers to how well an exercise fulfills its purpose. No two clients will take exactly the same route to reach an objective. Effectiveness is not just what researchers have said about an exercise or training method—it varies considerably among clients.

The bottom line to effectiveness is, "Will the exercise do what I want it to do for my client?" More specifically,

- What is the appropriate overload to challenge the desired fitness component?
- Does the stretch avoid excessive tension, and is the alignment such that the stretch is in the direction of the fibers and elongation of the muscle?
- For a strengthening exercise, is fatigue felt in the targeted muscles, and are they directly resisted by an external resistance such as free weights, equipment, elastic bands, or gravity?
- Is the exercise effective from the physiological point of view?
- What monitoring can be built into the design to track its effectiveness?

Risk

Careful risk analysis is inherent in any client-centered prescription. Details of doing a risk analysis are discussed in chapter 13.

Biomechanical Analysis of Exercise

Biomechanical analysis examines the method of execution of an exercise. We can apply biomechanical principles to optimize exercise benefits for our clients and at the same time attend to their limitations through biomechanical alterations of the exercise. Such analyses enable us to advise our clients concerning

- the best starting position for an exercise;
- the optimal speed for their objectives;
- the position of joints to isolate specific muscles;
- how to align the movement to the muscle;
- how to combine muscles for optimal results; and
- how to modify the leverage to gain a greater strength output.

The next section is guided by a number of biomechanical principles. The purpose, effectiveness, and safety of an exercise or sport skill may be affected by any or all of the following:

- Muscle length and force
- Direction of force application/alignment
- Biarticular (two-joint) muscle action
- Composition of forces
- Leverage and strength

Muscle Length and Force

The amount of force produced by a muscle is related to the physical length at which the muscle is held. How can you use this information to direct your prescription and optimize the results?

What Causes the "Sticking Point" in Weight Lifting?

A person working with weights will begin to feel weak at some point during the exercise. Getting the weight started and completing the last few degrees are the two usual sticking points. The maximum tension that can be generated in the muscle will occur when the muscle is activated at a length slightly greater than its resting length—up to about 120% of the resting length. When a muscle is shortened to about 50%-60% of its resting length, its force is minimal because actin and myosin filaments are doubled over and few cross-bridges are formed. As the muscle is elongated beyond 120% of the resting length, there is slippage of the cross-bridges, fewer are formed, and less force is generated (Edman 1992). As a result, your clients will feel weak at the ends of the range of motion. Select weights that they can lift through a full range of motion for the prescribed repetitions.

How Can Your Client Tap an Energy Reserve?

If your client is working with weights, a slight increase in the stretch of the muscle prior to the contraction will summon an energy reserve for increased performance. The reason is that the total tension or force generated in a shortening muscle receives a contribution from the passive (stretch) tension of the tendon and the connective tissue in the muscle (figure 10.6). This stored elastic energy or passive tension plus the voluntary muscular tension provide the total tension or force output. Your clients can apply this principle in their training or in their athletic activities by placing the joint in a preparatory phase (prestretched) prior to the power phase (e.g., the back swing of a batter or the squat of a volleyball spiker). This stored energy can be used only if the shortening contraction occurs within 0.0-0.9 seconds after the stretch and if the muscle is not lengthened too much (Komi 1992). With eccentric training, the force increases as the velocity of the lengthening contraction increases, up to a point where control is lost. These principles are the basis for plyometric training (chapter 11).

Direction of Force Application/ Alignment

Tension or force from a muscle is transferred through the tendon to the bone. The angle of attachment of the muscle dictates the direction of force application, which produces the movement (figure 10.7). Near the middle of the range of motion, the angle of insertion of the tendon usually directs more of the force perpendicular to the bone, resulting in its strongest position.

Force application is optimized when the muscle-tendon unit is directly aligned with the plane of

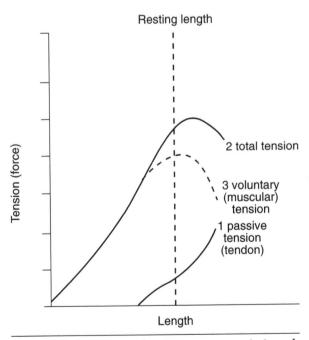

Figure 10.6   Relationship between muscle length and tension.

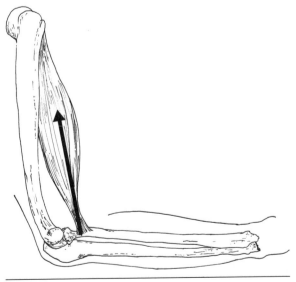

Figure 10.7   Direction of force application. Force increases as the angle between the tendon and the bone approaches 90 degrees.

movement. This can be seen with the prime movers for specific joint actions. In fact, careful alignment of the movement can emphasize the contribution from particular parts of a given muscle. With this information, you can personalize exercises for your clients. The external obliques are a good visual example. The muscle fibers run diagonally and therefore are most effective when pulling the trunk in the diagonal direction (such as in a curl-up with a rotation). In a straight curl-up, the external oblique muscle is not as effective—with spinal flexion, the pull of the muscle is at an angle to the action and the entire force is not utilized for the movement. Here are some other examples:

- **Cross-overs** (figure 10.8) using pulleys, tubing, or elastic bands are versatile exercises because it is easy to change the angle of the pull to suit the targeted muscle or the sport skill.

- The **pull down** exercise utilizes the latissimus dorsi. Different secondary muscles are pulled into play, however, if the bar is pulled down in front or behind the head. In front, the pectoralis major is employed because of the slight flexion. Pulling behind the head forces the shoulder joint backwards and activates the posterior deltoid.

- The **bench press** employs a horizontal movement of the shoulder joint and uses the sternal or horizontal fibers of the pectoralis major. With the incline bench press, the shoulder joint is angled upwards and activates the upper clavicular part of the pectoralis major.

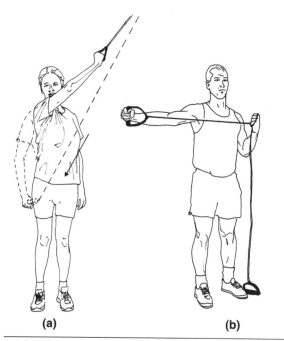

Figure 10.8 Cross-overs with different directions of force.

- **Rowing** action with any device may be done with elbows in or elbows out. With elbows in, the shoulder joints are extending to involve the latissimus dorsi and pectoralis major as prime movers. With the elbows up, the shoulder joints are horizontally abducting through contraction of the posterior deltoid, infraspinatus, and teres minor. A small change in alignment can make a significant shift in the purpose of the exercise.

Alignment of muscle action

Question: Which muscles are working in a side leg raise? What changes take place if the toe is pointing upwards? (Remember, the line of pull of a muscle across a joint will determine the functions of that muscle.)

Answer: The hip abductors lift the leg in a side leg raise. When the toe is pointed upwards, the task of lifting the leg has shifted to the hip flexors which are directly in the line of pull.

Biarticular (Two-Joint) Muscle Action

Biarticular muscles are those that cross two joints. They affect movement at both joints. You can apply this understanding to help clients stretch muscles from both ends, isolate muscles for conditioning, and perform aerobics more efficiently.

How Can a Biarticular Muscle Stretch From Both Ends?

Biarticular muscles are not long enough to allow a full range of motion simultaneously at both joints. If one of the two joints is moved to the end of its range of motion, the attempt to move the second joint to the end of its range will stretch the biarticular muscle nearer the second joint. For example, the hamstrings attach above the hip and below the knee. Once the knee is pulled tight to the chest, it is not possible to fully extend the knee because the hamstrings are too short. Attempting to extend the knee, however, will stretch the lower hamstrings. To stretch the upper hamstrings, extend the knee and rotate the pelvis forward as the trunk flexes. Hamstring strains are more common in the upper area of the hamstrings, suggesting that the latter stretch may be of greater value for prevention or rehabilitation. "Feeling" where the stretch is centered provides feedback that the biarticular principle is being used effectively.

Other biarticular muscles (and the joints they cross) that can be effectively stretched in this manner include

- Gastrocnemius (ankle and knee)
- Rectus femoris (knee and hip)
- Iliopsoas (hip and pelvis)
- Erector spinae (pelvis and spine)
- Levator scapulae (shoulder girdle and cervical spine)
- Triceps (shoulder joint and elbow)

Check the JAM Charts for joint movements (pages 170-174).

How Can We Isolate a One-Joint Muscle for Conditioning/Stretching?

If both ends of a biarticular muscle are brought closer together, the muscle is too short to exert a maximum force output, and therefore single-joint muscles can be isolated. This principle is used to isolate the abdominals in a curl-up. When the knees and hips are bent, the biarticular hip flexors (rectus femoris) are short and slack and do not contribute appreciably to the action. The work feels more difficult because the abdominals are being isolated. Adjustment of even one joint can shorten a muscle and decrease its involvement. For example, as the knee flexes during a resisted leg flexion exercise (figure 10.9), the hamstrings lose their force as their origin and insertion come closer together. The individual therefore

seeks help from the assistant movers for knee flexion. The JAM charts (end of chapter) indicate that these include the sartorious, gracilis, and gastrocnemius muscles.

In another example, the biarticular gastrocnemius (attaches above the knee) is more heavily activated during a standing calf raise than when it is shortened during a seated calf raise, thereby isolating the soleus (figure 10.10).

This method of isolation will also help you to analyze flexibility exercises. With the previous example of the gastrocnemius (two-joint) and soleus (one-joint), both muscles are stretched when the ankle is dorsiflexed. When the knee is straight, the gastrocnemius is maximally stretched; when the knee is flexed, the two-joint gastrocnemius is slack and the soleus stretch is optimized.

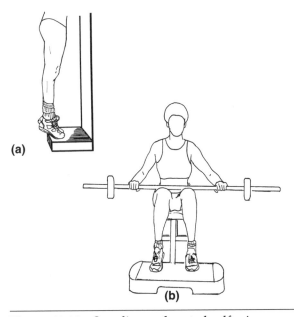

Figure 10.10 Standing and seated calf raises.

How Do You Get More Force From a Biarticular Muscle?

Prestretching a biarticular muscle can significantly improve its force output. For example, the flexor muscles of the wrist act as assistant movers for elbow flexion. When the wrist is slightly hyperextended during elbow flexion, the increased tension in these muscles contributes to the force of the movement. This is also seen in the leg flexion exercise (figure 10.9), in which the force of the hamstrings is improved when the pelvis is rotated forward and the muscle is elongated. Because greater resistance can be applied, the training results are increased. Caution your clients about excessive pelvic rotation in this exercise, which can increase

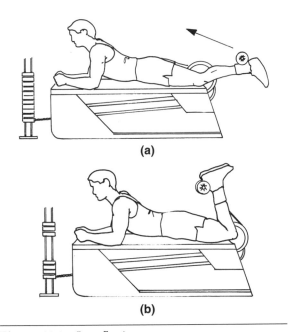

Figure 10.9 Leg flexion.

the lumbar curve and force the lower back muscles into contracture.

How Do Biarticular Muscles Increase Efficiency?

Two-joint muscles, particularly in the lower extremity, save energy by allowing concentric work at one joint and eccentric work at the adjacent joint. This mechanical coupling of joints allows for a rapid release of stored elastic energy (passive tension) (Hamill and Knutzen 1995). For example, in a vertical jump, the gastrocnemius concentrically plantar flexes the ankle. At the knee, which is extending, the gastrocnemius is eccentrically storing elastic energy. These joint couplings occur frequently in walking and jogging and reduce the work required from the single-joint muscles. *Closed kinetic chain exercises* (see chapter 11) that involve direct weightbearing utilize this mechanical coupling. They are quite useful, and clients wanting to strengthen their knee(s) would benefit by including this method of exercise design.

Composition of Forces

Try to visualize the combination of muscles involved in a particular joint movement. Using this visualization to teach your clients will direct their focus to the right muscles and provide them with helpful sensory feedback.

It is often possible to modify a movement in order to isolate a targeted muscle or muscle part. Joints do not always follow traditional movements. For instance, they may move halfway between flexion and abduction. Many sport skills or work tasks involve similar oblique movements. Think of a muscle as a string on a mannequin causing joint movement in the direction of the pull of the string. Each muscle acting on that joint is like a string pulling at a different angle. When more than one force is acting on the joint, you can apply the technique of *composition of forces* to help visualize the relative contribution of those muscles to the final movement.

Example:

The pectoralis major has two parts, combining the sternal (S) and clavicular (C) forces to produce a resultant force (R). This resultant force causes shoulder joint horizontal adduction (figure 10.11).

To use this technique,

- Draw (or visualize) the movement as an arrow. This is called the Resultant Force (R).
- Select, from the anatomical analysis, the two primary muscles causing the movement.

- Represent these muscle forces with arrows.
- The arrow heads indicate the direction of pull of the muscles. The length of the arrow depicts the relative strength of that muscle's involvement.
- Place the base of the two forces (S and C in this example) together on or near the point of attachment of the two muscles.
- Draw a parallelogram from the arrows.
- The diagonal of the parallelogram represents the composition of the forces—that is, the *resultant force*.

The final stage of this technique involves identifying which muscle you want to isolate. Alter the direction of the resultant force closer to the direction of that muscle. You can see in figure 10.11b that as the movement (R2) is angled more upward, the clavicular arrow becomes larger (C2). This means that the clavicular part of the pectoralis major is generating more force, effectively isolating it.

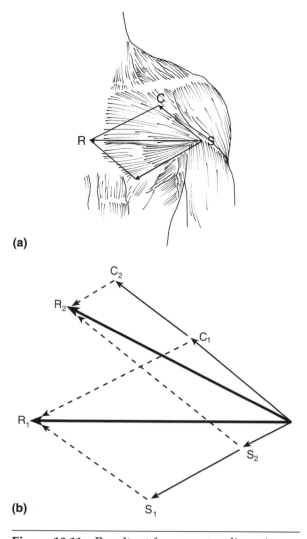

(a)

(b)

Figure 10.11   Resultant force: pectoralis major.

More examples of Composition of Forces:

■ Acting alone, the anterior and posterior parts of the deltoid flex and extend the shoulder joint respectively (figure 10.12). Their combined action (resultant) is shoulder joint abduction. When someone lifts an object by abducting the shoulder joint, she calls into play the anterior deltoid more heavily because the object is in front of the body. If she has a rounded shoulder posture, how would you modify the shoulder joint abduction to emphasize the posterior deltoid?

■ The two heads of the gastrocnemius, pulling in lateral and medial directions, together exert an upward force on the Achilles tendon and cause plantar flexion of the ankle (figure 10.13). Toeing-in will slightly pre-

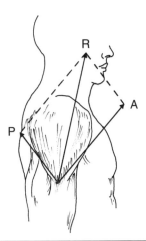

Figure 10.12 Resultant force: deltoid.

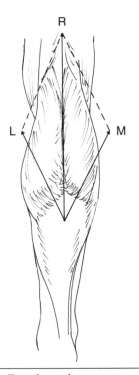

Figure 10.13 Resultant force: gastrocnemius.

stretch the lateral head of the gastrocnemius, allowing a small increase in the force output of that head during plantar flexion. Only the most avid body builders would want this advantage during an exercise such as a calf raise (figure 10.10).

■ The pull of the quadriceps on the patella guides the patella through the path of motion (figure 10.14a). Sometimes (figure 10.14b) the patella is directed laterally (R) by the quadriceps (Q) and patellar tendon (P)—particularly if the vastus medialis (M) is weak. This muscle imbalance can lead to inflammation on the posterior side of the patella.

■ A resultant force acting on the knee in a different direction (figure 10.15) is the pressure exerted on the back side of the patella from the quadriceps muscles (Q) and patellar tendon (P). As the knee flexes (as in a squat or a lunge), the resultant force increases (R_1 vs. R_2). Have your clients take precautions with the depths and applied loads during these type of exercises.

Leverage and Strength

Lever systems can help you modify exercises to optimize the efforts of your clients. If a client is having difficulty with an exercise or wants to make it more challenging, you can adjust the intensity by changing the lever system.

How Do You View the Body as a Series of Lever Systems?

To view the body as a series of lever systems, consider the joint as the fulcrum and the bones as lever arms that move around the fulcrum. Muscle contraction is the force applied to the lever (at the point where the tendon attaches to the bone), while the weight of the body

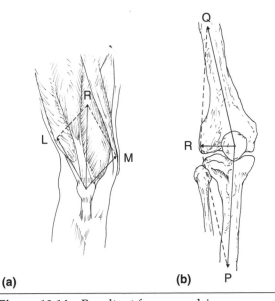

(a)   **(b)**

Figure 10.14 Resultant force: quadriceps.

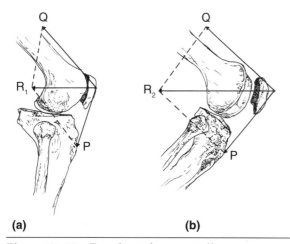

(a)   **(b)**

Figure 10.15   Resultant force: patellar pressure.

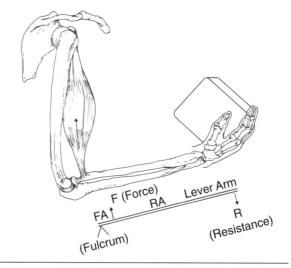

Figure 10.16   The arm as a lever system (e.g., third-class lever).

part(s) plus any external weight being lifted represent resistance to the force (figure 10.16).

The majority of levers in the body are third class, which means that the force is applied between the resistance and the fulcrum. The biceps acting around the elbow joint is an example of a third class lever. In figure 10.16, the elbow is the fulcrum, the radius is the lever arm, the biceps exerts the force, and the weight of the box and the forearm is the resistance.

The tendon of the biceps inserts to the radius just below the elbow. The distance from the fulcrum (elbow) to the force (biceps insertion) is called the force arm (FA). The distance from the fulcrum (elbow) to the resistance is called the resistance arm (RA) (figure 10.16).

adduction. In the foot, both invertors and evertors combine to plantar flex without rotation. A common effect of this synergistic muscle action is greater joint stabilization.

How Can You Adjust a Lever System to Modify the Difficulty of an Exercise?

You can modify the intensity or difficulty of an exercise by changing aspects of the lever system. Depending on your client's situation, you can adjust the resistance, force, force arm, or resistance arm.

The Resistance

If your clients are lifting weights or have load adjustments on their machines, it is easy to change the resistance. You can introduce (or change the thickness of) tubing or elastic bands. Water offers increased resistance and added safety element for joints. Increased resistance is the overload of choice when your client's goal is strength.

The Force

Force is the strength or the speed of the muscular contractions that cause a movement. Sometimes performing an exercise slowly demands more control and is more difficult than doing it more quickly. As your clients' muscular condition improves, they can generate greater forces in a more coordinated manner. Increased speed of

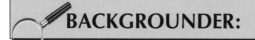

Synergists

Synergists are muscles that act together to create a resultant force. They can be separate parts of the same muscle, as when the anterior and posterior parts of the gluteus medius work together for hip abduction or the upper and lower trapezius muscles complement one another in shoulder girdle adduction. Synergists may also be opposing muscle parts that work together for one action but neutralize each other because of opposing roles. For example, wrist muscles that flex and abduct work in synergy with others that flex and adduct. The result is stronger wrist flexion with neither abduction or

movement is the overload of choice when your client's goal is muscular power. The speed adjustments on isokinetic and hydraulic machines (chapter 11) change the potential force outputs. Even aerobic machines like stairclimbers have similar setting options (i.e., slower speed settings generate greater force). With certain flexibility training methods, the isometric contraction phase of a PNF stretch (chapter 11) can modify the force of contraction, changing that element of the lever system and ultimately the effectiveness of the stretch.

The Force Arm

The distance between the joint and the insertion of the muscle (FA) cannot be changed, but it partially explains differences in performance among clients whose muscular conditioning (force) appears to be equal.

The Resistance Arm

Changing the distance between the joint and the resistance (RA) is the most versatile way to adjust the body's lever systems. As the resistance moves closer to the joint, the muscle will have an easier time moving it. The challenge is to recognize the parts of the lever system in question: Which joint is the acting fulcrum? What represents the resistance? What is the best way to shift the resistance arm? There are often multiple lever systems working at once, and you must identify the one most appropriate to adjust. The examples in table 10.8 illustrate the answers to these questions.

Anatomical and Biomechanical Analysis of a Weight Training Exercise

A full exercise analysis combines anatomical and biomechanical analyses. We must ensure that we meet our client's needs, account for any limitations, and validate the exercise design.

Table 10.8 Adjusting the Resistance Arm (RA)

EXERCISE	FULCRUM	RESISTANCE (R)	(RA) ADJUSTMENT
Curl-up	Lower back	Upper body weight	Arms above the head moves (R) away from the fulcrum—harder
Push-up	Shoulder joint	Weight of entire body	Done from the knees moves a reduced (R) closer to the fulcrum—easier
Dumbbell flies	Shoulder joint	Dumbbell & arm	Changing the angle of the elbow moves the (R)
Leg (knee) flexion/extension (machine)	Knee	Assigned weight & lower leg	Adjusting the position of the pad lower—harder
Standing knee lifts	Hip	Weight of leg (could use ankle weight or tubing)	Lift leg with an extended knee; (R) further from hip—harder
Bent-over rowing	Lower back (not shoulder joint)	Weight of upper body & barbell	Upright rowing brings (R) closer to lower back—less load on back structures

Maria worked as a sorter in the post office. She was interested in adding weights to her fitness program. Sometimes her shoulders tired at work, and she wanted to improve her shoulder endurance and prevent the injuries she had seen in some of her co-workers. Their injuries resulted from impingement (chapter 14), where the soft tissue between the head of the humerus and the acromion process of the scapula can be jammed.

One of the core exercises I designed for her was a lateral arm raise.

Anatomical Analysis

The purpose of the lateral arm raise is to develop the shoulders and upper back. The exercise effectively targets the deltoids and upper shoulder girdle muscles (table 10.9). Heavier weights and arms lifted above the horizontal can magnify the risk of impingement. Keeping the thumbs up provides the largest space for the tissues and a reduced risk. Since Maria had no shoulder problems, I expected that application of a progressive overload would bring the desired results with no com-

plications. I advised Maria to avoid rapid movements, especially much beyond the horizontal. If she began to feel any discomfort, she was to stop and ice her shoulder after the workout.

Biomechanical Analysis

The middle deltoid and supraspinatus have a direct line of pull for shoulder joint abduction. As the deltoid lifts the arm near to the horizontal, it is shorter and less strong. At this point, the shoulder girdle muscles play a more significant role.

The anterior deltoid assists with shoulder joint abduction. As Maria began to be fatigued, I noticed that she was lifting the weights a little more in front of her body to elicit more of the anterior deltoid. This change in alignment alters the composition of forces. Similarly, the thumbs-up position rotates the starting position of the shoulder, involving two more of the rotator cuff muscles (infraspinatus and teres minor). This change in alignment is not only a safety feature—it makes the lateral arm raise into a conditioning exercise for the rotator cuff. Since Maria's work required that

Table 10.9 Analysis of Lateral Arm Raises

PHASE	JOINT	MOVEMENT	CONTRACTION TYPE	MUSCLES
Up	Shoulder joint	Abduction Lateral rotation (thumbs up)	Concentric Isometric	Middle deltoid Supraspinatus Infraspinatus Teres minor
Up	Shoulder girdle	Upward rotation Abduction Elevation	Concentric	Serratus anterior Trapezius I & II Levator scapulae*
Down	Shoulder joint	Adduction Lateral rotation (thumbs up)	Eccentric Isometric	Middle deltoid Supraspinatus Infraspinatus Teres minor
Down	Shoulder girdle	Downward rotation Adduction Depression	Eccentric	Serratus anterior Trapezius I & II Levator scapulae*

*Pectoralis minor and trapesius IV are depressors and less effective in this exercise.

she raise her arms over her head, I encouraged her to use the thumbs-up position.

A lateral raise is a third-class lever where the fulcrum is the shoulder joint, the lever arm is the humerus, the primary force is the deltoid, and the resistance is the weight of the arm and the dumbbell. Increasing the bend of the elbow brings the resistance closer to the fulcrum, reducing the resistance arm and making the exercise easier. I encouraged Maria to use this position at the beginning. As she progressed, I began to have her straighten her elbows somewhat before changing the weight.

Effective exercise analysis allowed me to achieve the desired purpose of the exercise and to meet Maria's needs. You should always alter exercises—anatomically and biomechanically—in order to take your client's limitations into account.

Exercise Design

Just as a patient approaches the physician or pharmacist with the request, "Give me something for my . . .," clients approach exercise specialists requesting specific exercises to meet their needs. The proliferation of strength training technique seminars and exercise design workshops for aerobic leaders and personal trainers is a testament to the interest in exercise design (Griffin 1986b). Many people in the industry are on the verge of "design template syndrome" where every program they design starts to look the same! In contrast, we should be able to draw on a variety of exercises to personalize our prescriptions—particularly in the component areas of flexibility, muscular balance, and conditioning.

Exercise design may be compared to helping a client purchase a pair of running shoes. First, we need to analyze a shoe for its features. Knowing the requirements of our client, we try to match the features with their needs. We make final adjustments in size and width, and perhaps add a heel lift or extra arch support. The exercise design process is similar: After we analyze possible exercises, we select those that most closely match the needs of our client. We usually need to make modifications to improve the client "fit." And if the fit is still not right, we can still build the ideal exercise for our client from scratch!

The pinnacle of the prescription model is the "portfolio" of individual exercise designs. It is what we have to show our clients; it is from this that they expect results. Training methods and exercise equipment are the setting for the real actors—the individual exercises. The script for these actors starts with the design of the exercise and continues with adjustment of the prescription factors (FITT—Frequency, Intensity, Time, and Type of exercise) to suit the client.

Five-Step Approach to Exercise Design

The following method, which puts together the techniques learned in this chapter, is a simple five-step approach to guide you through this process of exercise design:

1. Identify the component and training method.
2. Target the muscle(s).
3. Determine the appropriate joint movements or position.
4. Design and/or modify.
5. Finish with a safety check.

Step #1: Identify the Component and Training Method

Sometimes you will have to take your client's vision and translate it into a physiological component. For example, your client may want to make it through his work day without low back pain. This may require exercises for stretching the hip flexors, lower back, and hamstrings; muscular endurance for the abdominals and gluteals; and some aerobic work. Your client's objectives may also involve multiple components. For example, someone who wants aerobic work but has a lower leg problem must deal with modifications of the aerobic task while rehabilitating the leg. As the client makes gains, the importance of some of the components may decrease (e.g., lower leg strength) while others may increase (e.g., cardiovascular endurance).

Careful selection of a training method (chapters 7 and 11) can assist in balancing several components. For your client with the lower leg problem, you might consider rowing, swimming, or circuit training with aerobic activities involving the upper body. For muscular conditioning, consider simple sets, closed kinetic chain exercises, or a calisthenic circuit utilizing surgical tubing. Even PNF stretching will develop isometric strength while improving joint flexibility.

Step #2: Target the Muscle(s)

Step #2 identifies the goal area of the body, then targets the primary muscle groups (figure 10.17).

In this step you must consider muscular balance and postural stabilizers. For example, someone who spends many hours at a computer has asked for exercises to

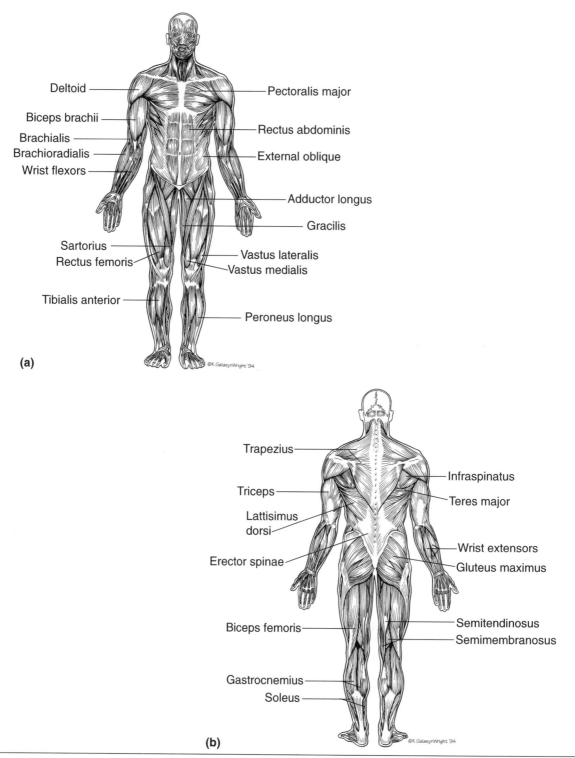

(a)

Deltoid

Biceps brachii

Brachialis

Brachioradialis

Wrist flexors

Sartorius

Rectus femoris

Tibialis anterior

Pectoralis major

Rectus abdominis

External oblique

Adductor longus

Gracilis

Vastus lateralis

Vastus medialis

Peroneus longus

©K.Galasyn Wright '94

(b)

Trapezius

Triceps

Lattisimus dorsi

Erector spinae

Biceps femoris

Gastrocnemius

Soleus

Infraspinatus

Teres major

Wrist extensors

Gluteus maximus

Semitendinosus

Semimembranosus

©K.Galasyn Wright '94

Figure 10.17   Front and rear view of adult male skeletal musculature.

help his baseball throwing ability. The exercise illustrated in figure 10.1b will strengthen the anterior chest and shoulder muscles used in throwing. However, these muscles are tight because of the constant computer posture. Targeted muscles must strike a muscular balance with their antagonists. Therefore your pre-

scription should include stretches for the active chest muscles and strengthening of the upper back and posterior shoulder muscles (i.e., posterior deltoid, latissimus dorsi, and trapezius).

Please note: Narrow targeting with muscle "isolations" is sometimes appropriate, but it may leave gaps in your client's program. Some machines can prevent muscles from working together naturally with other muscles as synergists or co-contractors. For example, there is little correlation between performance on isokinetic knee extension machines and functional performance in a weightbearing sport or activity that utilizes the quadriceps (Ellison 1993).

Step #3: Determine the Appropriate Joint Movements or Position

You can read the JAM (Joint-Action-Muscle) charts in reverse to determine the movement needed for an exercise design (see end of chapter). For example:

■ Use the Tri-Set system of training (chapter 11) to target the gluteus maximus. Table 10.14 (page 172) indicates that the gluteus maximus is a prime mover for hip extension and lateral rotation and an assistant mover for hip abduction. In step #4 you will see how to design three muscular endurance calisthenics that employ these hip movements, or a single exercise modified in three ways. The JAM charts are a reminder that multiple movements are required to fully challenge all fibers of a muscle.

■ A second example involves a client suffering from tension in the upper back. Step #2 targeted the upper trapezius muscles, levator scapulae, and the erector spinae of the cervical spine. Step #4 will design some static stretches for these muscles—but in what positions should the shoulder girdle and cervical spine be placed to stretch all of these muscles? Table 10.12 of the JAM charts (page 171) shows that the levator scapulae and trapezius I and II are responsible for shoulder girdle elevation, upward rotation, and some assisted adduction. Taking the opposite position will stretch these muscles, pulling origin and insertion apart. Table 10.17 shows the erector spinae would be stretched when the neck is flexed, laterally flexed, or rotated.

Step #4: Design and/or Modify

This system establishes the requirements before an exercise is selected. Your guidelines are the muscle actions or movements. You are not restricted to a menu of exercises. Let the creative juices flow!

In the first example, figure 10.18 suggests three calisthenics that work the gluteus maximus in (1) lateral rotation with extension tubing (dynamic); (2) extension (isometric); and, (3) abduction (dynamic). Dynabands could be used in all three exercises; or ankle weights used from a standing position in exercises 1 and 3; or the range of motion could be increased

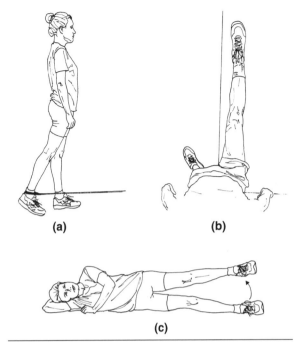

Figure 10.18 Strengthening exercises for the gluteus maximus.

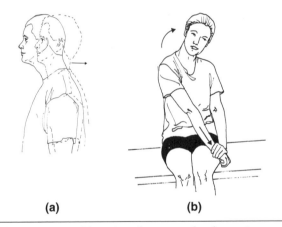

Figure 10.19 Exercises for upper back tension.

in all three movements. The more you know about your clients, the better you are able to meet their needs.

In of the second example (figure 10.19), the first exercise stretches both sides of the erector spinae, trapezius I, and levator scapulae. The second exercise focuses on one side at a time and stretches all four muscles. If your client is suffering tension at his computer work station, you could modify the second exercise to be done in a chair. Grasping the bottom of the chair seat, he would lean to one side with a lateral flex to the neck.

Step #4 may also involve refinement and modification of exercises. To generate creative ideas, consider changes in body position, joint angle, or range of motion; the addition of other body segments, stages of the exercise, or combining movements; or simulation of a work task or sporting skill.

Step #5: Finish With a Safety Check

After creating your design, scrutinize it for safety. Check for high risk in the design and later in the execution. Look for repetitive forces contributing to overuse; excessive force in the development of momentum; or forces applied when joints are not aligned. Modify the design further if the exercise has high injury risk.

Your client may already have some areas of weakness to which you need to be sensitive, such as muscle imbalances, joint instability, muscle tightness, or previous injuries. Chapter 13 examines safety and intervention in more detail.

A safe program is not simply the sum of the safety of individual exercises. The Program Design Template (table 10.10) identifies safety issues prominent at various segments of a program.

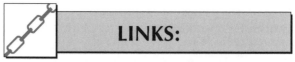

LINKS:

The "Weekend Warrior"!

A word of caution about the "weekend warrior," the impetuous client who charges from his week of sedentary living directly to the competitive playing field. He is a prime candidate for muscle or connective tissue injury caused by a rapid/forceful eccentric contraction. Avoidance is not the message he wants to hear, and a few cold stretches do little to prepare for the trauma. A longer warm-up integrating progressive eccentric actions similar to those in the sport will help. Also add a supplemental program to strengthen (eccentrically) the muscles used in the sport, particularly in preseason. Always include a critical evaluation of eccentric contraction patterns within your client's activity prescription.

What other counseling would be appropriate for this type of cleint? Why?

Table 10.10   Program Design Template

PRESCRIPTION	SAFETY ISSUE
Preparation (Warm-Up) Segment Range of motion (major joints are moved through their ROM)	• Increases joint lubrication & synovial fluid (protect) • Client's first check on how body feels before work • Some flexibility gains (stage 1)
Circulatory warm-up (light aerobic; same mode as CV work)	• Increases tissue temperature & synovial fluid in preparation for stretching • Gradual preparation for heart & circulatory system • Simulates joint mechanics with low trauma
Preparation (Warm-Up) Segment *(continued)* Stretch (emphasis on static stretching)	• Flexibility gains (stage 2) • Target muscles used, esp. if used eccentrically • Dynamic stretches for sport preparation
Transition (ease into next segment)	• Warm-up continues with a light overload in the activity to follow (start of progressive overload)
Aerobic Segment Progressive prescription	• Build-up gradually whether continuous or intervals • If intervals: adequate relief • Tear-down gradually; avoid final sprints or sudden stops (better CV adaptations permitted)

Table 10.10   *(continued)*

PRESCRIPTION	SAFETY ISSUE
Aerobic Segment *(continued)* Monitor	• Heart rate, perceived exertion, talk test, logging • Muscular tightness? Stretch as needed
Sport (sport specific)	Look for opportunities to: • Do a mini-warm-up and skill practice (esp. in inter-mittent sports such as baseball) • Stretch tight muscles • Tend immediately to minor injuries
Resistance Segment Progressive prescription	• Progressive overload & adequate relief (depends on training method) • Incorporate warm-up set(s) (e.g., 60% of training wt.) • Follow weight room safety rules (esp. spotting guidelines)
Specific training method (chapter 7)	• Follow method guidelines as prescribed
Muscle balance	• Check the balance (agonist & antagonist) of the program (i.e., need for specific muscle stretch or strengthening)
Monitor	• Muscular tightness? Stretch as needed • Differentiate between fatigue, soreness, & inflammation • Modify the exercise around minor injuries (incl. avoidance) • Ongoing check for correct breathing, speed of movement, base of support, and alignment such as pelvic stabilization and avoidance of extreme ROM
Cooldown Segment Stretch (emphasis on static stretching)	• Greatest flexibility gains (stage 3)—tissue is warm • Target muscles used, esp. if used eccentrically • Consider PNF if flexibility is a priority
Self check	• CV indicators (e.g., heart rate, depth of breathing, blood pressure) should be well down • Muscles should feel worked but not sore or tight • Any "hot spots" or minor injuries?—if so, ice them • Don't underestimate the therapeutic effect of a relaxing shower

JAM (Joint-Action-Muscle) Charts

Table 10.11 Shoulder Joint Muscles and Their Actions

MUSCLE	FLEXION	EXTENSION	ABDUCTION	ADDUCTION	MEDIAL ROTATION	LATERAL ROTATION	HORIZONTAL ADDUCTION	HORIZONTAL ABDUCTION
Anterior deltoid	PM		AM				PM	
Middle deltoid			PM					PM
Posterior deltoid		PM						PM
Supraspinatus			PM					
Pectoralis* major (cl)	PM						PM	
Pectoralis** major (st)		PM		PM			PM	
Subscapularis					PM		AM	
Infraspinatus						PM		PM
Teres minor						PM		PM
Latissimus dorsi		PM		PM				AM
Teres major		PM		PM	PM			

PM = Prime mover; AM = Assistant mover; * = clavicular   ** = sternal

Highlights

- A simple four-step approach to **anatomical analysis** of exercise looks at the following systems: (1) phases, (2) joints and movements, (3) types of contractions, and (4) muscles.

- The same muscle group is responsible for both the "up" and "down" phases of an exercise. It shortens on the way up with a concentric contraction, and lengthens on the way down with an eccentric contraction.

- A helpful visualization for exercise analysis is that muscles affect movement of the joints that they cross.

- The muscle group causing an action is named by that joint and action (if the contraction is concentric) (e.g., elbow flexors).

- **JAM charts** are quick reference charts indicating Joint, Actions, and Muscles. They facilitate the recall of the specific muscles that are responsible for the joint actions.

- The effectiveness of an exercise should be evaluated from an anatomical, physiological, and biomechanical point of view.

- The following biomechanical principles affect the execution, effectiveness, and safety of an exercise or sport skill: muscle length and force; direction of force application/alignment; biarticular (two-joint) muscle action; composition of forces; and leverage and strength.

- The force produced by a muscle is related to the length at which the muscle is held.

- The total tension or force generated in a shortening muscle receives a contribution from the

Table 10.12 Shoulder Girdle Muscles and Their Actions

MUSCLE	ELEVATION	DEPRESSION	ABDUCTION	ADDUCTION	UPWARD ROTATION	DOWNWARD ROTATION
Pectoralis minor		PM	PM			PM
Serratus anterior			PM		PM	
Trapezius I	PM					
Trapezius II	PM			AM	PM	
Trapezius III				PM		
Trapezius IV		PM		AM	PM	
Levator scapulae	PM					
Rhomboid	PM			PM		PM

Large muscles of the shoulder joint can influence shoulder girdle actions.

Table 10.13 Elbow and Radio-Ulnar Joint Muscles and Their Actions

MUSCLES	FLEXION	EXTENSION	PRONATION	SUPINATION
Biceps brachii	PM			AM
Brachialis	PM			
Brachioradialis	PM		AM	AM
Pronator quadratus			PM	
Pronator teres			AM	
Supinator				PM
Triceps brachii		PM		
Wrist extensors (posterior forearm)		AM		
Wrist flexors (anterior forearm)	AM			

Table 10.14 Hip Joint Muscles and Their Actions

MUSCLES	FLEXION	EXTENSION	ABDUCTION	ADDUCTION	MEDIAL ROTATION	LATERAL ROTATION
Iliacus	PM *					AM
Psoas	PM *					AM
Rectus femoris	PM *					
Pectineus	PM *			PM	AM	
Sartorius	AM		AM			AM
Tensor fasciae latae			PM		AM	
Gluteus medius			PM			
Gluteus minimus			AM		PM	
Gluteus maximus		PM	AM			PM
Semitendinosus		PM				
Semimembranosus		PM				
Biceps femoris (lh)**		PM				
Adductor longus				PM		
Adductor brevis				PM		
Adductor magnus				PM		
Gracilis				PM		
Six lateral rotators						PM

*These muscles may indirectly cause hyperextension of the lower back by tilting the pelvis forward; PM = Prime Mover; AM = Assistant Mover; ** LH = Long head.

passive (stretch) tension of the tendon and the connective tissue in the muscle.

- Force is optimized when a muscle-tendon complex is aligned directly in the plane of movement.

- **Biarticular muscles** cross two joints and affect movement at both joints. They are not long enough to allow a full range of motion at both joints at the same time.

- Two-joint muscles, particularly in the lower extremity, allow a rapid release of stored **elastic energy** if eccentric work is done at one joint while concentric work is done at the other.

- The technique of analysis involving **composition of forces** can be used when there is more than one force (muscle) acting on the joint in the same plane.

Table 10.15 Knee Joint Muscles and Their Actions

MUSCLES	FLEXION	EXTENSION	MEDIAL ROTATION	LATERAL ROTATION
Semitendinosus	PM		PM	
Semimembranosus	PM		PM	
Biceps femoris	PM			PM
Rectus femoris		PM		
Vastus lateralis		PM		
Vastus intermedius		PM		
Vastus medialis		PM		
Sartorius	AM		AM	
Gracilis	AM		AM	
Popliteus			PM	
Gastrocnemius	AM			

Table 10.16 Ankle and Foot Muscles and Their Actions

MUSCLES	DORSIFLEXION	PLANTAR FLEXION	INVERSION	EVERSION
Gastrocnemius		PM		
Soleus		PM		
Tibialis posterior*		AM	PM	
Peroneus longus*		AM		PM
Peroneus brevis		AM		PM
Flex digitorum longus*		AM	AM	
Flex hallucis longus*		AM	AM	
Tibialis anterior	PM		PM	
Peroneus tertius	PM			PM
Ext. digitorum longus	PM			PM
Ext. hallucis longus	AM		AM	

*These muscles also support the arch.

Table 10.17 Spinal Muscles and Their Actions

MUSCLES	FLEXION	EXTENSION	LATERAL FLEXION	ROTATION (SAME SIDE)	ROTATION (OPPOSITE SIDE)
Lumbar and thoracic spines					
Rectus abdominis	PM		AM		
External oblique	PM		PM		PM
Internal oblique	PM		PM	PM	
Psoas	AM	*			
Quadratus lumborum		AM	PM		
Erector spinae group		PM	PM	PM	
Deep posterior group		PM	PM		PM
Cervical spine					
Sternocleidomastoid	PM		PM		PM
Scaleni group	AM		PM		
Erector spinae group		PM	PM	PM	
Deep posterior group		PM	PM		PM

*The psoas may pull the spine into hyperextension without balance from the abdominals, especially if the iliacus tilts the pelvis forward.

PM = Prime Mover; AM = Assistant Mover

- Muscles that act together to create a resultant force are called **synergists**.
- Changing the distance between the joint and the resistance is the most versatile way of adjusting the body's lever systems.
- The **Five-Step Exercise Design** model is as follows:
  1. Identify the component and training method.
  2. Target the muscle(s).
  3. Determine the appropriate joint movements or position.
  4. Design and/or modify.
  5. Finish with a safety check.
- **Program design** provides overall perspective to the exercises and activities. As with exercise design, program design must have safety in mind.

Chapter 11

Personalized Prescription for Muscle Balance and Conditioning

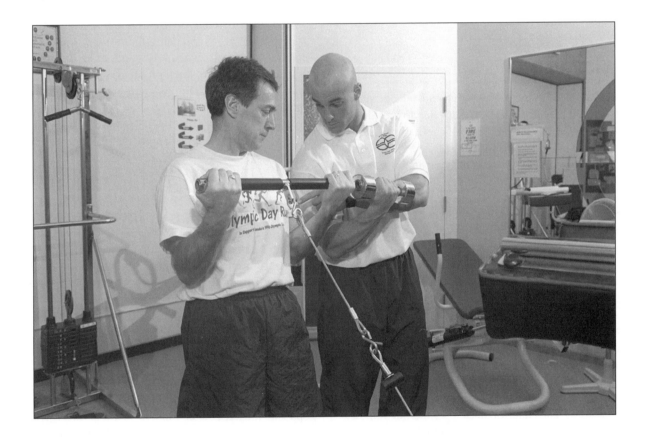

- The Practical Value of the Muscle Balance and Approach

- Tightness vs. Length: Implications of Imbalance

- How to Analyze Muscle Imbalance

- Personalized Prescription

- Prescription Factors (Including Muscular Conditioning Methods)

- Matching Resistance Equipment to the Client

- Program Demonstration and Follow-Up

Muscle balance includes muscle tightness, flexibility, strength, and endurance as these factors work together to provide support and movement. Muscle balance is a holistic approach to muscular fitness.

Although not a new concept, muscle balance is a new approach to solving problems. It gets right to the heart of your clients' needs, whether they are athletes, fitness enthusiasts, or are recovering from injuries.

The Practical Value of the Muscle Balance Approach

A client's problem may not be with a single component of fitness. When we study only one component, we get a very limited view of a person's needs and the potential solutions. As an alternative, this chapter introduces prescription for muscle balance. Based on applied anatomy, muscle balance provides an understanding of the major muscles of the body and the joint actions they produce.

An Example

Your client plays recreational baseball and complains of some discomfort when raising his arm to throw. Because the shoulder felt weak, he had initiated a strengthening program for his shoulders and chest, with no apparent improvement. Your initial observations include a rounded shoulders posture and well-developed chest muscles. This is a classic example of muscle imbalance that needs an integrated approach to prescription. Many of the major upper body muscles internally (medially) rotate the shoulder. Throwing the ball powerfully employs these muscles. The external (lateral) rotators, however, are relatively small. The stronger and tighter internal rotators involved in throwing are overpowering the weaker external rotators. In baseball, the magnitude and speed of this force is significant. The rounded shoulders are the result of this imbalance and a contributing cause of the shoulder pain. The single component approach used by the client to strengthen the shoulder actually increased the imbalance. The anterior muscles (internal rotators) need to be lengthened, and the external rotators (pos-

terior) need improved strength and muscular endurance. This is the muscle balance approach.

Using the Muscle Balance Approach

Muscle balance relates to everyday concerns. A loss of muscle balance may be reported as a pain or a general feeling of fatigue or tightness. During screening, you may recognize muscle imbalance from poor posture or poor alignment (chapter 5). Repetitive activity can use certain muscles excessively and underuse opposing muscles. A client's job may demand a prolonged position or repeated movements.

Imbalance may be the underlying cause of headaches or low back discomfort. Most clients will approach you with relatively vague initial concerns. They may speak of aches and pains, or an area of their body that does not feel particularly good, or an old injury that keeps emerging. Such problems are usually multifaceted: they are not limited to strength, flexibility, or endurance, but may involve strength of one muscle group and flexibility of an opposing muscle group. You need to take an integrated approach to best serve your clients.

Tightness vs. Length: Implications of Imbalance

A joint is a pivot point or a fulcrum whose position is constantly affected by the pull of the muscles around it. A key to structural balance is equal pull by opposing muscles. Joint alignment and posture are affected by these forces. Figure 11.1 shows a loss of structural alignment when a tight muscle overpowers a longer muscle.

Muscle length testing (chapter 5) can determine if the muscle length is limited or excessive. If the muscle is short, it will restrict normal range of motion. Muscles that are too short are usually strong and hold the opposite muscle in a lengthened position. Excessively long muscles are usually weak and allow adaptive

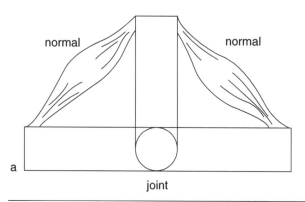 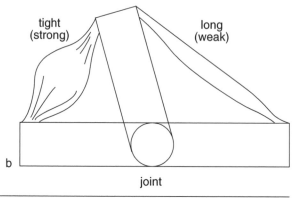

Figure 11.1 Muscle balance: (a) joint in structural balance, (b) joint misaligned—muscle imbalance.

shortening of antagonists (Kendall, McCreary, and Provance 1993).

Muscles can be imbalanced in several ways. They can have unmatched levels of flexibility, strength, contracture, or a combination of the above.

Imbalance Resulting From Tight Muscles

Flexibility is the range of joint motion; *muscle tightness* is the range of muscle length. For muscles that pass over one joint, these two measures are very similar. For muscles that pass over two or more joints (e.g., gastrocnemius, hamstrings, rectus femoris, erector spinae), the range of muscle length will be less than the total range of motion of the joints over which the muscle passes. For example, the knee must be flexed to permit a full range of hip flexion because the hamstrings are too tight if the knee is straight.

Often there is tightness in the most active muscle group, which overpowers the more passive, longer opposing muscle group. For example, you should always examine the lower leg balance of clients who are runners. Without proper stretching, constant use of the calf muscles will cause tightness. Calf stretching will help prevent alterations in the running mechanics and subsequent injuries.

Imbalance Resulting From Weak Muscles

Muscle weakness has many causes. Even in active people, certain muscles are seldom overloaded. If weakness is due to lack of use, prescribe specific exercises for those muscles. If it is due to overwork, fatigue, or strain, prescribe rest—at least in the short term. Relieve the stress before prescribing additional muscular work. With the runner in the previous example, strengthening the anterior shin would prevent problems resulting from unmatched levels of calf strength.

Imbalance Resulting From Muscle Contracture

Commonly known as muscle spasms, muscle contracture also can cause imbalance. Contracture may result from injury, prolonged shortening, or weakness in the opposing muscle. These continued involuntary contractions usually respond to application of heat or cold and progressive static stretching.

Clients who suffer from chronic low back pain are often diagnosed as having "back spasms." Traditional treatments include rest, ultrasound, various forms of heat, and massage. Although these treatments may relieve symptoms, they do not address the cause of the underlying muscle imbalance.

Imbalance Resulting From Combinations of Strength, Length, and Spasm

You need to prescribe both strengthening and stretching for total body balance. A reduction of tightness may be needed before certain strength exercises can be properly performed, or vice versa. Therapeutic exercises to strengthen weak muscles and stretch tight muscles are the most effective and lasting means by which muscle balance is restored or maintained.

Lower back spasms are often caused by weakness of opposing muscles. In the earlier example, the weakness would be in the abdominals around the trunk and the gluteus maximus and hamstrings around the pelvis. Traditional treatment, which is passive, would actually leave the client with *two* weak muscles: the abdominals and the lower back muscles! When pain subsides and the traditional treatment has relieved some inflammation and spasm, you would start your client on abdominal strengthening exercises (with precautions for the back—see chapter 15). As in one of the case studies in chapter 12, tight hip flexors can place added pressure on the lower back.

How to Analyze Muscle Imbalance

Clients are not going to say that they have muscle imbalance. But you can make a correct judgment if you ask the right questions.

The Joint Stress Cycle

Failure to recognize the loss of muscle balance may lead to acute injury, or can be the underlying cause of chronic overuse injury. Figure 11.2 is a generalized model of how muscle imbalance can induce injury.

The *joint stress cycle* works like this: If your client has a muscle imbalance, such as tight anterior chest muscles (including shoulder internal rotators), there will often be a malalignment (e.g., rounded shoulders). These muscles lose flexibility, and the joint becomes progressively more stiff until the muscle is in constant partial contracture; it has progressively less endurance and strength. At this point, a person will alter his mechanics—for example, he may throw a ball with a distinct sidearm style. But the adjustments themselves cause additional problems, creating a vicious circle of pain and misalignment.

How do you know if your client is within this joint stress cycle? *Most* clients, whether active or inactive, are somewhere on the cycle! It is your job to decide where your client is on the cycle.

Where Is Your Client on the Joint Stress Cycle?

Start by obtaining a client history of musculoskeletal problems. Use the questionnaire on page 179 to gather the client's answers and to record your own observations. This information will help you get your client out of the joint stress cycle.

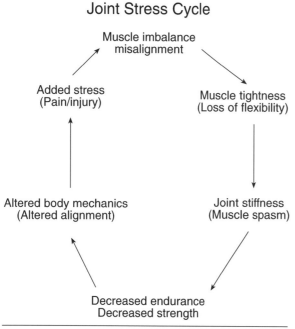

Joint Stress Cycle

Figure 11.2   The joint stress cycle.

Muscle Balance Assessment

Select assessment items only after you and your client together have decided on priorities. Chapter 5 describes and interprets the following assessments:

- Postural assessment (including static/dynamic foot alignment and longitudinal arch assessment)
- Muscle length assessments
  1. **Upper body**: pectoralis minor, pectoralis major (sternal), shoulder internal rotators, shoulder external rotators
  2. **Lower body**: hip flexors, hamstrings, gastrocnemius, tibialis posterior/soleus (ankle range of motion)
- Forward trunk flexion

Because muscle imbalance adds stress to joint support structures and can lead to poor posture and injuries, early detection is important. Faulty body mechanics, as determined by postural screening, should be confirmed by the muscle tests. Postural analysis will indicate which muscle length tests to perform. Interpretation of muscle length tests, in turn, provides a measurable starting point for client-centered prescription.

Personalized Prescription

The goals of training for performance, rehabilitation, or fitness may differ, but muscle balance is important for all. Objectives for muscle balance usually include stretching tight muscles, strengthening weak muscles, reducing spasms, building muscular endurance, or improving posture.

Muscle balance is the cornerstone of the client-centered approach to the integration of fitness components (i.e., muscular endurance, strength, and flexibility). A muscle must be long enough to allow a normal range of motion and be short enough to provide joint stability. Therapeutic exercises to strengthen weak muscles and stretch tight muscles are the means by which muscle balance is restored.

Remember, muscles that are too short are usually strong and hold antagonists in a lengthened and weakened position. Table 11.1 shows (for the lower body) the progression from postural assessment to the identification of probable areas of muscle imbalance, and provides guidelines for exercise design.

Refer to "Opposing Muscles" (page 180) to determine muscle pairs and to aid you in designing exercises based on the muscle testing.

Chapter 12 presents two case studies that illustrate the progression from postural analysis to selection of muscle length test items and on to a personalized prescription.

Prescription Factors (Including Muscular Conditioning Methods)

After assessing (chapter 5) a client's muscle tightness (flexibility) and weakness (strength and endurance), we can personalize the training program by using a simple FITT formula: Frequency, Intensity, Time (duration), and Type (mode).

Muscle Tightness (Flexibility)

Flexibility is an often neglected component of physical fitness. It is not just an improvement of joint range of motion (ROM)—it improves muscle relaxation, muscle

JOINT STRESS QUESTIONNAIRE/OBSERVATIONS

1. Do you currently have any pain? _____

2. If so, in what joint/area do you feel the pain? _____

   In what positions do you feel the pain? _____

   During what movement do you feel the pain? _____

3. Does your occupation or fitness activity overuse one body segment? _____

4. Do you feel you are currently overtraining? _____

5. Do you feel tight anywhere? _____

   Is this felt during/after activity? _____

6. Do you get tired (muscularly) more easily than you used to? _____

7. Have you experienced a loss of strength? _____

8. Are you compensating in your movements to avoid pain or loss of strength? _____

9. Are things getting worse? _____

10. What do you think is causing this "problem"? _____

    How could it be alleviated? _____

Watch your client during a workout. Look for altered body mechanics, stiffness, or postural faults, then answer these questions:

11. Did you notice any altered body mechanics, stiffness, postural faults, etc., when your client walked in? _____

12. Did you notice any altered body mechanics, stiffness, postural faults, etc., when your client was active? _____

13. Can any altered body mechanics, stiffness, postural faults, etc., be accounted for because of acute symptoms from current or chronic injuries? _____

14. Based on the questions and initial observations, where is your client on the joint stress cycle?

    _____

Assessment *(chapter 5)*: Perform a postural screening particularly on the area of greatest concern. Perform muscle length testing to determine whether the muscle length is limited or excessive.

Objectives: Establish specific objectives and a plan for exercise design and monitoring.

Table 11.1 Exercise Design From Muscle Testing: Lower Body

POSTURAL FAULT	MUSCLES IN SHORTENED POSITION	MUSCLES IN LENGTHENED POSITION	EXERCISE IMPLICATION
Flexed knee	Popliteus Hamstrings at knee	Quadriceps Soleus	• Stretch knee flexors • Stretch hip flexors if tight; may contribute
Medially rotated femur (often associated with pronation of foot or toeing in, see Backgrounder below)	Hip medial rotators	Hip lateral flexors	• Stretch hip medial rotators • Strengthen hip lateral rotators
Knock-knee	Tensor fascia lata Lateral knee joint structures	Medial knee joint structures	• Stretch tensor fascia lata
Postural bowlegs	Hip medial rotators Quadriceps Foot everters	Hip lateral rotators, popliteus, tibialis posterior and long toe flexors	• Strengthen hip lateral rotators
Ankle pronation	Peroneals & toe extensors	Tibialis posterior & long toe flexors	• Strengthen inverters and muscles supporting the arch
Ankle supination	Tibialis (esp. posterior)	Peroneals	• Strengthen peroneals

BACKGROUNDER:

Opposing Muscles

Joint (movement direction)

Foot/ankle—

Anteroposterior	Dorsiflexors (tibialis anterior, peroneus tertius)	Plantarflexors (gastrocnemius, soleus)
Lateral and rotary	Tibials (tibialis anterior and posterior)	Peroneals (peroneus longus and brevis)

Knee—

Anteroposterior	Flexors (hamstrings, gastrocnemius)	Extensors (quadriceps)

Hip—

Anteroposterior	Flexors (iliopsoas, rectus femoris, pectineus, tensor fascia latae, sartorius)	Extensors (gluteus maximus, hamstrings)
Lateral	Abductors (gluteus medius, tensor fascia latae)	Adductors (add. longus/brevis/magnus, gracilis, pectineus)
Rotary	Internal rotators (gluteus minimus, tensor fascia latae)	External rotators (gluteus maximus, six external rotators)

Trunk—

Anteroposterior	Flexors (rectus abdominis, external oblique)	Extensors (erector spinae, deep posterior spinal group)
Lateral	Lateral flexors—left oppose right (quadratus lumborum, external and internal oblique, erector spinae group)	Same
Rotary	Rotators to the same side (internal oblique, erector spinae group)	Rotators to the opposite side (external oblique, deep posterior group)

Pelvis—

Anteroposterior	Forward tilt (hip flexors, trunk extensors)	Backward tilt (trunk flexors, hip extensors)
Lateral	(Gluteus medius and minimus)	(Quadratus lumborum, external oblique)

Shoulder joint—

Anteroposterior	Flexors and horizontal adductors (anterior deltoid, pectoralis major)	Extensors and horizontal abductors (posterior deltoid, latissiums dorsi, teres major)
Lateral	Abductors (deltoids, supraspinatus)	Adductors (latissimus dorsi, teres major, pectoralis major)
Rotary	Internal rotators (subscapularis, teres major)	External rotators (infraspinatus, teres minor)

Shoulder girdle—

Vertical	Elevators (trapezius 1 & 2, levator scapula, rhomboids)	Depressors (trapezius 4, pectoralis minor)
Lateral	Abductors (serratus anterior, pectoralis minor)	Adductors (trapezius 2, 3, & 4, rhomboids)
Rotary	Lateral rotators (trapezius 2 & 4, serratus anterior)	Medial rotators (pectoralis minor, rhomboids)

Elbow—

Anteroposterior	Flexors (biceps brachii, brachialis, brachioradialis)	Extensors (triceps brachii, anconeus)

Radio-ulnar—

Rotary	Pronators (pronator quadratus, pronator teres, brachioradialis)	Supinators (supinator, brachioradialis, biceps brachii)

Wrist—

Anteroposterior	Wrist flexors	Wrist extensors
Lateral	Abductors (radial side)	Adductors (ulnar side)

balance, and preparation for activity. Lack of flexibility is often the cause of musculoskeletal injuries, low back pain, and headaches.

The effectiveness of a stretch is related to the behavior of the connective tissue and muscle when under stress. Limitation to ROM is due 47% to joint structure, 41% to muscle fascia, and 10% to tendons (Brooks 1993).

Factors in Stretching Prescription Effectiveness

In prescribing any exercise for your client, consider the following factors that directly affect the quality of stretch:

- Duration of the applied force (how long to hold a stretch)

- Intensity of the applied force (how hard to push a stretch)
- Temperature of the tissue (related to pre-stretch warm-up)
- Degree of relaxation of the muscle (amount of tension in a muscle)
- Type of applied force (e.g., ballistic, static, PNF)
- Alignment of muscle fibers to be stretched (direction of pull on the muscle)

Other prescription factors you should considered in your client's program design are

- number of exercises (within the flexibility program),
- number of repetitions (number of times the same stretch is performed),
- other activities within the workout (aerobic, strengthening, sports, etc.), and
- frequency of workouts (how often the flexibility program is done per week).

Controlling the Prescription Factors

By prudent selection and control of the prescription factors, you can increase the quality of your client's stretches.

Duration, Force, and Temperature

A stretch of relatively long duration and low force at elevated tissue temperatures will provide an effective permanent stretch (*plastic deformation*) (Sapega et al. 1981). If the duration of stretch is short, the intensity of force is high, and the tissue temperature is normal or cold, the muscle-tendon structure will return quickly to its original length (*elastic deformation*) and much of the benefit of the stretch is lost. Warming up for stretching has replaced the notion of stretching to warm up. If your client has significant tightness, he will benefit from a prewarmed, long, static stretch routine done frequently and without the ballistic effect of other activities.

Relaxation

Attempting to stretch muscles in spasm may cause injury. Connective tissue can be stretched effectively only if the muscle is relaxed. Strain is most often felt around the tendon of the muscle if it has tension. Heat, light aerobics, loosening, or ROM exercises can provide some relaxation, particularly if your client has come directly from an environment of repeated movements or static posture, such as sitting at a computer terminal. The mode of training can also affect the state of relaxation. For example, PNF (Propriocep-

tive Neuromuscular Facilitation) involves a phase of isometrically contracting the muscle to be stretched. The proprioceptor is sensitive to the isometric tension, producing a reflex inhibition of the muscle, less resistance to stretch, less discomfort, and a greater range of motion. But remember—if the muscle-tendon structure is inflamed, rest may be the best prescription.

If the alignment of the muscle-tendon structure is directly in the line of the stretch (or movement), the tensile stretch (or force application) is optimized. Pay special attention to alignment detail when you demonstrate the program to your client.

Program Parameters

A well-rounded flexibility program, or conditioning program, should include at least one exercise for each major muscle group. When postural screening and muscle length testing will led to greater emphasis on (or avoidance of) certain muscle groups, you can provide the appropriate overload in the form of additional/ isolation stretches, more repetitions, longer duration, more frequent sessions, or a change of stretching technique. Heyward (1998) suggests two to six repetitions of each exercise for a minimum of three days a week, with the duration of stretch from 10 to 60 seconds.

Your prescription should include the stretch specific to the area of tightness, the proper positioning and execution of the stretch, and the method of stretching best suited to your client.

Flexibility Training Methods

Hartley-O'Brien (1980) discusses two approaches to improving flexibility: decreasing the resistance to the stretch, and increasing the strength of the opposing muscle. Decreasing resistance to the stretch can be accomplished by either increasing the connective tissue length or attaining a greater degree of relaxation in the target muscle. Table 11.2 describes the appropriate stretching techniques for each approach.

You must have thorough knowledge of your clients before you can determine the best approach for their situation. A client who has a competitive sport once or twice a week probably has tight muscle-tendon structures, whereas a previously inactive client may lack the strength of opposing muscles to pull the joint through a larger range of motion. If your client's objective is to attain a ROM that allows an ease of daily function or improved posture, static stretching may be the best training method.

Most types of flexibility training fall into three categories: static, dynamic (ballistic), and proprioceptive neuromuscular facilitation (PNF).

Table 11.2   Stretching Techniques

APPROACH	TECHNIQUE

(1) Decrease resistance to the stretch
   a) Lengthen connective tissue
 	
   b) Relax stretch reflex of targeted muscle
	a) Warm-up (include light aerobics), massage, loosening, dynamic stretching
	b) Static stretch with brief intermittent isometric contractions, relaxation techniques

(2) Increase strength of opposing muscles a) Resistance training of opposing muscles (muscle balance)	a) Isolation of specific muscle(s) and isometric or concentric contractions
(3) Combined approach	

Active Loosening

Relaxation, or the absence of muscular tension, must exist before a stretch is attempted. Reduced tension can assist stretching out connective tissues. ***Active loosening*** can relieve muscle tension and promote relaxation (Kuprian 1982). Active loosening exercises include rhythmic swinging of the limbs, active shaking of the limbs, or rotating the torso or limbs.

Many athletes know the effects of shaking the extremities in order to loosen particular muscles. A sprinter never gets into the starting blocks without thoroughly loosening her legs and arms. She shakes her legs while in a slight straddle position, as if she were trying to throw her legs away. She shakes her arms while standing with the upper body slightly inclined and the arms hanging loosely. Loosening exercises facilitate more rapid recovery from stress through a facilitated blood flow. Failure to loosen up leads to an early loss of strength, slowing of movements, and fatigue (Eitner 1982).

Other examples of effective loosening exercises include

- lifting the shoulders and allowing them to fall;
- lying on the upper back, supporting the waist with the hands, shaking the legs in the air;
- standing, twisting trunk to the left and right (avoid excessive momentum, and avoid if any history of back problems);
- standing, leaning against wall with outstretched arms, swinging each leg back and forth;

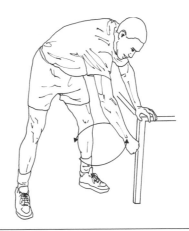

Figure 11.3   Active loosening.

- lying supine with knees bent, shaking the legs (especially calves and hamstrings);
- standing, one arm leaning on a table, letting other arm swing in a circle by rocking body weight in a circular pattern (figure 11.3).

Static Stretching

Static stretching involves controlled elongation of an antagonistic muscle by placing it in a maximal position of stretch and holding it. The golgi tendon organs (GTOs) in the muscle's tendon are sensitive to the tension of a static stretch. The GTO's signal to relax overrides the muscle spindles' signal to contract. The muscle spindles need a few seconds to adapt to the lengthened position before they decrease their discharge. The reflex contraction of the muscle to be stretched lessens, and the muscle is more relaxed and prepared to stretch. Recommendations for the optimal time for holding the stretch range from as short as 3 seconds to as long as 60 seconds (Knott and Voss 1985). Assuming muscle temperature is elevated, Sapega et al. (1991) suggest a 30 second duration. If the stretch time is reduced to 15 seconds, 2-4 repetitions should be completed. Static stretching can be either active or passive.

Active Static Stretching

Active static stretching is accomplished by moving the agonist muscle to the end of its ROM, and holding it in that position with an isometric contraction of the agonist muscles—without other aid. For example, to stretch the anterior chest and pectoralis minor muscles (figure 11.4), contract the posterior shoulder girdle and shoulder joint muscles. This type of stretch is especially useful for people whose ROM is limited by the strength of the agonist muscles. You will recognize these clients by noting a large difference between their active ROM and an assisted (passive) ROM. Active static stretching may also be effective after strength training or heavy eccentric work when a forced stretch may elongate the fibers excessively.

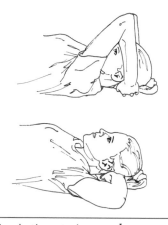

Figure 11.4 Active static stretch.

Passive Static Stretching

In *passive static stretching*, an outside agent applies the force. This form of stretching is effective when the ROM is limited by soft tissue extendibility. Its effect on warmed muscle is to lengthen the connective tissues passively. The outside force may be provided by pressure or held traction, external leverage, or support of a partner.

■ *Pressure or held traction.* This technique is used in a side-lying quadriceps stretch where the heel is pulled towards the buttock (figure 11.5). The stretch should be gently and gradually increased.

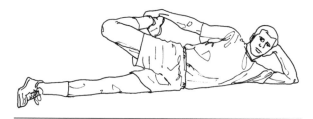

Figure 11.5 Passive static stretch (pressure / traction).

■ *External leverage.* This can be seen in figure 11.6 in which the shoulder internal rotators are elongated by the position of leverage in the doorway.

■ *Support of a partner.* The partner assists the stretch beyond an active ROM but must remain in close communication with the client and carefully control the stretch intensity. Figure 11.7 shows a partner hamstring stretch.

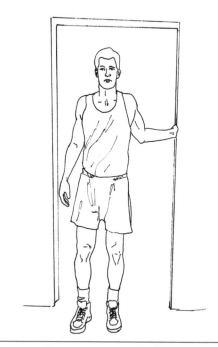

Figure 11.6 Passive static stretch (external leverage).

Dynamic Stretching

Active, bouncing movements initiated by contraction of the agonist muscle produce a quick stretch of the antagonist muscle. If uncontrolled momentum becomes a factor in the stretch, it is referred to as a ballistic stretch. Ballistic stretching can cause overstretching, resulting in microtears within the musculotendinous unit. Connective tissue has a safe elastic range; but if stress exceeds a yield point, small tears will occur. Repetition of such microtrauma can cause inflammation (chapter 13). The tearing can also lead to

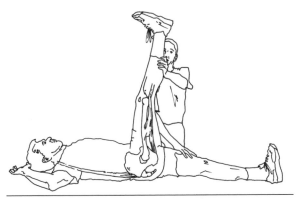

Figure 11.7 Passive static stretch (support of a partner).

formation of scar tissue, with a gradual loss of elasticity. The risk of injury is higher with this type of stretching than with others, and is dependent upon the intensity and velocity of the stretch, and the temperature of the muscle (Alter 1996).

However, many sports require dynamic/ballistic movements. Since ballistic stretching is functional and does increase ROM (Hartley-O'Brien 1980), it is reasonable to integrate it into athletic training programs as long as the ballistic stretches correspond to actions required by the sport. If you prescribe this type of stretching for a client, target the specific muscle to be stretched, establish safe alignment, and avoid excessive momentum. Dynamic stretching should follow static stretching, and only after the body temperature is sufficiently warm. Dynamic stretching should consist of rhythmic actions similar to those in the client's sport. Start with small movements and gradually increase the range of motion.

Proprioceptive Neuromuscular Facilitation (PNF)

PNF stretching invokes neurological responses that facilitate stretching. It works by generating a force/tension (generally an isometric muscle contraction) in the muscle that stimulates the golgi tendon organs, which then inhibit the muscle spindles and relax the muscle. Prior to the stretch, have your client hold an isometric contraction against a resistance at the end of the limb's ROM for about 6-10 seconds. The static stretch that follows also stimulates the golgi tendon organs to further relax the muscle to be stretched. Your client should repeat the sequence several times, to allow for a greater reflex inhibition and thus a greater stretch.

PNF Methods

McAtee (1993) summarized the common PNF procedures as follows:

- *Hold-relax (HR)* employs an isometric contraction of the antagonist at the limit of the initial ROM, followed by a period of relaxation. Then the limb actively moves further in the same direction against minimal resistance through the new ROM to the new point of limitation. The strong isometric contraction is thought to recruit more muscle fibers and then fire the inverse stretch reflex, relaxing the target muscle and permitting further stretch (Osternig et al. 1990). HR is effective when ROM has decreased because of muscle tightness on one side of a joint.

- *Contract-relax (CR)* is similar to HR. You provide resistance as the client attempts to move the limb to the initial limit of the ROM of the target muscle. Since your resistance prevents the limb from moving, his muscles contract isometrically. Then your client relaxes, and you again move the limb passively beyond the initial limit. CR is preferred to HR when ROM is good and when motion is pain-free.

- *Contract-relax, antagonist-contract (CRAC)* is similar to CR, except that after the isometric contraction, the client actively moves the limb into the new ROM. This active contraction of the antagonist is thought to relax the target muscle (called reciprocal inhibition), thereby allowing a better stretch (Voss, Ionta, and Myers 1985).

- *Manual Isometric Stretch* is a modification of a PNF, utilizing the relaxed state of the muscle immediately following an isometric contraction. Have your client manually resist the contraction of a muscle in the mid-range of movement for 6-15 seconds, then move the muscle into a passive static stretch, allowing enough time for connective tissue elongation and neuromuscular relaxation. The following two exercises may be performed as manual isometric stretches of the shoulder.

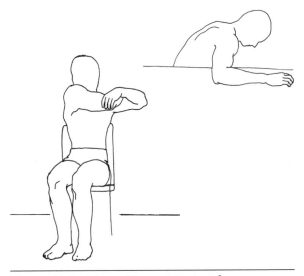

Figure 11.8 Manual isometric stretches.

Advantages and Client Suitability of PNF Stretching

PNF is considered an advanced method of stretching, both for the client and for exercise specialists, who have varying levels of skill in its application. It has a number of advantages and is well suited for certain clients:

- Specific benefits are associated with the PNF method used (see PNF Methods).
- ROM gains, especially passive mobility, have been equal to or greater than with other stretching methods.
- It produces strength, muscle balance, and joint stability.
- Increased relaxation of the muscle allows greater stretch of the connective tissue.
- Because it generally requires a partner, it gives you an opportunity to increase rapport with your client.
- It can be used to stretch any muscle in the body.
- It provides an excellent opportunity to motivate your client.
- It is popular with therapists because it approximates "natural" movements.
- PNF can be adapted to be done without a partner.

Despite all these pluses, use PNF with caution. Because it may produce excessive tissue stretch, PNF stretching should be performed only with the supervision of a knowledgeable and experienced exercise specialist.

Muscle Weakness

Excessively long muscles usually permit an excessive range of motion. Treat this instability and weakness with specific therapeutic exercises.

Every muscle is a prime mover (agonist) in a specific action, and each muscle has an opposing muscle (antagonist) (see Backgrounder, page 180). Maintaining this simple balance is the objective of resistance training whether your client is primarily concerned with fitness, health, or performance. The client's needs dictate the design detail.

Factors in Muscle Conditioning Prescriptions

Consider the following prescription factors for any conditioning exercises you prescribe:

- The broad goal (fitness, health, or performance)
- The muscular component (strength, endurance, power, hypertrophy)
- The muscle groups to be trained for muscle balance or specific needs (e.g., sports)

- The design/selection of specific exercises to satisfy the above factors
- The training method
- The selection of equipment (see pages 193-198)
- The order of the exercises
- The starting loads for each exercise
- The training volume (i.e., load × sets × reps) and rest periods
- The guidelines for progressive overload

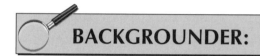

BACKGROUNDER:

Basic Facts About Strength Training

- **Strength** is the maximum force generated during muscle contractions.
- Strength can be exerted without joint movement (isometric) or with joint movement (isotonic).
- **Power** is the ability to exert strength quickly.
- **Muscular endurance** is the ability to apply force repeatedly or sustain a contraction for a period of time.
- **Muscle hypertrophy** refers to an increase in muscle size.
- A **repetition** is the completion of a designated movement through a full range of motion. A **set** is a specified number of repetitions attempted consecutively. **Intensity** is the power output of an exercise and is dependent upon the resistance and the speed of the movement.
- Low-repetition, high-resistance weight training favors strength and hypertrophy gains.
- Low-resistance, high-repetition training favors muscular endurance gains and possibly some aerobic gains if rest periods are brief.
- High speed specific tasks can enhance power outputs.
- With a **concentric contraction**, the muscle shortens as it exerts a force to overcome a resistance. With an **eccentric contraction**, the muscle lengthens as it exerts a force.
- A **closed kinetic chain** exercise involves the foot or hand being in contact with the ground or some other surface. The ankle, knee, and hip joints form the kinetic chain for the lower extremity. Here the forces begin at the ground and work their way up through each joint.

Controlling the Prescription Factors

To be genuinely client-centered, you must control each prescription factor to meet specific client needs.

Progressive Overload

The universal principle of conditioning is *progressive overload*, that is, a periodic increase in workload that increasingly overloads the muscle group. The correct amount of overload depends on your client's objectives and training level. The challenge is to shape the overload to suit your client by manipulating the prescription factors according to the principle of specificity—namely, that gains in muscular fitness are specific to the muscle group, training method, and exercise volume.

Components, Training Methods, and Equipment

Chapters 5 and 6 discuss components of muscular fitness. Training methods (e.g., simple sets, pyramid, circuit) and equipment (e.g., constant, variable, or accommodating resistance) are covered later in this chapter.

Muscle Groups, Specific Exercises, and Order

Arrange your selection of muscle groups, specific exercises, and order so that successive exercises do not involve the same muscle group. Knowing the purpose and benefit of each exercise can help avoid overworking a particular body area (chapter 10). Large-muscle, multiple-joint exercises generally should precede small-muscle, single-joint, isolation exercises. This will avoid early fatigue and poor performance later in the workout. Have your client work on areas of weakness or imbalance while he is still fresh. For the large muscle exercises, have him do a warm-up set with less weight. Performing one exercise for each muscle group promotes a balanced development and helps prevent overuse injuries. For example, a frequent cause of shoulder rotator cuff injury is overtraining of the upper chest muscles and undertraining of the upper back and posterior shoulder muscles.

Exercise Volume

Exercise volume is one of the most important prescription factors. The intensity or load must be heavy enough to cause temporary discomfort and momentary muscle fatigue. For combined strength-endurance improvements, the resistance should be about 75% of the maximum load your client is able to lift. Baechle (1994) indicates that most people can complete 8-12 repetitions with about 75% load. If your client is a beginner or is training at high intensity, one or two sets are sufficient to produce excellent benefits. Prescribe a frequency of three days per week for strength development. At least two days per week are necessary for maintenance. Detraining will occur when frequency is less than one day per week.

Muscular Conditioning Methods

Your selection of muscular conditioning methods is important in shaping the prescription to meet your client's needs, time constraints, experience, motivation, and level of condition. Your design can become quite distinctive when you manipulate prescription factors within a system.

Simple Set System

The simple set system consists of one or more sets of each exercise. It usually demands 8-12 repetitions with a weight that elicits a point of momentary failure. A simple set system can be performed at any resistance, for any number of repetitions or sets, to match the goals of the client. This system is very versatile, allowing the beginner and advanced client enough variation to suit their needs.

Pyramid System

The pyramid system begins by working a specific muscle group using a relatively light weight so that about 10-12 repetitions can be performed. After each set the weight is increased so that fewer and fewer repetitions can be done, until only one or two repetitions can be performed. The resistance is then progressively decreased each set, and the session ends with a set of 10-12 repetitions (see example below). The system can be modified to do any number of reps for the desired number of sets and is favored by many body builders for its potential hypertrophy gains. The first half of the pyramid is called the *light-to-heavy system*. The reverse *heavy-to-light system* is preferred over the former in producing strength gains (Fleck and Kraemer 1987). For example:

SETS	REPS	WEIGHT
1	10	
1	8	
1	6	
1	4	
1	1-2	
1	4	
1	6	
1	8	
1	10	

Superset System

The superset system uses several sets of two exercises performed one after the other with little or no rest. The two exercises are for the same body part but are for antagonistic muscles. For example, you might follow a bench press with rowing exercise, arm curls with triceps extensions, or leg curls with leg extensions. Have your client rest for one or two minutes after both exercises are complete, then complete the remaining two to five sets. The repetitions are usually limited to 8-10. Supersets can lead to significant increases in strength (Riley 1982); and, if your client is fit and motivated, they can reduce his workout time by letting him pack more exercises into a given training session.

A variation of the superset system uses one set of several exercises for the same muscle group performed one after another with little rest. For example, this may include bench press, military press, and incline flies; or one set of lat (latissimus dorsi) pull-down, seated rowing, and bent-over rowing. This variation is also effective in improving muscular strength and hypertrophy.

Table 11.3 prescribes a sample superset program. Do the first set of exercise 1(a), followed immediately by the first set of exercise 1(b). Rest one to two minutes, the go on to second sets of 1(a), 1(b). Follow this format for the prescribed number of sets and reps.

Tri-Set System

A tri-set is a group of three exercises for the same body part, one done after another with little or no rest between exercises or sets. Use tri-sets to work three different muscle groups, to work the same muscle from three different angles, or to work the same area of the muscle (from the same angle). Three sets of each exercise are usually performed. Fleck and Kraemer (1987) report that tri-sets are good systems to increase local muscular endurance. A tri-set might include lateral raises, arm curls, and triceps extensions all working the upper arms and shoulder area

Table 11.3   Superset Program

EXERCISES	REPS (SETS)	EXERCISES	REPS (SETS)
1(a) Leg extensions (quadriceps)	10-8-6 (3)	4(a) Bench press (pectoralis major)	10-8-6 (3)
1(b) Leg flexions (hamstrings)	10-8-6 (3)	4(b) Lat pull-down (latissimus dorsi)	10-8-6 (3)
2(a) Resisted hip abduction (hip abductors)	10-8/leg (2)	5(a) Dumbbell flies (anterior deltoid & pectoralis major)	10-8 (2)
2(b) Resisted hip adduction (hip adductors)	10-8/leg (2)	5(b) Reverse flies (posterior deltoid & latissimus dorsi)	15-15 (2)
3(a) Standing toe raise— calf machine (gastrocnemius)	8 to 12 (1)	6(a) Standing barbell curl (biceps)	10-8 (2)
3(b) Seated barbell toe raise (soleus)	15 to 20 (1)	6(b) Dips (triceps)	up to 15 (2)

but distinctly different muscles. A tri-set for the same muscle group (different angles) may comprise decline flies, bench presses, and incline flies.

Plyometrics

While weight training can produce gains in strength, the speed of movement is limited. Since power combines strength and speed, many athletes need to train to decrease the amount of time it takes to produce muscular force. A form of training that combines speed of movement with strength is plyometrics.

Principles of Plyometrics

Plyometric training comprises rapid eccentric lengthening of a muscle followed immediately by rapid concentric contraction of that muscle to produce a forceful explosive movement. The increase in explosive power comes in part from the storage of elastic energy within the pre-stretched connective tissue tendon. The concentric contraction can be magnified only if the preceding eccentric contraction is of a short range, and is performed quickly and without delay (Voight and Tippett 1994). Plyometrics emphasizes this speed of the eccentric phase and control in dynamic movements.

Examples of plyometric exercises for the lower extremity include hops, bounds, and depth jumping. In depth jumping, your client jumps to the ground from a specified height and then quickly jumps again as soon as she makes ground contact. For the upper extremity, you can prescribe medicine balls or other weighted equipment.

A Sample Plyometric Circuit

One benefit of plyometric training is that it can be organized into circuits. The following program (figure 11.a) describes a high volume circuit designed to improve both vertical and linear power patterns (Chu 1992).

Guidelines for Using Plyometrics

Plyometrics is a very valuable tool, but you must use it judiciously according to the tolerance levels of your clients. Take care to demonstrate all movements, provide adequate recovery, avoid overtraining, and match the activity to your client's abilities. The following guidelines will help you avoid injuries and maximize your clients' improvement:

- An extended warm-up and gradual buildup should precede each workout. Plyometrics involves a lot of eccentric (i.e., ballistic) actions, and the muscles must be stretched and exposed to light eccentric movements in the warm-up.

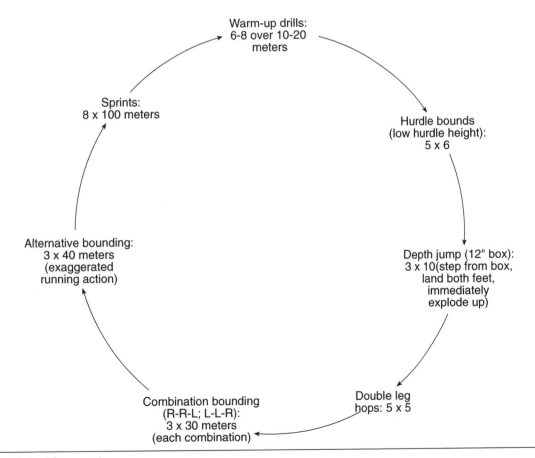

Figure 11.9 Plyometrics program.

- The greater the intensity, the longer the recovery. This guideline applies both between sets during the workout and between workouts.

- Proper technique and explosive intensity are important. Stop the exercise if your client's form begins to fail.

- Train specific movement patterns for specific activities.

- You can modify prescription factors for progressive overloads by increasing the number of exercises; increasing the number of repetitions and/or sets; or decreasing the rest periods between sets. Discourage use of ankle or wrist weights, as they may cause excessive momentum.

- Careful observation, monitoring, and testing of your client will provide important feedback for motivation and progression.

- Frequency should be no more than three times per week in the preseason (higher volume), and less during the season (higher intensity).

- Plyometrics at the end of a workout should be shorter and less stressful that at the beginning, as your client is partially fatigued.

Circuit Weight Training System

Chapter 7 described circuit training under Aerobic Training Methods (page 101). Circuit weight training consists of a series of resistance exercises in a multiple station system: approximately 10-15 repetitions of each exercise, at a resistance of 40%-60% of maximum (RM), with 15-30 seconds rest between exercises (Fleck and Kraemer 1987). Design the circuit to meet specific goals or use available equipment. This is a very time-efficient method of developing strength and endurance (with some aerobic benefits). Heyward (1998) presents a sample circuit weight training program in figure 11.10.

Systems That Are Extended Forms of Other Systems

Some systems of resistance training are extensions of other systems or can be employed within an existing system. They allow further manipulation of the prescription factors that allow individual needs to be addressed. The following are examples of such extensions.

Split Routine System

Developing hypertrophy is a time-consuming process for body builders. Not all body parts can be covered in

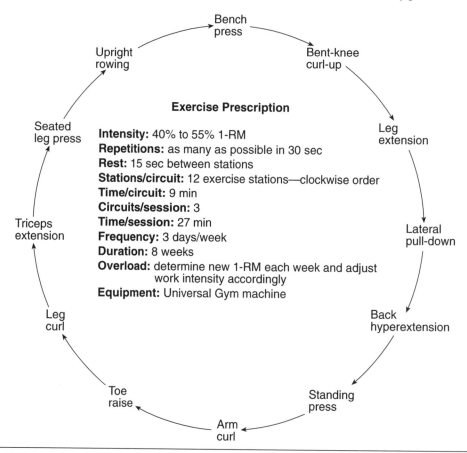

Exercise Prescription

Intensity: 40% to 55% 1-RM
Repetitions: as many as possible in 30 sec
Rest: 15 sec between stations
Stations/circuit: 12 exercise stations—clockwise order
Time/circuit: 9 min
Circuits/session: 3
Time/session: 27 min
Frequency: 3 days/week
Duration: 8 weeks
Overload: determine new 1-RM each week and adjust work intensity accordingly
Equipment: Universal Gym machine

Figure 11.10   Circuit weight training.
Reprinted, by permission, from V. Heyward, 1991, 1998, *Advanced Fitness Assessment and Exercise Prescription*, 2nd ed., Champaign, IL: Human Kinetics, 124.

one training session. The split routine system trains various body parts on alternate days—arms, legs, and abdomen on three days per week, for example, and chest, shoulders, and back on alternate days. Variations in this example may allow a reduction of training days. Calder et al. (1994) found that split routines (four sessions/week) produced similar results to whole routines (two sessions/week) over five months of training. The increased time for recovery helps reduce overuse injuries and overtraining and allows for a more intense training level.

Exhaustion Set System

Momentary failure is the point at which another full repetition is not possible—that is, the set has been done to exhaustion. You can incorporate sets to exhaustion into almost any training system. This system appears to recruit a large number of motor units and to produce significant strength gains (Baechle 1994). An added "burn" can be achieved by performing five or six partial repetitions after exhaustion.

The weight used to reach momentary failure is called a repetition maximum (RM). If eight repetitions of 150 lb are done to exhaustion, the 8 RM is 150 pounds. If you have assessed your client's 1 RM (chapter 5), the following chart can estimate a prescription for intensity (% of 1 RM) and number of repetitions that will elicit momentary failure (Fleck and Kraemer 1987):

> 60% 1 RM = 15 to 20 RM (i.e., 15 to 20 repetitions to exhaustion at 60% 1RM)
> 65% 1 RM = 14 RM
> 70% 1 RM = 12 RM
> 75% 1 RM = 10 RM
> 80% 1 RM = 8 RM
> 85% 1 RM = 6 RM
> 90% 1 RM = 4 RM
> 95% 1 RM = 2 RM
> 100% 1 RM = 1 RM

Forced Repetition System

The forced repetition system allows you to work very closely with your client. After a set to exhaustion, help your client determine just the amount of weight that will permit her to do three or four additional repetitions. By demanding stimulation from a partially fatigued muscle, this approach is well-suited to clients who want increased strength and muscular endurance.

The Prescription Factors for Resistance Training chart (table 11.4), although only a guideline, shows how manipulation of prescription factors can affect the specificity of training effects.

For example, a client interested in general conditioning may have a prescription outline as follows:

- Goal: Fitness, general conditioning
- Component: Strength-endurance
- Muscle groups: All major muscle groups (10-12)
- Specific exercises: Ten to twelve basic exercises for all major muscle groups, plus selected exercises for areas of weakness or imbalance
- Training method: Simple sets (i.e., set-rest-set)
- Equipment: Stack weights and free weights
- Order: Complete large muscle, multi-joint exercises (all sets) before small muscle, single-joint exercises; do a lighter warm-up set for each large muscle exercise.
- Starting Loads: Seventy-five percent of maximum
- Training Volume: Two sets; 8-10 repetitions; 60-90 seconds rest between sets; slow-moderate speed; 3 days/week.
- Progressive Overload: Increase repetitions up to 15; then increase load by 10% while reducing reps to 8; reassess after 6-8 weeks.

The American College of Sports Medicine (1990) has recommended guidelines for the development of muscular fitness in healthy adults. They include strength training of a moderate intensity, sufficient to develop and maintain a healthy level of fat-free weight (FFW). As a minimum, they recommend one set of 8-12 repetitions of 8-10 exercises that condition the major muscle groups, at least two days per week. Muscular strength and endurance are the most common component goals for fitness and health programs. Further examples and case studies are found in chapter 12.

Matching Resistance Equipment to the Client

Prescription for resistance training employs

- a type of resistance or method of loading;
- ergonomics—the interface between client and machine; and,
- the selection of a training method with assignment of personalized prescription factors.

We have already established that decisions about exercises selected, the method of training, and factors such as sets, reps, rest, and intensity must be client-centered. We must also make some important decisions—in consultation with our clients—about the best method

Table 11.4 Prescription Factors for Resistance Training

PRESCRIPTION FACTOR	STRENGTH	STRENGTH-ENDURANCE	MUSCULAR ENDURANCE
Time (duration of 1 set)	< 10 seconds	10-30 seconds	30-60+ seconds
Energy source	98% ATP-PC	50% ATP-PC 50% LA	LA & O2
Intensity/load	90-100% max. (*)	75-90% max. (*)	50-75% max. (*)
Repetitions	1-5 (*)	5-15 (*)	> 15 (*)
Sets	3-6 (**)	2-5 (**)	1-3 (**)
Rest (between sets)	1-3 minutes (*)	15-90 seconds (*)	0-60 seconds (*)
Rate (speed)	Slow, controlled	Slow-moderate	Moderate
Method of progression	Load	Reps then load	Reps or sets

(*) Fine-tune within this range for your client.
(**) Start at lower end of range and work up.

of resistance, the type of equipment, and the interface of that equipment with the client (ergonomics).

Which Is the Best Workout: Free Weights or Machines?

Most fitness centers have several types of machines along with free weights and benches. Moreover, resistance equipment is increasingly popular in the home market. The best workout for your client will be with the equipment that meets his needs. Table 11.5 presents the advantages and disadvantages of free weights and machines.

Types of Resistance

Any type of resistance will affect muscle conditioning. This section examines the advantages and client suitability of specific types of resistance: body weight, free weight, constant resistance, variable resistance, hydraulics and pneumatics, electronics, isokinetics, and others.

Gravity

Gravity is an ever-present force: it's constant, and it's free. What a wonderful asset for an exercise designer! We need only remember that it works in only one direction—down.

Body Weight

Body weight remains the most versatile source of overload and is truly "client-centered"! It represents a load that often reflects the real demands placed on the body. Lifting your body weight or a segment of your body demands a concentric contraction of the muscles (i.e., shortening of the muscle under tension). The lowering action involves an eccentric contraction of the same muscles (i.e., lengthening of the muscle under tension). Examples include chins, dips, curl-ups, aerobic floor exercises, calisthenics, plyometrics, etc. The Gravitron is a specialized piece of equipment that uses a percentage of your body weight to do exercises such as chins and dips. Body weight resistance is well-suited to clients recovering from an injury (chapter 14).

Free Weight

Dumbbells and barbells are probably the oldest and most easily understood forms of resistance. Bars come in five-, six-, and seven-foot (Olympic) lengths, and are straight, cambered, or angled for arm curl work (EZ Curl). A stable adjustable-incline bench allows a large range of exercises and joint angles. Free weights may be the obvious choice for the client who has no access to a larger facility, has a limited budget, and limited space at home. Free weights are also the method of choice for many body builders interested in muscle

Table 11.5 Advantages and Disadvantages of Free Weights and Machines

ADVANTAGES	DISADVANTAGES
Free Weights • Can be tailored to specific demands of individual client; permit unlimited variety of exercises • Supporting muscles also used; should assist with muscle balance • May be more effective in increasing muscle mass (O'Hagan et al., 1995)	• Safety is a consideration for the novice (i.e., proper execution and slippage) • A spotter is needed with heavier weights • There is a learning curve where technique may initially impair performance
Machines • Isolation of a single large muscle group • Greater safety since they guide the movement; remove the concern for balance; more difficult to cheat • Easier to use; appropriate for beginners; guide clients through full range of motion • Ease of changing loads (e.g., pin placement) • Move quickly from one exercise to another; well-suited for circuit training • Certain machines may be able to adjust resistance to suit the force output; control speed of movement; dictate type of muscle contraction; simulate a sport skill; or provide electronic feedback	• Restricted to predetermined movement patterns (i.e., less versatile) • Restricted to predetermined joint angles • Cost and space restrict home use • Loss of balance of movement and supportive muscle action • Do not teach coordinated power movements often needed for sports • Client fit. Many machines (esp. home models) have insufficient adjustments to comfortably and safely fit a small or large client

isolation and hypertrophy. They lend themselves to single-joint exercises such as the biceps curl, and to multi-joint exercises such as a squat. Free weights are categorized as constant resistance (i.e., weight does not change through the range of motion). As with calisthenics, the muscles work concentrically when lifting and eccentrically when lowering. Safety is a consideration for the novice, such as when the client hits a sticking point with no spotter. Proper instruction and supervision are critical (see spotting guidelines later this chapter).

Machine—Constant Resistance

Constant resistance machines generally duplicate free weight exercises and offer both the concentric and eccentric contractions. Although the machine may alter the direction of motion required, the resistance is still the movement of weight against gravity. One popular machine is the "multi-gym," with stations for different major muscle groups. The cable system employed simply redirects gravity; and with some cable crossover alignments a person can cut in half the stack resistance, permitting the exercise of smaller muscle groups in more gradual increments.

Machine—Variable Resistance

Variable resistance equipment is designed around the principle that the force a muscle produces during contraction is not constant. In fact, muscles produce the greatest force in the middle of the range of motion and the least force at either extreme (Wolkodoff 1989). Most often a cam-shaped pulley alters the effective resistance of the weight stack to match the strength curve of the muscle. Some believe that such equipment provides particularly high training efficiency: with optimal resistance through a full range of motion, the client can get an intense workout quickly. One of the difficulties with cam equipment is that no two people are alike in their muscle strength curves, so the machines are built for an average force curve. Nonetheless, many clients prefer the comfortable lift provided by variable resistance equipment. Devices such as springs, rubber bands, or sliding fulcrums increase the resistance through the range of motion, which is not how most muscles actually work. Through hands-on experience, you should get acquainted with the feel of different brands of variable resistance equipment. Also look for devices that limit range of motion and that allow users of different size to fit comfortably and safely. Equipment examples include Nautilus, David, Polaris, Cybex, and Eagle.

Hydraulics and Pneumatics

Alternatives to weight stacks include hydraulics and pneumatics. *Hydraulics* use a cylinder of compressed water or oil to vary the resistance. They offer concentric-concentric work where the muscles on the one side of the joint raise the weight, and the antagonist muscles on the other side of the joint pull it down. These machines are time-efficient, since only half the number of machines is needed. One advantage is reduced muscle soreness for the novice exerciser; a disadvantage, however, is that many daily activities and sport skills involve eccentric contractions. *Pneumatics* use compressed air and make the muscle work eccentrically (i.e., muscle is developing tension while it is being elongated). Hydraulic and pneumatic machines differ from weight stacks in that the client does not have to deal with overcoming the inertia of the weight or the momentum created once the machines are moving. They are quite safe, good for higher-speed training, and can be adapted for clients interested in sport training. Equipment examples include Hydra-Gym and Keiser.

Electronics

Computerized equipment can offer a number of different exercise modes: isometrics, isotonics, or isokinetics. Usually linked with an integrated display panel, the detail and immediacy of the feedback is very motivating.

Isokinetics

Isokinetic machines mechanically control the speed of movement. The resistance is accommodating and matches the force produced by the muscle group throughout the entire range of motion. Although some hydraulic and pneumatic machines simulate isokinetics, they allow some acceleration through the initial range of motion (O'Hagan et al. 1995). This may not be a problem for some people; but electronic resistance

machines, particularly the dynamometers, provide true isokinetic conditions. Some electronic machines provide resistance only during concentric contractions, while others offer resistance during both concentric and eccentric phases. Advantages of isokinetic devices include accommodating forces, reduced muscle soreness (concentric only), display feedback, collection of data, high- or low-speed training, and development of muscular power, strength, and endurance (Heyward 1998). They also offer a great deal of safety, since resistance dissipates with the onset of pain, injury, or fatigue. Machines with high-speed settings are appropriate for clients training for sports with high-speed skills (e.g., football or track). Disadvantages include cost, accessibility, need for motivation, and a constant-speed action that is not natural to most activities. Equipment examples include Cybex, Orthotron, Omnitron, Kin-Com, and Hydra-Gym.

Other

Other types of resistance are possible: elastic bands/ tubing, water, and manual resistance.

■ **Elastic.** Surgical tubing or commercial bands (e.g., Dynaband) come in a variety of thicknesses that offer a range of resistance. The effective resistance increases as the device is elongated. By carefully positioning both your client and the secured end of the tubing, you can obtain a variety of movements and joint angles. For about a dollar, you can supply your client with a personal home gym or a hotel workout! Elastic has a short life, however—beware of breakage or release while it's under tension. Some home multi-gyms use various thicknesses of tubing as a basis of resistance.

■ **Water.** In water, gravity and impact are non-issues. The medium controls speed and offers a natural, accommodating resistance. Your client can vary the resistance by trying different body segments, body positions, or specialty devices. The enveloping resistance allows for an endless combination of joint angles, and simple/complex movements. Water exercise is particularly appropriate for older clients and those suffering from arthritis or joint problems.

■ **Manual resistance.** You can simulate many of the principles of exercise machines by working as a training partner. Knowing what muscles cause specific joint movements, you can position yourself to provide manual resistance. If the resistance is greater than your client's force, the contraction will be eccentric; if it equals that of the client, it will be isometric; if less than the client's force, it will be concentric. You can also control the speed of movement to simulate isokinetic training. A creative exercise specialist can mold the nature of the resistance to the direct needs of the client.

Application and Alignment of Resistance

Do not leave the interface between your client and his equipment to chance. It is not the machine's job to know the proper alignment, stabilization, range of motion, and application of resistance—it is yours.

Is the Path of Motion Defined by the Machine the Same As Your Client's Path of Motion?

Many machines have a guided range of motion that may cause problems for smaller or larger clients. If seats and lever arms cannot be adjusted and your client looks or feels unnatural throughout the movement, the machine path is probably unsuitable. Always ascertain the following:

- A correct position of the joint before the exercise begins
- A safe end point to the range of motion (the machine may have a range-limiting device)
- A smooth arc of motion of the joint

Monitor your client carefully for these three checks, especially during spinal movements and shoulder rotations. New technology is addressing this issue. Some Pec Decks (e.g., Cybex) now employ a dual axis technology that allows clients to determine their own optimal arc of movement and range of motion. You should monitor the path of motion even when using low-tech body weight resistance. For example, take care that your client does not go too low during dips and excessively hyperextend her shoulder.

The ankle, knee, and hip joints form a kinetic chain. When the foot is stabilized or fixed, this kinetic chain is closed. An open kinetic chain exists when the foot is not in contact with the ground or some other surface. Knee flexion and extension using a machine are examples of open kinetic chain exercises. In a closed kinetic chain, the foot is weightbearing: the forces begin at the ground and work their way up through each joint. There is an advantage in having forces absorbed by various anatomical structures rather than simply dissipated as in an open chain.

Is the Direction of Force Application Safe and Optimal?

It is important to find a direction of movement that generates maximal muscular force (see chapter 10). Always determine if the force angle allows for the maximum resistance to be lifted.

With pulley systems, tubing, or water, your role involves establishing the correct body position for your client. The purpose of the exercise will significantly affect the line of pull and the position of the joints. The example in the previous chapter (figure 10.2, page 147) shows the line of pull and the position of the shoulder considerably different in three similar exercises.

Similarly, the use of various angles on an incline bench can be used to isolate targeted muscles when using free weights. For example, a 10-degree decline on the bench when doing flies can help a body builder focus on the lower fibers of the sternal section of the pectoralis major. A 45- degree incline will swing the emphasis to the clavicular section of the pectoralis major.

Does the Equipment Allow Proper Alignment Between the Machine's Fulcrum and the Center of the Moving Joint?

If the fulcrum of the machine does not align with the center of the moving joint, that joint will experience additional shearing force (making it slide apart) that increases more rapidly than the resistance on the machine (Hamill and Knutzen 1995). Clients with previous injuries to that joint are at significant risk. The following examples illustrate this problem on various pieces of equipment.

- Many Pec Decks have their pivot points in front of the shoulder, forcing the shoulder girdle to abduct significantly and decreasing the effectiveness of the exercise.
- The knee is particularly vulnerable to shearing forces. Joint alignment on leg extension machines is critical. Correct placement of shin pads (not too low) and a resistance varied by a cam reduces knee stress and optimizes strength gains.
- The Leg Curl machine involves similar issues. An angled bench that elevates the pelvis will help maintain alignment of the lower back as the knee flexes.
- Users of Hack Squat machines should be aware that, since the pelvis and back are quite stationary (unlike a regular squat), the knees are placed under greater shearing stress.
- Abdominal machines are particularly difficult because there are multiple pivot points that change throughout the range of motion. Actions that have the trunk flexed well forward creating an "L" position increase lower back

stresses (Hamill and Knutzen 1995). Crunching downwards or bringing a tucked lower body upwards are preferred movements if no pain is present. Some say that this movement focuses the intensity of contraction to the lower abdominals. More importantly for people with low back problems, this movement appears to present less compression on the discs of the lower back.

Program Demonstration and Follow-Up

First impressions about the prescription begin in the demonstration stage and continue to be reinforced through all the stages of monitoring.

Table 11.6 outlines the stages and activities from the time we meet our clients for the program demonstration until the late program follow-up.

Encouraging an Experiential Approach

You can encourage an experiential approach to the program demonstration and follow-up by designing situations that offer all the ways adults like to learn (Fitness Ontario 1983). Here are four different learning styles, each followed by an example:

■ **Learning by doing:** Your client learns by performing a series of abdominal exercises at a very slow and controlled pace, rather than the faster pace to which she is accustomed.

■ **Learning by observation:** You ask your client to comment on specific items she noticed—for example, "How did the slow exercises feel? Was there more energy required to perform the series slow or fast?"

■ **Learning by knowing the theory:** This is a combination of your client's experience and observations—you ask, for example, "What does this mean about the next time you will do sit-ups?"

Table 11.6 Stages in the Program Demonstration and Follow-Up

STAGES	ACTIVITIES
Program designed and follow-up established (already complete)	Reassessment of client goals, values, motivational interests and levels, fitness assessment results.
Reconnect: Recreating and further building a positive climate	Give clients permission to be themselves. Show pleasure in what they are doing. Provide protection from negative forces, e.g., negative self-talk, interruptions, intimidating atmosphere.
Program demonstration	Ensure clients' needs are being met. Base delivery of the information on clients' preferred learning style. Use an experiential learning approach.
Program clarification	Determine level of comfort and understanding. Modify if necessary.
Follow-up—early stage	Make appointment for connection in 2-3 days. One-week appointment.
Follow-up—mid to later stages	Time frame one week to two months. Extrinsic motivators? Program adjustments? Movement towards intrinsic motivators.

■ **Learning by applying the information to individual situations:** Have your client consider how this information will apply to other exercises he executes. "What would be the best way to perform muscle endurance exercises? Where else can this information apply?"

Base the amount of information you share with your client on his current stage of learning as well as on his preferred learning style. In the beginning stages, focus on giving only the important points. As your client becomes more experienced, you will be able to offer more alternative exercises, with your client making his own selection.

Exercise Demonstration

Demonstrating an exercise is both an art and a science. It requires a balance between your technical knowledge and your people skills. With practice, you will learn to alter the technical aspects to suit each client's personality and learning style.

Use the Exercise Demonstration Checklist on page 198 to ensure that your demonstration will be successful. The chart serves only as an outline—once you have reviewed the information in the rest of the chapter, adapt this model as appropriate.

The Science of Exercise Demonstration

There are four primary steps in an effective exercise demonstration:

1. Focus on overall body posture. Orient your client toward "setting" herself into a good body position prior to any exercise.

2. Focus on exactly where you want your client to begin and end each movement, and how the body should be positioned in both phases. For example, when beginning a bench press, your client should press her lower back into the bench, feet on the bench (if possible, hands slightly wider than shoulder with apart, etc.).

3. Give alignment and "feeling" cues to assist in the execution phase of the exercise. For example, when doing side-lying lateral leg raises, show how the hips are aligned one on top of the other, raising to approximately 45 degrees, knees facing forward, etc.

4. Focus on quality vs. quantity. This refers to the number of repetitions your client performs *correctly* and the speed at which they occur.

Spotting is an important component of exercise demonstration. *Spotting* refers to the visual and physical aspects of monitoring clients as they execute exercises. Visual spotting is done for all exercises, while physical spotting is used primarily in weight training. Watch for correct body alignment, signs and symptoms of fatigue, signs of discomfort, control of movements, and the direction of the exercise energy. Assist the client to complete more repetitions, make technique corrections, or complete the range of motion. Spotting the client provides an excellent opportunity to monitor good form. Table 11.7 lists the major spotting guidelines for monitoring technically sound mechanics.

The Art of Exercise Demonstration

Imagine that you are demonstrating a squat. Each of the following statements reflects the five stages of the Exercise Demonstration Checklist, and is accompanied by a critique for the designated stage.

■ **Pre-demo.** "By doing the squats on a regular basis, you will be better able to lift yourself up from a chair and be able to walk further without fatigue." This first step reflects a bit of salesmanship. You need to *sell the benefits* and show your client how the exercise is relevant to him.

■ **Demonstration.** "Stand with feet shoulder-width apart, and with your arms on the chair for support like this . . ." You are the role model. Yet you must be sensitive to your client's style of learning—tactile, auditory, or visual (as in this example).

■ **Client trials.** "As you bent your knees to lower your body, your knees moved beyond the line of your toes initially, but then you pressed your hips further back as you lowered your body and realigned . . ." Your focus is on your client's behavior. Leave him with a feeling of success and an idea of how to do better.

■ **Communication.** "If I understand you correctly, you feel that doing 15 repetitions of the squats is too many at this time. Is that correct?" Whether you use paraphrase, as in this example, or some other counseling technique (see chapter 1), you must make time for high-quality, one-on-one discussions with your client.

■ **Follow-up.** "Which part of the program are you most looking forward to? Are there any areas of the program you are unsure of or want to clarify?" Ask for your client's feelings. If you have rapport with him, you will gain valuable insights. Knowing that you are there for him gives him the confidence for greater autonomy.

EXERCISE DEMONSTRATION CHECKLIST

1. Pre-demonstration

    ———— Any related experience with this exercise?

    ———— Describe purpose of exercise (include fitness benefits and relevance to stated needs and wants).

2. Demonstration

    ———— Describe, in detail, directions for exercise execution.

    ———— Physically demonstrate the exercise: a) start/finish positions, b) execution.

    ———— State exercise precautions.

3. Client trials

    ———— Set client up to start, and position yourself as a spotter.

    ———— Feedback: a) Focus on behavior, b) single correction, and c) positive language.

    ———— Determine starting prescription levels.

4. Communication

    ———— Climate setting

    ———— Eye contact

    ———— Terminology at appropriate level for clien.

    ———— Paraphrasing/active listening

    ———— Use of open- and closed-ended questions

5. Follow-up

    ———— Probe to determine client's learning from session.

    ———— Probe to determine client's feelings/concerns; modify if necessary.

    ———— Encourage use of self-monitoring techniques.

    ———— May suggest progressions to encourage independence.

Table 11.7 Spotting Guidelines to Monitor Lifting Techniques

AREA	SPOTTING GUIDELINES
Upper body	(1) Position yourself close to the client where you have the most effective position for assistance. (2) Assist the client with heavier weights to bring the weight to the starting position. (3) Position your hands on the barbell. (4) Position your hands at the joint which is immediately below the weight during dumbbell exercises. (5) Assist the client at the end point of a movement during the final reps.
Lower body	(1) See Upper body (1) (2) Assist the client to bring the weight to the starting position for squats and lunges. (3) Position your hands just above the waist for squats and lunges. (4) Position your hands on the machine or the involved limb for pulley, machine, or hand exercises. (5) Assist the client at the end of a movement or if the speed decreases due to fatigue.
Trunk	(1) Use the assistance of gravity by using incline or decline positions of the bench. (2) Teach a pelvic stabilization to minimize lower back curvature and strain. (3) Manually assist when client has difficulty with correct movements. (4) Manually assist at the ends of normal range of motion once fatigue has occurred.

Monitoring Progress

The following guidelines will assist you in monitoring progress:

- Clients interested in strength gains will continually want to increase their load.
- Monitoring girth measures will track gains in hypertrophy.
- Clients working on strength-endurance should increase their reps up to about 15, then increase the load and drop the reps back down. As their condition improves, they may decrease the rest between sets.
- Clients working muscular endurance should use repetitions or sets as a method of progression. Decreasing rest time between sets can further challenge this component.
- Monitoring total poundage per workout will easily demonstrate improved work capacity.
- Program cards that allow quick recording of these factors can save time and encourage regular recording.

Highlights

- The symmetry of muscle balance plays an integral role in preventing injuries and maintaining normal biomechanics.
- Muscle balance is the cornerstone to the integration of muscular fitness components in a client-centered approach.
- With attention to alignment criteria and careful observation, you can detect faulty posture that may produce strain.

- There is a very effective and functional process that flows from postural analysis to the selection of muscle length testing items and on to a personalized prescription.

- A client with forward chin, cervical lordosis, and a tight neck would benefit from exercises designed to stretch the neck extensors and strengthen the neck flexors.

- A client with rounded shoulders and tight pectoralis minor and major should stretch those muscles and strengthen the shoulder extensors, external rotators, and scapular adductors.

- A client with lumbar lordosis and anterior pelvic tilt, who tests positive for tight erector spinae and hip flexors, can alleviate lower back stress with exercises that (1) stretch the back extensors and hip flexors and that (2) strengthen the abdominals and hip extensors.

- The quality of a stretch and the effectiveness of a flexibility program depend upon duration, intensity, temperature, relaxation, type of force, alignment, number of exercises, number of repetitions, and frequency.

- Any prescribed conditioning exercise must consider goal, component, muscles, exercises, method, equipment, order, load, volume, and method of progression.

- In selecting equipment, consider the best method of resistance, the type of equipment, and the interface of that equipment with your client (ergonomics).

- There are various types of resistance: gravity (including body weight, free weight, constant resistance machines, and variable resistance machines); hydraulics/pneumatics; electronics (including isokinetics); and others including elastic, water, and manual resistance.

- The stages in the program demonstration include

  1. program design and follow-up,
  2. further building of a positive climate,
  3. program demonstration,
  4. program clarification,
  5. follow-up—early stage, and
  6. follow-up—mid to later stages.

- You can encourage an experiential approach to learning by designing situations that offer all the ways adults like to learn: by doing; by observation; by knowing the theory; and by applying the information to one's own situation.

- The art and science of exercise demonstration involve balancing your technical knowledge with your people skills.

- There are five primary steps in an effective exercise demonstration: pre-demonstration, demonstration, client trials, communications, and follow-up.

Muscle Balance and Conditioning Case Studies

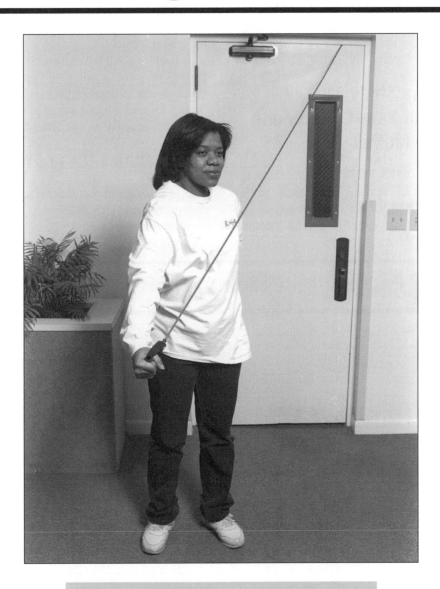

- Case Study #1: Thirty-Seven-Year Old Working Mother

- Case Study #2: Forty-Five-Year-Old Weekend Warrior

Inherent in the concept of musculoskeletal fitness are the inseparable qualities of alignment and muscle balance. Counseling (part 1), assessment (chapter 5), and prescription (chapter 11) are directed toward preservation or restoration of good body mechanics in posture and movement.

Screening for common postural faults provides a direction for follow-up muscle testing. The prescription goals of training for performance, rehabilitation, or fitness may differ, but the need to maintain muscle balance is important for all. Setting objectives for muscle balance usually centers around stretching tight muscles, strengthening weak muscles, reducing spasm, building muscular endurance, or improving posture.

Two studies will illustrate this progression from postural analysis to selection of muscle length test items and on to a personalized prescription. The case studies (as well as chapter 5) detail a number of muscle tests. You can pursue this area further through the resources listed for chapters 5 and 11.

Case Study #1: Thirty-Seven-Year-Old Working Mother

Rose was a 37-year-old bank teller with two children aged three years and 18 months. She did not exercise regularly. Rose suffered from headaches caused by neck tension and pain. She wanted to exercise at home,

and could devote 25 to 30 minutes, 4-5 days per week, to her program. Her primary objectives were to improve upper body endurance and eliminate neck pain.

Assessment

A cursory check of Rose's posture, with particular attention to upper torso alignment, revealed some areas that warranted further examination. I felt that an apparent lack of balance could be confirmed with some muscle tightness assessment.

The postural assessment (table 12.1) helped to fine-tune the priorities.

I observed no significant problems with Rose's feet, knees, or pelvis, but I did note the following misalignments: depressed chest; increased cervical curve; forward shoulders; palms rotated medially; scapulae abducted; and a forward head.

Interpretation (Case #1)

The combination of postural faults just described often creates neck and shoulder tension and discomfort, because the weight of the head is supported by the

Table 12.1 Postural Assessment Chart—Case #1

Feet		Pronated		Supinated		Arch		Toe in/out		
Knees		Rotational-patella		Hyper-extended		Flexed		Bowlegs		Knock-knees
Pelvis		Anterior tilt		Posterior tilt		Lateral tilt		Rotation		
Chest	X	Depressed		Elevated		Rotational ribs		Abdomen protruding		
Spine		Lumbar lordosis		Flat		Thoracic kyphosis	X	Cervical lordosis		Scoliosis
Shoulder		Low		High	X	Forward	X	Rotational palms		
Scapulae	X	Abducted		Adducted		Winged		Elevated		
Head	X	Forward		Tilt		Rotation	for.	Chin		
Other	X	Neck Tension Headaches								

posterior muscles rather than the skeletal system. Strengthening of the anterior neck muscles (sterno-cleidomastoid) can help restore balance.

The shoulder girdle and neck musculature are linked. It was clear to me that muscle length testing could help determine the underlying cause of Rose's rounded-shouldered posture. The pectoralis minor exerts a forward and downward pull on the front of the scapula and may alone cause the roundness. Tightness of the pectoralis major will contribute to the forward pull of the shoulders and may cause an internal rotation of the shoulder as seen by the palms facing backwards. Because Rose was relatively untrained, I suspected weak and overstretched posterior scapular adductors (trapezius and rhomboids), and a depressed chest (which often accompanies rounded shoulders).

Chapter 5 described procedures for muscle length assessments for the pectoralis minor, pectoralis major (sternal-S), shoulder internal rotators, and shoulder external rotators. The "normal" values quoted for the tests are conservative: any deviation from them deserves attention. Here is what I found for Rose:

- Pectoralis minor: moderate tightness, left and right.
- Pectoralis major (S): left and right arms 5 degrees off table.
- Shoulder internal rotators: left and right forearms 10 degrees off table.
- Shoulder external rotators: normal ROM.

Prescribing for Rose

It seemed clear that Rose's forward chin, cervical lordosis, and a tight neck would benefit from exercises designed to stretch the neck extensors and strengthen the neck flexors and that her rounded shoulders should respond to stretches for tight pectoralis minor and major and to strengthening exercises for shoulder extensors, external rotators, and scapular adductors (see Opposing Muscles, pages 180-181).

Several exercises are beneficial for both areas, with simple training methods appropriate for the home environment. Static stretching is the suggested method for lengthening the tight muscles. Isometric exercises, tubing, and calisthenics are the appropriate strength training techniques. I prescribed these exercises for Rose, as described in Exercise Design Summary—Case #1 on page 204.

Follow-Up

Weekly phone conversations with Rose seemed very promising. She managed daily to devote nearly an hour to her prescription. She liked the convenience of working out at home and the easy-to-follow program. I joined her for a workout in the third week and was amazed at her rapid increase in muscular endurance, especially in the posterior shoulder area. However, the dull ache in her neck had not disappeared. My concern at this point was that Rose might be overtraining and perpetuating the symptoms.

I didn't want to discourage Rose from her exercise habit, but some modifications were necessary. We designed a workout log to track the volume of work and any symptoms. She agreed to exercise only three days per week for 30 minutes. To maintain an adequate overload, I moved her up to heavier tubing and substituted bent-over flies with some newly acquired dumbbells for the supine scapular retraction exercise. We selected a starting weight that brought Rose to fatigue by the eighth to tenth repetition on the first set.

I scheduled a reassessment in five weeks to judge the effectiveness of the prescription for Rose's posture and muscle balance. Continued weekly phone calls confirmed a reduction in neck pain and tension headaches.

Prescriptions are rarely a straight highway to success. But with regular monitoring and follow-up modifications, the journey can resume in the right direction.

Note: If your clients are seeking gains in strength-endurance, select a starting weight that brings them to fatigue by the eighth to tenth repetition on the first set. Adjust the weight, if necessary, and have them do as many repetitions as possible on the second set. Refer to table 11.4 for progressions and other guidelines.

Case Study #2: Forty-Five-Year-Old Weekend Warrior

Kevin was a divorced 45-year-old broker who worked long hours. He played old-timers hockey once a week for six months of the year. He suffered from moderate low back discomfort and occasional sciatica. He had just joined a local fitness club and was willing to commit to three 50-minute workouts per week. He wanted to lose fat from the trunk area and improve the condition of his back.

Assessment

Kevin was concerned about his back and trunk region. An overview of his posture revealed some areas to examine further. His prolonged stress and sitting posture at work were obvious concerns. To confirm an apparent lack of balance, I assessed the strength and

Exercise Design Summary—Case #1

ASSESSMENT

Postural fault	Muscles in shortened position	Muscle in lengthened position
Forward head lean and forward chin Cervical lordosis	Erector spinae, deep posterior (cervical) Trapezius 1	Sternocleidomastoid

EXERCISE PRESCRIPTION

Stretch neck extensors

Chin tuck Pull head straight back keeping jaw and eyes level. 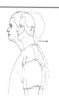	**Lateral neck stretch** Grasp arm and pull downward and across body while gently tilting head. 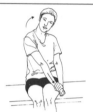

Strengthen neck flexors

Resisted neck flexion Facing forward with finger tips on forehead, bend head forward through a full range. Give moderate resistance. 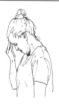	

ASSESSMENT

Postural fault	Muscles in shortened position	Muscles in lengthened position
Rounded shoulders Internal rotation of shoulder joint Scapular abduction	Pectoralis major Subscapularis Pectoralis minor, serratus anterior	Latissimus dorsi Infraspinatus, Teres minor Trapezius 2, 3, & 4 and rhomboids

EXERCISE PRESCRIPTION

Stretch pectoralis major, minor, and internal rotators

Shoulder internal rotator stretch Keep palm of hand against door frame, elbow bent at 90 degrees. Turn body from fixed hand until a stretch is felt.	**Supine wand thrust** 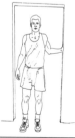 Hold wand with involved side palm up, push with un-involved side (palm down) out from body while keeping elbow at side until you feel a stretch. Then pull back across body, leading with uninvolved side. Be sure to keep elbows bent.

(continued)

EXERCISE PRESCRIPTION *(continued)*
Stretch pectoralis major, minor, and internal rotators *(continued)*

Door frame pec stretch

Keep palm of outstretched horizontal arm against door frame. Turn body until a stretch is felt. Vary the level of the arm.

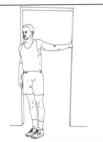

Strengthen shoulder extensors, horizontal abductors, external rotators, and scapular adductors*

Resisted diagonal shoulder extension

Grasp tubing with arm reaching above shoulder and across body. Gently pull downward and away from your body. Return slowly to starting position.

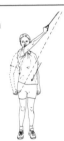

Resisted shoulder external rotation

Using tubing, and keeping elbow in at side, rotate arm outward away from body. Be sure to keep forearm parallel to floor.

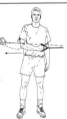

Supine scapular retraction

With fingers clasped behind head, pull elbows back while pinching shoulder blades together.

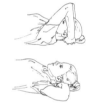

*For clients who prefer dumbbells, upper back strengthening exercises may be replaced with bent over flies or reverse flies.

*For stack-weight users, rowing and pull-downs could be substituted.

*For clients seeking gains in strength endurance, select a starting weight that brings them to fatigue by the 8th to 10th repetition on the first set. Adjust the weight, if necessary, and have them do as many repetitions as possible on the second set. Refer to the Strength-Endurance Prescription Factors Chart for progressions and other guidelines.

tightness of the muscles that attach to the spine and pelvis.

Postural Assessment

The postural assessment (table 12.2) helped to fine-tune the priorities.

Kevin's postural chart showed nothing significant at the feet, knees, shoulder, scapulae, or head. I did note the following misalignments: an anterior tilt to the pelvis; a protruding abdomen; and an increased curvature to the lower back with accompanying discomfort.

Muscle Balance Assessment

Muscle testing showed tightness in the 1-joint hip flexors (the iliopsoas crosses only the hip) and 2-joint

hip flexors (the rectus femoris crosses both hip and knee). Further assessment revealed some tightness of the hamstrings; a progressive unassisted curl-up test (chapter 5) revealed weak abdominals; and a modified trunk forward flexion assessment disclosed low back tightness.

Chapter 5 describes procedures for muscle length assessments for hip flexors, hamstrings, and forward trunk flexion. As was true with the previous example, any deviation from the "normal" values given for these tests should lead to further investigation. The observations I made for Kevin are as follows:

■ Hip flexors: one-joint and two-joint hip flexors tight; tensor fascia latae also tight.

Table 12.2 Postural Assessment Chart—Case #2

Feet		Pronated	Supinated		Arch		Toe in/out		
Knees		Rotational patella	Hyper-extended		Flexed		Bowlegs		Knock-knees
Pelvis	X	Anterior tilt	Posterior tilt		Lateral tilt		Rotation		
Chest		Depressed	Elevated		Rotational ribs	X	Abdomen protruding		
Spine	X	Lumbar lordosis	Flat		Thoracic kyphosis		Cervical lordosis		Scoliosis
Shoulder		Low	High		Forward		Rotational palms		
Scapulae		Abducted	Adducted		Winged		Elevated		
Head		Forward	Tilt		Rotation		Chin		
Other	X	Back Discomfort Sciatica							

- Hamstrings: 80 degrees (normal).
- Forward trunk flexion: hamstrings normal; short muscles in lower back (no roundness).

Interpretation (Case #2)

The increased lumbar lordosis had caused the weight of the upper body to settle on the lower back, aggravating any low back problems. Although it is common in such cases to see exaggerated curves in the thoracic and cervical regions (to compensate for the lumbar curve), Kevin did not exhibit such symptoms. The anterior tilt to his pelvis, in conjunction with the lumbar lordosis, is very common and likely resulted from one or several muscle imbalances. Tight hip flexors pulled his pelvis forward and down—a condition often associated with short spinal extensors, which also contribute to anterior pelvic tilt. Weak and perhaps overstretched abdominals are not sufficient to withstand such forces. I decided that strengthening the hip extensors (gluteus maximus and hamstrings) would resist the pull of the very strong hip flexors.

Prescribing for Kevin

Because Kevin had lumbar lordosis and anterior pelvic tilt, and tested positive for tight erector spinae and hip flexors, he could alleviate his lower back stress with exercises that stretched the back extensors and hip flexors, and that strengthened the abdominals and hip extensors. The chart on page 180 is a useful reference for muscle pairs.

The exercise design began with therapeutic exercises for the lumbar lordosis, followed by exercises for the related anterior pelvic tilt. The methods of training included static stretching for muscle tightness. To strengthen the abdominals, Kevin started with only the resistance of gravity and body weight. For the hip extensors, I suggested that he add resistance from tubing or from the appropriate machines at the fitness club.

Follow-Up

I had an opportunity to talk with Kevin during most of his club visits. The first four weeks of his program

Exercise Design Summary—Case #2

ASSESSMENT

Postural fault	Muscles in shortened position	Muscles in lengthened position
Lumbar lordosis	Erector spinae, deep posterior (lumbar)	Abdominals

EXERCISE PRESCRIPTION

Stretch back extensors

Supine knees to chest—stretch Pull both knees in to chest until a comfortable stretch is felt in lower back. Keep back relaxed. 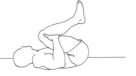	**Seated back stretch** Sit on the edge of a chair with legs spread apart. Tuck your chin and slowly bend downward. Relax in a comfortable stretch. Return slowly. 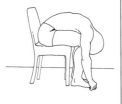

Strengthen abdominals

Curl-up—Level 1 With arms at sides tilt pelvis to flatten back. Raise shoulders and head from floor. Return in a controlled fashion. 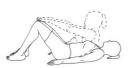	**Abdominal crunch** With legs over foot stool or chair and arms positioned behind head, tilt pelvis to flatten back. Raise head and shoulders from floor. 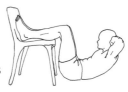

ASSESSMENT

Postural fault	Muscles in shortened position	Muscles in lengthened position
Anterior pelvic tilt	Iliopsoas, rectus femoris, pectineus, tensor fascia latae	Gluteus maximus Hamstrings (possibly)
Sciatica	Piriformis	

EXERCISE PRESCRIPTION

Stretch 1- and 2-joint flexors, piriformis

One-joint hip flexor lunge Slowly push pelvis downward until a stretch is felt on front of hip. 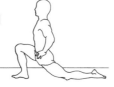	**Side lying quad stretch** Pull heel in toward buttocks until a comfortable stretch is felt in front of thigh. Add a posterior pelvic tilt. 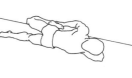

(continued)

EXERCISE PRESCRIPTION *(continued)*	
Stretch 1- and 2-joint flexors, piriformis *(continued)*	

Wall lean stretch

With arm against wall, slowly lean hips toward wall with other arm supporting trunk.

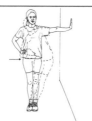

Supine piriformis stretch

Cross legs with involved leg on top. Gently pull opposite knee toward chest until a comfortable stretch is felt in the buttock/hip area.

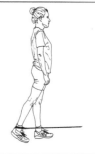

Strengthen hip extensors

Supine hip thrusts

Start in supine position with lower leg vertical and pillow under head. Slowly raise buttocks, keeping stomach tight.

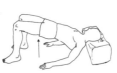

Resisted hip extension

With tubing around involved ankle and opposite end secured in door jam, bring leg backwards, keeping knee straight.

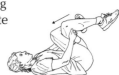

Note: Stack weight leg extensions or other machines may be substituted to strengthen hip extensors.

preceded the start of his hockey season. After a guided demonstration and three workouts on his own, I introduced some aerobic intervals that simulated the shift changes for his hockey. I explained that the aerobic activity would have an added benefit for his back.

Since he enjoyed the aerobic intervals, we continued them throughout the hockey season using different equipment for a cross-training effect (see chapter 7). A month into the season, Kevin began coming in only twice a week as opposed to three times as prescribed. This would not have been a concern had not Kevin indicated that his home workouts had pretty much dropped off.

Kevin was in an "action stage" (see chapter 1), and his risk of relapse was high. I could tell he felt guilty about the transgression, but I reassured him that this was a normal state of affairs and our job now was to deal with the lapse. With his two club aerobic workouts and weekly hockey, he was pleased with the cardiovascular improvements he was feeling. However, he was taking two days of rest after his hockey because his back felt tight and fatigued. Although he agreed that he needed to do the muscle balance exercises more frequently, Kevin admitted that he had little motivation to follow his home program. We came up with two

modifications. First, I linked Kevin up with one of our apprenticing personal trainers for an additional 15 minutes per visit of guided strengthening and stretching similar to his prescribed exercises. To deal with the tightness created by the hockey, I gave him five stretches—specifically adapted to the bench in his locker room—that he agreed to do before and after each game.

Client-centered prescription involves carefully listening to your client's feedback and modifying the path as necessary in response. It often involves side trips and doubling back, but it always moves in the direction of better health for your client.

Highlights

- These case studies have illustrated how to use **postural assessment charts** (tables 12.1 and 12.2), and how to use information gained from **muscle length assessments** (chapter 5).

- Both studies showed the importance of **follow-up** and **reassessment**, and provided examples of modifications made in a prescription in order to adjust to the client's particular circumstances.

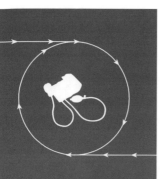

PART V

Design Issues for Special Populations

Our understanding of the effects of physical activity on human health has advanced in recent years, not only among fitness professionals but also in the general population. Consequently, fitness consumers increasingly want specific results, more choices, and more guidance about how to exercise. Many of us—whether clinical kinesiologists, personal trainers, physical therapists, athletic trainers, chiropractors, physical educators, or fitness specialists in private or community settings—have noted the lack of resources for guiding these informed consumers.

Part V looks at prescription situations that merit special consideration. Many of our clients are recovering from or have a history of orthopedic injury. One focus of Part V is on overuse injuries and exercise prescription for injury recovery and prevention. Another focus is on specific prescriptions for stretching and strengthening.

The final chapter provides activity recommendations for special populations with chronic conditions. Since certain types of physical activity may aggravate health conditions, this chapter includes a list of "red flags" that can alert us to such aggravations. The chapter specifically discusses arthritis, diabetes, exercise-induced asthma, and hypertension.

Chapter 13

Preventing and Treating Overuse Injuries

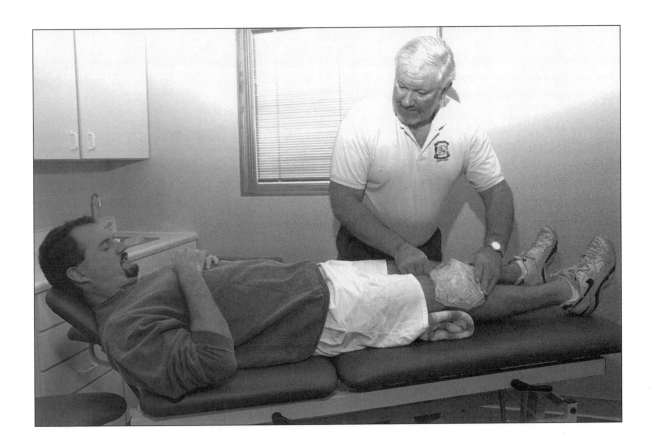

- What Are Overuse Injuries?
- Recognition of Overuse
- Factors Contributing to Overuse Injury
- Intervention and Prevention of Overuse Injuries

The most important outcome of safety and early intervention is prevention of injury. We must understand the mechanism of injury, the risk factors that contribute to injury, and the steps involved in exercise prescription to help a client recover.

Exercise has risks, and our clients' adherence to their programs depends on their avoiding injury. Flare-ups of preexisting injuries can be major obstacles. Careful supervision and appropriate intervention can provide early detection of risk factors that contribute to overuse injuries.

What Are Overuse Injuries?

The most common types of fitness injuries—and as many as 50% of all sports injuries—are caused by repetitive microtrauma (Hess et al. 1989) in which soft tissue becomes inflamed or cellular tissue degenerates. The damage can be cumulative, resulting in ligament strains, joint synovitis, muscle myositis, or tendinitis. Injury occurs most often when the tendon has been strained repeatedly until it is unable to endure further tension.

Musculotendinous Structure

Tendons consist primarily of collagenous fibers (70%) embedded in a gel. *Endotendons,* which are connective tissue sheaths surrounding fibrils of collagen, carry blood vessels and nerves. The most external sleeve is called the *peritendon,* which is like an elastic sleeve allowing free movement of the tendon against surrounding structures. Muscle and tendon function as one unit. Injury may occur at any point along this muscle-tendon unit: in the muscle belly, in the tendon, at the musculotendinous junction, or at the tendon-bone attachment.

Chronic overuse injury occurs with repetitive use rather than with an acute stretch or blunt traumatization—it is the cumulative effect of thousands of repetitive cycles. Generally there are two kinds of fitness/sports activities that lead to overuse damage: (1) endurance activities, and (2) those associated with repetitive actions. The common element of the culprit activity is involvement of eccentric muscle contractions and the development of *delayed-onset muscle soreness (DOMS).* Microscopic evaluation of the early stages of an injury have shown tearing of the muscle and connective tissue fibers and swelling (Wanhol et al. 1985).

Tendinitis and Inflammation

Tendinitis is among the most common overuse problems (see examples in chapter 14). It is an inflammatory response within the tendon as a result of microstructural damage to the collagen fibers. The tendon is particularly vulnerable because the force of a contracting muscle is transmitted through the tendon; microtearing occurs because the collagenous fibers are not very elastic (see The Terms of Structural Biomechanics, page 213).

Treatment of tendinitis involves rest and avoidance of the repetitive motion causing the irritation. Immediate and frequent icing is a very effective way to reduce inflammation and pain. Tendinitis and anti-inflammatory treatment are outlined in chapter 14.

Recognition of Overuse

Though inflammation is required for proper healing, an excessive or prolonged inflammatory response can become self-destructive. It is important to ask clients about pain and to be alert for signs of pain while they are exercising.

The Initial Session

The initial counseling session should establish past injuries, current pains, and potential causes of injury. In many cases, your clients will approach you after they have started on their program and experienced some discomfort.

Effective questioning and probing is critical to determine your client's needs. With your client, fill out the Pain Questionnaire on page 214 to establish a history and possible causes of the pain.

Catching Pain Early

Clients do not always take pain seriously, and some will mask it until it becomes acute. When a movement is performed repeatedly and the tendon becomes irritated and inflamed, it is time for action. During movement your client may indicate a feeling of pain, warmth, possible swelling, or crepitus. Crepitus is a crackling sound similar to the sound of rolling hair between the fingers by the ear. To insure early intervention so that problems will not become serious, watch carefully for these symptoms of overuse.

The series of events that lead to overuse injury are remarkably predictable (O'Connor, Sobel, and Nirschl 1992). Figure 13.1 illustrates the vicious recurring spiral of overuse injuries.

You must interrupt this spiral of overuse to prevent tissue degeneration and to promote proper healing. Clients should seek help when they first experience pain, whether at an initial meeting or later during their program. Watch for symptoms of overuse and opportunities to intervene when there has been any of the following:

- A change in execution (e.g., joint alignment)
- A change in the client's interface with equipment (e.g., set-up/starting position; change of shoes)
- Failure of execution with no spotting
- An increase in load or intensity
- Omission of warm-up or cooldown

- Resumption of training after a period of inactivity
- Addition or deletion of exercises from the original prescription
- A change in location of workouts (e.g., surface) or environment (e.g., temperature)
- Addition of supplemental activity such as a sport

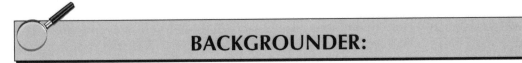

BACKGROUNDER:

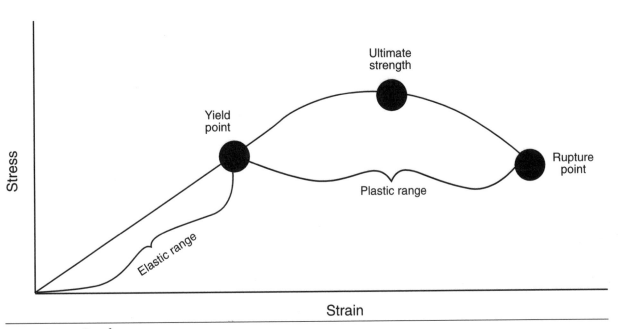

Stress-Strain Graph

The Terms of Structural Biomechanics

Resilience - Ability of tissue to *vigorously* return to its original size when unloaded.

Damping - The characteristic of tissue to return to its original size *less vigorously* than it was deformed (i.e., loss of energy).

Absorbed strain - If loading goes into the plastic range, a considerable amount of energy may be lost (dissipated during permanent deformation).

Strain - Deformation; changes in tissue size, shape, length.

  Tensile—pulling apart (e.g., tendon, ligament, muscle).

  Shear—sliding apart (e.g., joint surfaces, L5-S1, epiphyseal plates).

  Compression—pressure (e.g., intervertebral disc, cartilage).

  Stress—reaction forces to external loads set up within the tissues (e.g., stress created in bone, ligament and tendon within the arch of the foot to support body weight).

Elasticity - Ability to return to original dimension immediately.

Plasticity - Ability to retain changes in size or length when load is removed.

Stress-strain curve (load deformation) - The deformation (strain) increases proportionally to the stress resisting the load. The muscle-tendon complex has properties of elasticity up to a point (elastic range), after which permanent deformation (plastic range) and ultimately a rupture will occur.

PAIN QUESTIONNAIRE

1. Do you have any current pain? _____

2. What are the symptoms? _____

3. How long have you had these symptoms? _____

4. Have you had any past, related conditions and what treatment was provided? _____

   _____

   _____

5. In what joint/area do you feel the pain? _____

6. In what positions do you feel the pain? _____

7. During what movement do you feel the pain? _____

8. Do you feel the pain more or less before the activity? _____

9. Do you feel the pain more or less after the activity? _____

10. How long does the pain last? _____

11. Do you get tired (muscularly) more easily than you used to? _____

12. Have you experienced a loss of strength? _____

13. Are you compensating in your movements to avoid pain or loss of strength? _____

    _____

14. Do you feel tight anywhere? _____

15. Have you changed your prescription? _____

16. Have you recently increased your exercise volume or intensity? _____

17. Have you changed your location of exercise, type of equipment, or other conditions?

    _____

18. Have you recently changed shoes or are your shoes worn? _____

19. Is the injury (pain) getting worse? _____

20. What do you think is causing this "problem"? _____

21. How could it be alleviated? _____

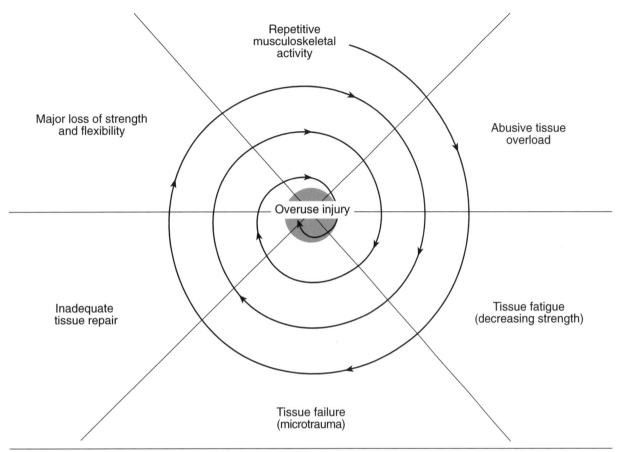

Figure 13.1   Spiral of overuse injuries.

 BACKGROUNDER:

Common Sites of Overuse Tendon Injuries

Overuse injuries to the muscle-tendon are common to many fitness activities and sports used for conditioning purposes. So much so, in fact, that some of the injuries have taken on more common names such as: Tennis elbow, Swimmer's shoulder, and Jumper's knee. The following information lists the common sites of overuse tendon injuries (Hess G.P. et al. 1989).

Tendon	Common name
Adductor brevis, gracilis, pectineus, iliopsoas	"Groin pull"
Achilles	Achilles tendinitis
Patellar	"Jumper's knee"
Common wrist extensor tendon	"Tennis elbow" (lateral epicondylitis)
Common wrist flexor	"Golfer's elbow" (medial epicondylitis)
Supraspinatus	"Swimmer's shoulder"—impingement
Other rotator cuff tendons (infraspinatus, teres minor, subscapularis)	Rotator cuff tendinitis
Tibialis posterior	"Shin splints"

Responding to Pain

You must carefully evaluate the pain associated with an overuse injury. Nirschl (1988) has described a pain phase scale for overuse injuries. This pain scale is useful for initial assessment and as a way to monitor a program's rate of progress.

LINKS:

Pain Scale for Overuse Injuries

Phase #1 Stiffness or mild soreness after activity. Pain usually gone within 24 hours.

Phase #2 Stiffness or mild soreness before activity that is relieved by warm-up. Symptoms not present during activity but return after, lasting up to 48 hours.

Phase #3 Stiffness or mild soreness before activity. Pain partially relieved by warm-up. It is minimally present during activity but does not alter activity.

Phase #4 Pain more intense than phase #3. Performance of activity altered. Mild pain noticed with daily activities.

Phase #5 Significant (moderate or greater) pain before, during, and after activity, causing alteration of activity. Pain with daily activities but no major change.

Phase #6 Pain persists even with complete rest. Pain disrupts simple daily activities and prohibits doing household chores.

Phase #7 Phase #6 pain that also disrupts sleep consistently. Pain is aching in nature and intensifies with activity.

Factors Contributing to Overuse Injury

Our clients get hurt because of the inherent structure and mechanics of their bodies (intrinsic) and because of their environment or type of training (extrinsic). Table 13.1 lists intrinsic and extrinsic factors that can contribute to overuse injuries.

Intrinsic Factors

Intrinsic factors are biomechanical characteristics unique to an individual. Always screen clients as discussed in chapter 5, and carefully follow up after your prescription to monitor any potential risk. It also can be useful to do some mental sleuthing based on your client's history of injuries—you may uncover an intrinsic predisposing factor that has not been corrected.

For example: Overpronation of the ankle produces a whipping action on the Achilles due to the excessive range of motion. These torsion forces may be related to degenerative changes to the tendon (Achilles tendinitis). Clement, Taunton, and Smart (1984) reported that almost 60% of injured runners overpronated. Careful observation of the Achilles and subtalar joint while your client is standing and walking should reveal a pronation problem. A medial wearing pattern on the heel of your client's shoe is additional evidence.

Excessive pronation has also been linked to higher incidence of shin splints due to the increased stretch of the tibialis anterior. In fact, torsion of the tibia that comes with pronation makes it difficult for the patella to track evenly during gait. Patella Femoral Syndrome can result (see chapter 14).

Extrinsic Factors

Training errors are the primary extrinsic factor associated with overuse tendon injuries. Clement, Taunton,

Table 13.1 Risk Factors That Contribute to Overuse Injuries

INTRINSIC	EXTRINSIC
Malalignment	Training errors (excessive/repeated force)
Muscle imbalance	Equipment
Inflexibility	Environment
Muscle weakness	Technique
Instability	Sports-imposed deficiencies

and Smart (1984) identified training errors in 75% of tendon injuries and overuse syndromes. Changes in duration, intensity, or frequency of activity are common mechanisms of extrinsic overload. Sports can overload musculoskeletal systems in predictable patterns. For example, sports involving throwing may leave the external rotators of the shoulder fatigued from continual eccentric deceleration of the arm. This chronic fatigue leads to a loss of flexibility, weakness, and eventual injury (figure 13.1).

Fitness activities also follow patterns of overuse. Initial studies of high-impact aerobic dance revealed a high incidence of lower-extremity injuries (Griffin 1987): the inherent repetitive overload causes fatigue, loss of strength, and microtrauma to the tibialis posterior, soleus, and gastrocnemius. Without continuing rest and ice treatment, tissue repair is inadequate and subsequent performance is painful, weak, and restrictive. People in this situation suffer from shin splints or Achilles tendinitis.

You can usually trace training errors to repetitive force that contributes to overuse, and/or to excessive force in the development of momentum.

Overuse

There are two common mechanisms of overuse injury:

1. **Abusive tissue overload** that causes acute macrotrauma may initiate a tendinitis that is resistant to healing and continues as an overuse injury.
2. **Repetitive submaximal tissue overload** can lead to microtrauma with incomplete cellular repair and subsequent deterioration of connective tissue.

The aerobic dance craze in the 1980s reinforced the overuse cause of injury. Repeated studies (Hamill 1991; Marti 1988; Richie, Kelso, and Bellucci 1985; Rothenberger 1988; Vetter 1985) showed that

- The reported mechanism of injury was most often a repetitive high-impact force and/or sharp increases in injuries occurring when the frequency of workouts was greater than four times per week.

Momentum

You should develop the ability to spot high-momentum movements that place clients at risk. Since momentum is the product of velocity × mass, momentum is high when a large part of the body moves rapidly. A joint experiences even greater forces as

- the mass of the moving part is further away from the joint (longer lever); or
- the movement goes to the end of the range of motion.

At risk during actions such as these are the joint capsule, musculotendinous unit, and other soft tissue structures. The following design illustrates progressive increases in exercise momentum.

Example: Triceps Kickbacks (dumbbells)

Level A. Upper arm stays by side of body; elbow extends and returns. (Small body part; short lever; momentum low but depends on weight used.)

Level B. At the end of elbow extension, the entire arm extends at the shoulder; return. (Additional arm weight provides greater momentum; greater range of motion; and longer lever.)

Level C. Same as level B with a rotation of the spine as the weight is lifted higher. (As shoulder reaches end of its range of motion, momentum forces trunk to rotate; addition of any speed to force a heavy weight up would create dangerous torque strain on the back.)

Level C takes the range of motion of the shoulder and elbow beyond a safe point. The high-momentum actions described introduce a repeated tensile stretch to the muscle-tendon unit, including the lower back.

Always stress quality of motion. Every individual has a unique *stop point* for each joint, linked to muscle tightness and muscle strength. This is the point in a joint's ROM that, for motion to continue, would require involvement of another joint. Identifying the stop point requires a learned "intuitive inhibition"; you can help your clients discover these stop points by carefully observing excessive movement as they exercise.

You should also evaluate your clients' *eccentric contraction patterns*. Eccentric contractions generate the greatest muscular forces. Very great strain is placed on connective tissue when it is elongated under tension, creating considerable potential for microtearing. Eccentric contractions occur when

- muscles attempt to counter the force of momentum by slowing down the action—examples

The buildup of momentum is very common in fitness activities, and many movements are contraindicated. To test your skill of recognizing momentum but also the risk it may present, try the following quiz.

Momentum Quiz

For each of the following exercises identify

A. how the momentum is produced (mass × velocity) and

B. possible adverse effects.

EXAMPLE:

Full neck circles

A. The head is quite heavy; if done quickly, momentum will affect the neck.

B. Facet joints of the cervical spine will be jammed during the hyperextension phase; may affect the neck arteries.

1. Straight-leg speed sit-ups

A.

B.

2. Stepping down and up quickly from a high aerobic step (bench)

A.

B.

3. Full squat with barbell

A.

B.

Answers:

1.A. All mass above the hips is being raised and lowered rapidly.

1.B. Hip flexors are exerting a strong anterior pull on the pelvis and lower back.

2.A. Body weight and gravity combine on the down phase.

2.B. The ankle (Achilles), knee, and possibly the back may be injured if client has a forward bend posture.

3.A. Body and barbell weight and gravity combine on the down phase.

3.B. Knees and possibly back can be injured if form is poor.

include ballistic arm action, especially with hand weights; and the follow-through action during racquet sports;

■ muscles attempt to counter the force of gravity—examples include any lowering of a limb or of the body, such as the lower body's strain during the support phase of running (figure 13.2).

Eccentric overload is evident in the high incidence of lower leg injuries during many aerobic weightbearing activities (Styf 1988; Grana and Coniglione 1985; Richie, Kelso, and Bellucci 1985). Eccentric patterns also appear in dynamic front lunges, which require many eccentric contractions to counteract the force of gravity—gastrocnemius, soleus, and tibialis anterior to control the speed of ankle dorsiflexion; quadriceps to control knee flexion; gluteus maximus and hamstrings to control hip flexion; and probably the erector spinae, which controls the downward tendency of spinal flexion.

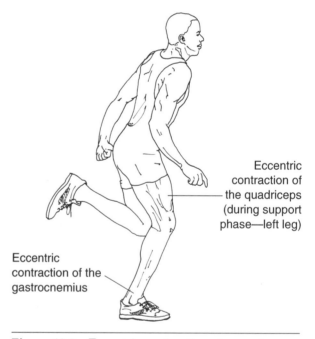

Eccentric contraction of the quadriceps (during support phase—left leg)

Eccentric contraction of the gastrocnemius

Figure 13.2 Eccentric contractions in running.

Intervention and Prevention of Overuse Injuries

Overuse injuries can be very discouraging to our clients. To optimize their quick (and permanent) return to their programs, we should encourage the following three-step progression: healing and hardening; fitness and focus; risk control.

Exercise Guidelines
Step One: Healing and Hardening

Recurrent injury often results from incomplete rehabilitation. Healing involves collagen deposit and vascularization through rehabilitative exercise and cardiovascular conditioning. At first, exercise enhances tissue oxygenation, minimizes atrophy, and aligns collagenous fibers to increase tissue strength. Soon after an injury, have your clients

- limit excessive stretching of damaged tissue;
- do isometrics (progressing from submaximal) at different joint angles;
- start with mid-range isotonics (daily), completing about 30 repetitions in two to three sets (may start with no weight).

During this stage, your clients should limit the range of motion to that in which they remain pain-free.

As your clients heal, have them progress to

- full effort on isometrics;
- isotonics in full ROM—gradually increasing weight by 10% to 20% and reducing repetitions initially, then gradually increasing them again;
- a minimum frequency of three exercise sessions per week;
- use of rubber tubing or elastic bands (if you deem it appropriate);
- incorporation of ROM exercises and moderate static stretching to regain muscle balance and to treat muscles that have tightened because of compensation;
- light cardiovascular exercise that does not traumatize the injured tissue (e.g., aquafitness, hand ergometry, stationary bicycle).

Step Two: Fitness and Focus

Steps two and three, as well as some of the hardening phases of step one, are as much a prescription for prevention as for rehabilitation. The progression for overuse intervention is relevant regardless of whether your client is in pain, at risk, or just trying to avoid injury. General body conditioning—including cardiovascular, strength and endurance, muscle balance, and flexibility—enhances rehabilitation of any injury and will decrease the chance of its recurring. Introducing

exercises specific to the injury, however, can provide neurophysiological stimulus and help (re)develop proprioceptive skills.

During step two, follow whichever of these guidelines are specifically appropriate to your client:

- Include full ROM strengthening, reaching momentary failure at the end of each set.
- Insist on a minimum exercise frequency of two or three times per week.
- Select other resistance equipment (e.g., isokinetic, hydraulic, variable-resistance).
- Use heavier/thicker tubing or bands to isolate movements/muscles.
- Include partner-resisted exercise and PNF (proprioceptive neuromuscular facilitation) with client-specific static stretches.
- Add activities specific to the client's sport or usual training activities (e.g., interval training; muscle isolations; drills for agility, speed, and skill).
- If the client is involved in a power-oriented eccentric activity, progressively build the eccentric strength and power of the involved muscle groups (e.g., eccentric Achilles exercises).

Step Three: Risk Control

Reexamine your client's history and assessment to uncover specific intrinsic and extrinsic risk factors for (re)injury. Controlling these forces is the objective of step three.

Minimizing Extrinsic Risks

Avoiding training errors can be the single most effective way to minimize extrinsic risks. In a typical exercise prescription, the client follows a format that may start with a warm-up, lead into cardiovascular activity (balanced by some muscular conditioning), and finish with a cooldown. Copy and use the checklists on page 220 to insure that each of these program segments is free of training errors.

Minimizing Intrinsic Risks

Intrinsic risks are the biomechanical or structural risks that each client brings to the exercise prescription. Always make it an objective of your prescription to correct malalignments, muscle imbalances, joint instability, and muscle tightness or weakness. A prescription must assess intrinsic risk to be truly client-centered.

RISK CONTROL CHECKLIST

Warm-Up

____ Use smooth, dynamic ROM movements—reaching as far as the muscle comfortably allows.

____ Avoid forced, prolonged, or rapid movements of the back.

____ Avoid hyperextension of the neck or lowering the head below the heart.

____ Avoid excessive reps with arms above shoulders; control arm speed.

____ Introduce and progress low-impact movements to raise temperature and heart rate.

____ After some warming, statically stretch the muscle groups to be used in the workout.

____ Add supplemental stretches if muscles are tight or sore, or if expecting higher intensity than usual.

____ Progress to pre-aerobic level (lower end of target heart rate).

____ If workout is to be high eccentric, build eccentric overloading gradually.

Cardiovascular

This checklist is particularly relevant if your client is unconditioned, just returing from a layoff, or moving up to the next level.

____ Avoid excessive stress, especially to the lower body, by using intervals, pyramids up and down, split routines, or a circuit.

____ Know the "stop point" where the feeling of burn replaces momentary fatigue (especially in eccentric work).

____ Check for excessive pronation, forefoot weight bearing, turning with foot planted.

____ Minimize impact shock by encouraging light feet and resilient knees, providing low-impact alternatives, and ensuring that footwear and floor surface are appropriate.

____ Intensity and duration are the training errors linked most closely to overuse injury. Look for signs of overtraining (e.g., decreased performance, lethargy, early fatigue, elevated heart rate).

____ A few minutes of cardiovascular cooldown are important for circulatory adjustments, and one of the best opportunities for gains in flexibility—hold static stretches for up to 30 seconds.

Muscular Conditioning

____ In designing a program, consider previous injuries to structures providing joint stability (e.g., include avoidance or rehabilitation).

____ Remember momentum and gravity as forces with which to contend.

____ Avoid excessive knee or back flexion, lifting arms with palms forward, and allowing hip extension to force the back into increased lumbar lordosis.

____ Remember that progression may be rapid initially, then level off.

____ Intervene with help or with an exercise alternative when technique or condition appear to be a problem.

____ Suggest beginning with a light set and following with static stretch of the muscle(s) used (especially if used eccentrically).

____ Think *muscle balance*—remember, the cardiovascular activity has already worked selected muscles.

Cooldown

____ Relieve anticipated muscle tightness that may result from eccentric work—e.g., in quadriceps, calves, and erector spinae.

____ Stretch tight postural muscles—e.g., anterior chest, hip flexors, hamstrings.

____ Be sure client is relaxed and cool before heading back to daily routine.

LINKS:

"Too Painful to Jog"

A 35-year-old female has approached you about some pain she has recently felt in her Achilles and just below her patella. She had been jogging 20-25 min/session, 2-3 days/week for the last five weeks and had been asymptomatic. Five days ago she went for a 2-hour volleyball tryout after a regular jog. The pain escalated over the next three days to the point where it was too painful to jog.

The repetitive eccentric motion of the volleyball activity was sufficient to cause irritation to the muscle tendon unit of the Achilles and patellar areas. A normal initial inflammatory process has taken place; icing and rest are advised until the symptoms disappear. In the interim, an aquafit program, upper body resistance work with some tubing, and some therapeutic exercises for her lower legs will refocus on some new and some parallel goals until she can resume jogging. Some counseling about overuse may be warranted.

This approach has dealt with the extrinsic causes of the injury and will probably get the client back to jogging within a reasonable time. However, you have not yet addressed the potential for reinjury due to a possible structural weakness (intrinsic). Once the discomfort has subsided, examining your client's muscle balance/alignment (chapter 5) will identify weak links and provide a basis for therapeutic exercise prescription.

You can combine these activity suggestions to correct intrinsic needs with guidelines emerging from the extrinsic causes of injury to design the core prescription for your client. From this point, progress with your client through the three steps of the overuse intervention progression: Hardening, Fitness, and Risk Control.

Highlights

- The muscle-tendon complex has properties of elasticity up to a point (elastic range), after which permanent deformation occurs.

- **Tendinitis** is an inflammatory response to microstructural damage of the collagen fibers.

- **Overuse injuries** may be caused by

    1. intrinsic factors unique to your client, such as malalignment and muscle imbalance; or

    2. extrinsic factors including training errors, technique, and environment.

- **Training errors** can usually be traced to

    1. excessive force in the development of momentum; or

    2. repetitive force contributing to overuse.

- The greatest muscular forces are generated through eccentric contractions; more strain is placed on connective tissue when it is elongated under tension.

- Watch for an opportunity to intervene early in an overuse situation, such as at times of increases in intensity or loading, changes to surface or environment, change of shoes, beginning of a new activity, or resumption of training after a period of inactivity.

- **Overuse Intervention** Progression:

    1. Healing and hardening

    2. Fitness and focus

    3. Risk control

- Use intervention techniques when approaching clients to provide support, safety, or modification. Watching and correcting your clients' technique will provide opportunities to teach, motivate, and prevent injury.

Chapter 14

Exercise Prescription for Injury Recovery and Prevention

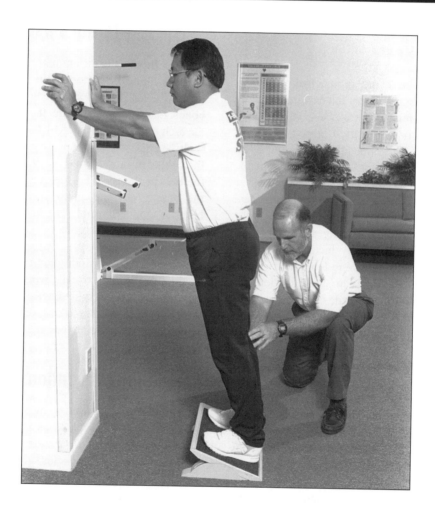

- Anti-Inflammatory Treatment
- Plantar Fasciitis
- Achilles Tendinitis
- Shin Splints
- Patellofemoral Syndrome

- Hamstring Strain
- Lower Back Pain
- Rotator Cuff Tendinitis (Impingement Syndrome)

This chapter should help anyone who works with clients recovering from, or having a history of, orthopedic injury. You will find a brief description and a background in functional anatomy for each of the conditions listed above, along with probable causes and strategies for prevention. You will find specific exercise designs for stretching and for strengthening injured tissues.

Anti-Inflammatory Treatment

Inflammation can hamper reconditioning in many overuse injuries. Prevention or elimination of inflammation must be a priority both before and during exercise prescriptions.

Revision and Rest

The first step is to correct any biomechanical abnormality or training error that may have caused inflammation—e.g., work-related overuse, continuation of a sport while injured, or aggravation caused by poorly designed exercises. The affected muscles must be allowed to rest, sometimes for several weeks depending on the pain. Andrish and Work (1990) suggest stopping the offending activity until the pain subsides, usually in about one to two weeks. At that time, your client may gradually resume training at about half the previous intensity and gradually increase the effort over three to six weeks. Returning too quickly is the most common reason injuries recur. Pay attention that the warm-up and cooldown include complete stretching to the affected area.

Cryotherapy

The use of cold (cryotherapy) is not only effective immediately after an injury or flare-up; it should be continued as long as inflammation persists. Ice causes local vasoconstriction and slows metabolic activity; it relieves pain and muscle spasm. When your client has joint pain, stop all painful activities immediately. Stop the workout early and use the time to ice the joint. Continue with two or three cold treatments per day, lasting 8-10 minutes each. Curwin (1984) recommends that ice be applied at the end of every activity session and more frequently when the tendinitis is acute.

Medications

Aspirin or ibuprofen may also help ease symptoms if your client has no medical contraindications. When inflammation is acute, have your client take the medication regularly (without exceeding the label limit). If inflammation persists or worsens, your client should see a physician.

For this type of injury, several acronyms have emerged (e.g., RICE). Adding a P to the phrase introduces the awareness of prevention not just treatment to the equation: **PRICE (Prevention, Rest, Ice, Compression, Elevation).** Relative rest is obviously protective. But always design activities your clients can do to enhance healing and maintain fitness, not simply avoid certain activities. For example, if your client has a running injury, running in water with a flotation belt can be an effective alternative.

Plantar Fasciitis

Plantar fasciitis is inflammation of the strong tissue that runs along the bottom of the foot and connects the heel to the base of the toes. Along with the muscles and bones, this connective tissue, the plantar fascia, forms the arch of the foot (figure 14.1). The plantar fascia is multilayered fibrous connective tissue. It arises from the calcaneus and forms five divisions that insert on the ball of the foot. By tensing like a bowstring on the plantar surface of the feet, the plantar fascia helps to support the arch. The Achilles tendon attaches from the calcaneus to the soleus and gastrocnemius muscles.

What starts as a slight pain in a client's heel may gradually build. It is usually worse the first step of the morning and can be quite intense when the area bears weight such as with walking or running. A sufferer may limp or bear weight on the lateral side of the foot to ease the pain.

Cause and Prevention

Plantar fasciitis is caused by overstretching the fascia. Alignment problems such as overpronation or low arches may contribute. Pressure on the fascia may be due to weak foot muscles—including the small intrinsic muscles in the foot and other muscles in the lower leg such as the flexor digitorum and tibialis posterior. Tight gastrocnemius and soleus muscles can also cause fasciitis by keeping the Achilles tendon tight, thereby making the ankle less flexible and forcing the plantar fascia to absorb more weight. Any activity in which the weight is taken on the ball of the foot—such as high impact aerobics, basketball, sprinting, tennis, or bounding—can create excessive pull on the fascia.

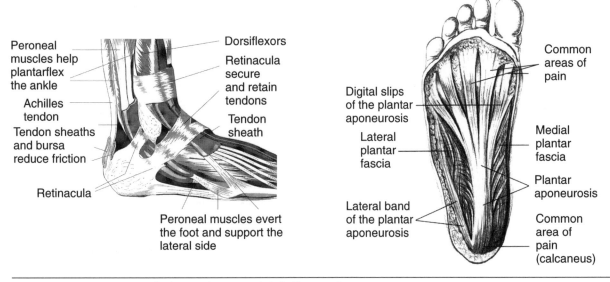

Figure 14.1 Anatomy of plantar fascia and Achilles tendon.

Massaging with ice for five to seven minutes can be effective. Apply cold packs for up to 20 minutes (Rizzo 1991). Before advising clients to be fitted for an orthotic, help them look for good supportive footwear with distinct arch support, strong heel cup, and full sole cushioning. A heel lift may also be needed. Although people with plantar fasciitis should avoid some high trauma activities, other activities such as recline cycling, swimming, pool running, rowing machines, or circuit weight training should not produce discomfort. Anything that produces pain should be avoided. Walkers should decrease their mileage, avoid hills, and look for a softer surface.

Stretching Guidelines and Prescription

Gentle, prolonged stretching should be pain-free. Stretching exercises should focus on the Achilles tendon and the soleus and gastrocnemius muscles. Figure 14.2a shows a soleus stretch with the rear knee bent to further elongate the Achilles.

A simple wedged heel-cord box (figure 14.2b) can facilitate stretching (Tanner and Harvey 1988). Your client can achieve more complete fiber elongation by using variations such as straight knees or toes inward/outward.

Massage and foot manipulation can help relax tight, rigid connective tissue in the foot itself and in the intrinsic muscles. Have your injured client do stretching at least twice a day.

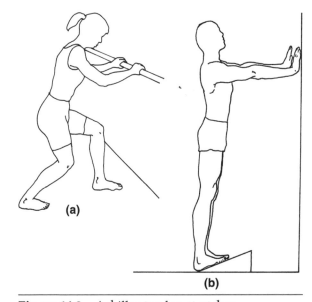

Figure 14.2 Achilles tendon stretches.

Strengthening Guidelines and Prescription

Weak foot muscles may not be able to support the dynamic structure of the foot. Strong muscles are required to help maintain a sound arch and withstand the sometimes three- to five-fold load increase placed on the plantar fascia when, for example, the foot is landing during a moderate downhill run (Batt and Tanji 1995). Once the foot is pain-free and flexibility is returning, your client should begin strengthening

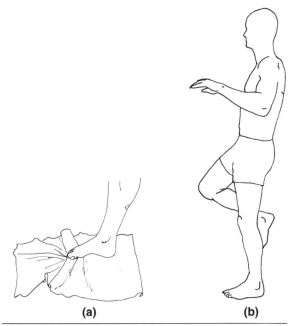

Figure 14.3 (a) Toe curls with towel. (b) Single leg balance.

exercises. By using her toes to pull a towel (figure 14.3a) or to grasp a marble, your client can condition the intrinsic muscles of her foot and the toe flexors that help support the arch. Daily practice of this exercise may still take six weeks to improve the foot's configuration.

Balancing on one leg will help strengthen and reacquaint the lower leg muscles with the proper support alignment (figure 14.3b).

Before you permit resumption of full intensity activity, prescribe a progression using closed kinetic chain (weightbearing) exercises including the ankle, knee, and hip (chapter 11).

Achilles Tendinitis

Achilles tendinitis is inflammation of the tendon, its sheath, or the bursae (figure 14.1). Your client may describe pain located two to five centimeters above the calcaneus (Prentice 1994). In early, mild tendinitis, the foot loosens up at the beginning of activity but the pain gradually increases. More advanced, chronic Achilles tendinitis causes pain when your client climbs stairs or walks normally; it escalates with activity and subsides with rest; and may be accompanied by weakness during plantar flexion. Morning stiffness, poor flexibility, and swelling/tightness of the calf muscles are common symptoms.

Cause and Prevention

Racquet sports players and longer distance runners are particularly susceptible to Achilles tendinitis. The com-

bination of repetitive microtrauma from these activities and excessive pronation is particularly risky. Insufficient stretching or rapid overstretching can lead to damage. The injury is often slow to heal because of poor vascularization in the lower part of the tendon (Myerson and Biddinger 1995). Have your clients avoid repetitive, weight-bearing dorsiflexion, particularly during high-impact eccentric contractions of the calf muscles such as the push-offs required by many sports. Once you have established the cause, prescribe specific changes to prevent further aggravation. Use cryotherapy immediately after the injury or flare-up, as well as into the reconditioning and management stages. Initial conservative management of mild to moderate Achilles tendinitis should involve a decrease in activity by at least 50%. Examine your client's running shoes for proper heel fit. If other biomechanical problems exist (chapter 5 and 13), consider adding a 1/4- to 1/2-inch heel lift or referring your client for orthotics. Low-impact activities such as cycling, rowing, swimming, low-impact aerobic dance, or most weight training—as long as they do not produce pain—can help your client maintain aerobic conditioning. Limit any toe push-offs.

Stretching Guidelines and Prescription

Your client should begin gentle, passive stretching as soon as pain allows. Have her stretch the Achilles tendon with a static dorsiflexion—knee straight (gastrocnemius) and bent (soleus) (figure 14.2a). Turning the toes slightly inward during stretches shown in figures 14.2a and b will enhance the Achilles stretch.

If these stretches create pain, have your client use partial or non-weightbearing ankle dorsiflexion stretches. Figure 14.4 shows a seated ankle dorsiflexion using tubing or Dynaband. This stretch may also be performed with a bent knee.

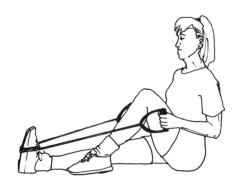

Figure 14.4 Seated tubing dorsiflexion.

Strengthening Guidelines and Prescription

Begin with light progressive resistance exercises for the calf muscles. One easy method is to work against tubing or an elastic band by placing the foot in the loop and pressing down (starting position as in figure 14.4). Dynamic plantar flexion with weights or a machine may start in a seated position (figure 14.5). Single leg balancing (figure 14.3b) and standing toe raises are fully weightbearing with a closed kinetic chain (chapter 11).

The final progressive stage prior to returning to activity should include progressive eccentric strengthening. This may be initiated with standing toe raises (figure 14.6), moving rapidly into plantar flexion

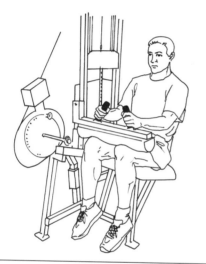

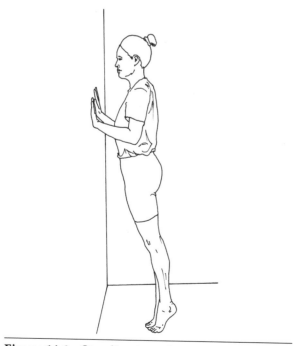

Figure 14.5 Seated heel lift.

Figure 14.6 Standing toe raises.

from a slow decent. A progression of this exercise involves performing it on the edge of a stair and allowing the heel to lower.

Shin Splints

Shin splints, or more precisely medial tibial stress syndrome (**MTSS**), is an inflammation of the fascia, tendon, periosteum, bone, or combination of these along the posterior medial border of the tibia (figure 14.7). The pain can range from a slightly uncomfortable dull ache to an intensity that makes weight bearing difficult.

Sometimes referred to as **posterior shin splints**, MTSS is probably associated with fatigue tear of fibers of the tibialis posterior muscle at its insertion into the periosteum of the tibia (Torg, Vegso, and Torg 1987). Shin splints are an overuse condition common to people who start a weightbearing training program too vigorously, to jumpers (e.g., volleyball, basketball, high-impact aerobics), and to runners logging more than 30 miles per week.

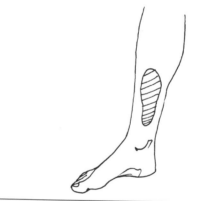

Figure 14.7 Pain location for shin splints (medial tibial stress syndrome).

Occurring in the upper anterior shin, **anterior shin splints** are aggravated by overuse of the tibialis anterior, and in some clients may reveal a stress fracture (Fick, Albright, and Murray 1992).

Cause and Prevention

MTSS pain is in the muscles that are active during the first 80% of the stance phase, such as the tibialis posterior and the flexors of the toes (Prentice 1994). The subtalar joint normally goes from a supinated position at heel strike to a pronated position during midstance, then returns to supination during push-off. Hyperpronation during midstance places these muscles under significant stress—they will contract eccentrically (lengthening) to try to stabilize, but eventually the point of attachment (origin) will become inflamed.

Other factors sometimes related to MTSS include a tight Achilles tendon, running on hard surfaces, progressing too rapidly in training, logging exceptionally long training hours, muscle imbalance between weak shin and strong calf muscles, and improper footwear. If a biomechanical abnormality or training error is the cause, it must first be corrected. Allow the affected muscles to rest, sometimes for several weeks depending on the pain. Use this time to ice (8-10 minutes, two or three times/day) and perhaps to investigate the need for orthotics or to ensure that the shoe is well-cushioned in the heel and insole. Andrish and Work (1990) suggest stopping the offending activity until the pain subsides (usually about one to two weeks), resuming training at about half the previous intensity, and gradually working up to previous levels over three to six weeks. Returning too quickly is the most common reason shin splints recur. Be sure your client pays close attention to warm-ups and cooldowns, ensuring complete stretching of the lower leg. Consider prescribing cross-training, particularly with non-weightbearing exercise such as swimming, stair-climbing, cycling, rowing, or low-impact aerobic classes. If your client is a die-hard jogger, direct her to the grass or flat bark-covered trails and increase mileage before increasing intensity throughout the recovery.

Stretching Guidelines and Prescription

Inflammation of the tibialis posterior and flexors of the toes causes tightness and decreased flexibility. Stretching exercises should target these muscles as well as the gastrocnemius, soleus, tibialis anterior, and peroneals. After some aerobic exercise to warm the muscles, your client should do static stretches several times, holding all the stretches at least 30 seconds and holding stretches for the Achilles tendon up to 60 seconds. The heel cord box as shown in figure 14.2b is very effective. The bent knee position aids in stretching the tibialis posterior as well as the soleus.

Figure 14.4 utilizes surgical tubing (or Dynaband) to stretch the calf muscles. The peroneal muscles on the lateral side of the calf are the ankle evertors, and can be stretched by wrapping a Dynaband around the lateral side of the foot and pulling the ankle into inversion (figure 14.8). Your client should relax at the end of the range of motion to feel the stretch.

Using the Dynaband or a hand (figure 14.9), pull the foot up behind, bringing the heel to the buttock. This shifts the stretch to the front of the shin to reach the tibialis anterior.

Toe curls with a towel (figure 14.3a) will strengthen the flexors of the toes and the tibialis posterior as

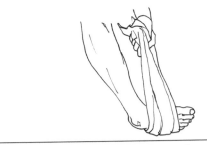

Figure 14.8   Dynaband peroneal stretch.

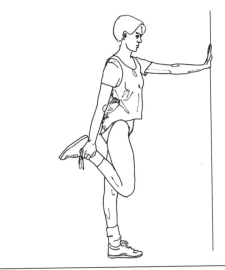

Figure 14.9   Heel to buttock stretch.

well as strengthening the arch to minimize hyperpronation.

Strengthening Guidelines and Prescription

The affected muscles in shin splints usually show signs of weakness and early fatigue. Start a strengthening program when the pain is minimal. The anterior muscle groups are very often weak and out of balance with the posterior plantar flexors. Movements as simple as seated or standing toe lifts or drawing the alphabet with the feet usually present enough of an overload for the early stages of conditioning. The opposite foot, a partner's resistance, or surgical tubing can all be used to create added resistance to this dorsiflexion.

Clients with MTSS (posterior shin splints) should also strengthen their ankle evertors and invertors. A uniplane wobble board, which is simple to build (figure 14.10), can be used with the foot aligned with the half-cylinder keel under the board. Have your client rock back and forth in a controlled manner, touching the right edge then the left edge. Although a well-cushioned shoe is mandatory for a return to training, most of the rehabilitation exercises will provide greater benefit if done with bare feet.

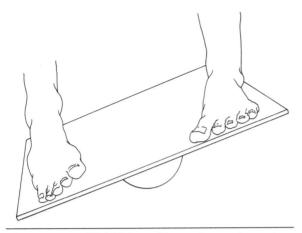

Figure 14.10   Wobbleboard inversion and eversion.

Patellofemoral Syndrome

The patella moves up and down within a groove at the front of the femur (figure 14.11). Deviation from this aligned tracking produces **patellofemoral pain** resulting from irritation behind the patella and wearing of the articular cartilage.

Clients may complain of pain in the front of the knee when they sit in a car or at the movies, kneel or squat, get up from a chair and start walking, or go up or down stairs. The pain may appear at the beginning or end of a workout, and may result in swelling or fullness in the knee. Other symptoms may include giving way, popping, catching, or locking (Doucette and Goble 1992). Patellofemoral syndrome is one of the most common knee complaints, accounting for 57.5% of the knee injuries in one group of runners (Taunton et al. 1987). It occurs most often in women, in the young, and in those who are active in running or in court sports such as basketball and tennis.

Cause and Prevention

Improper alignment and tracking of the patella is a major cause of patellofemoral pain (figure 14.11c). Your clients may notice such pain especially as they run up hills or straighten their knees with weights. Causes of poor tracking include the following:

■ Deficiency of supporting and stabilizing muscles. Kneecap motion is guided by the quadriceps, particularly the vastus medialis. This muscle may be less resistant to fatigue than the vastus lateralis, creating an uneven pull on the patella (Prentice 1994).

■ Tightness of supporting structures. If the vastus lateralis or the lateral retinaculum (figure 14.11a) are tight, lateral tilting or tracking of the patella may occur. Because the iliotibial band is connected to the lateral retinaculum, its tightness may affect tracking during flexion. Both the hamstrings and the gastrocnemius cross the knee joint, and tightness can increase patellar pressure. Tight hamstrings increase knee flexion and can change lower leg mechanics. A tight gastrocnemius muscle can limit dorsiflexion and produce excessive subtalar motion (Galea and Albers 1994).

■ Structural alignments. Wide hips and knock-knees may contribute to lateral tracking of the patella (Prentice 1994). An awareness of this alignment problem can help you direct your client to alternate activities or reduce the prescription load. Excessive pronation of the foot usually causes a rotation of the tibia, which may result in increased lateral pull on the patella. Orthotics may be appropriate.

■ Besides poor tracking, patellofemoral syndrome may be caused by acute trauma, chronic repetitive stress such as running, sudden increases in workloads or mileage, uneven or hilly terrain, or poor running shoes.

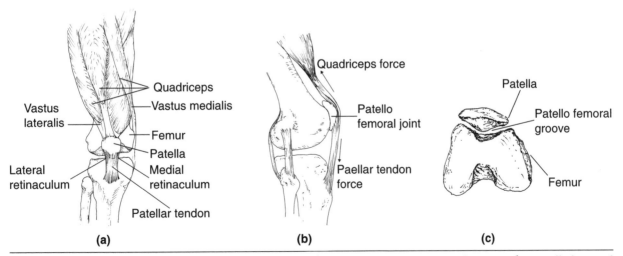

Figure 14.11   Anatomy of the patellofemoral joint with (a) anterior knee joint (b) forces on the patellofemoral joint and (c) patellofemoral tracking.

Have your client replace running shoes that are older than a year, have more than 500 miles on them, or look worn out on the soles or broken down on the uppers.

Ask at-risk clients if they have changed their intensity, distance, or terrain. Have them stay away from hills, switch to lower impact aerobic activities, or decrease mileage. When a client has knee pain, stop all painful activities for at least two to four weeks. Aspirin or ibuprofen may help ease symptoms, as may icing.

Stretching Guidelines and Prescription

Tightness in a number of muscles may contribute to patellofemoral pain: vastus lateralis, iliotibial band, hamstrings, and gastrocnemius. Stretching the quadriceps (including vastus lateralis) can decrease patellofemoral compression during dynamic activities. However, stretching this muscle may be contraindicated if pain exists past the 70 degree position of knee flexion. From a prone position, your client should flex one knee to the end of the active ROM. If there is no pain, she should then reach back and grasp the ankle with the opposite hand and continue gently to increase the knee flexion (figure 14.12a). If she has difficulty reaching her ankle, you can passively assist the stretch.

To stretch the iliotibial band, your client stands with legs crossed. The affected leg is close to an adjacent wall or table and behind the other leg. She then moves

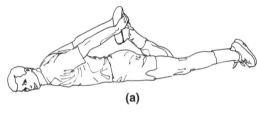

(a)

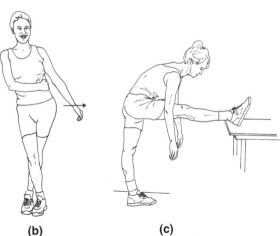

(b)   **(c)**

Figure 14.12   (a) Vastus lateralis stretch. (b) Iliotibial band stretch. (c) Hamstring stretch.

her pelvis toward the table, keeping the back leg straight (figure 14.12b).

To stretch the hamstrings, your client places one leg on a table with knees straight. While holding her back straight, she bends forward from the hips to a point of tension. After about 20 seconds, she lowers slightly, tilting the pelvis forward and holding for another 10-15 seconds (figure 14.12c). The gastrocnemius can be stretched effectively with exercises shown in figures 14.2 and 14.4.

Strengthening Guidelines and Prescription

To guarantee a safe return to normal activities, your client must fully regain strength in the injured leg. Have her do the following exercises every second day, and stop if there is any pain or she is unable to do the exercise correctly. Most people do well by progressing from about 5 to 15 repetitions, then adding a second set and building from 10 to 15 reps. She should allow a minute or two between sets, depending on her stage of recovery, eventually building to four or five sets. Exercises to strengthen the vastus medialis will promote a return to muscular balance and increase the medial stabilization of the patella.

Start with end range extensions (figure 14.13a), in which your client reclines with a firm pillow or rolled towel under her knee to create about 30 degrees of flexion. With her hip slightly rotated laterally and the opposite knee flexed, she then straightens her knee and holds for 10 seconds. Small ankle weights can increase resistance.

Exercises with the foot in a fixed position on the ground (closed chain exercises) are especially functional because they use common movement patterns and act to control the body's momentum (eccentric contractions) as well as to teach kinesthetic awareness. Closed kinetic chain exercises are favored in therapeutic exercise prescription, particularly for the knee (Prentice 1994). Closed kinetic chain exercises include leg press, partial squats, stepping, stationary cycling, and plyometrics. Two specific examples of closed chain exercises are forward lunges (figure 14.13b) and step-downs (figure 14.13c).

In a forward lunge, your client steps forward about 2-3 feet from a standing position, keeping the knee over the foot and not allowing the front knee to flex more than 90 degrees. At the same time, she lowers the back knee until it is 4 to 6 inches from the floor. She returns to an upright position and alternates legs. As her strength increases, she can hold small hand weights.

In a step-down, she stands sideways on a bottom step or aerobic step box with the injured leg nearest the

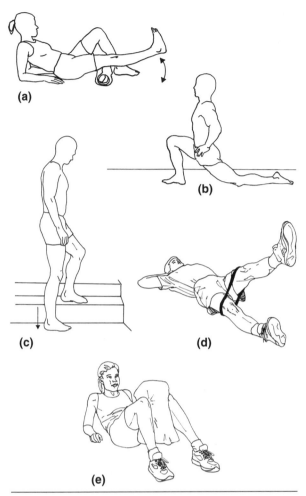

Figure 14. 13 (a) End range extensions. (b) Forward lunges. (c) Step-downs. (d) Straight leg raises with tubing. (e) Inner thigh pillow squeeze.

stair. Slowly she bends the injured knee until the opposite foot lightly touches the ground, then slowly straightens it. As she progresses, she may add hand weights or use higher steps.

Working with a wobble board (figure 14.10) can strengthen supporting muscles of the lower leg.

Open chain exercises (the foot is free), such as provided by isokinetic knee extension equipment, can isolate a muscle such as the vastus medialis by using ROM stops for the last 30 degrees of extension. They can also introduce higher speed contractions under stabilized conditions, which may be appropriate for athletes.

Rubber tubing or Dynabands can also be used, especially when knee movement is still painful. From a lying position, with the tubing around both legs just above the knee, your client performs straight leg raises to strengthen hip flexors (figure 14.13d).

Finally, since most of the vastus medialis originates from the tendon of the adductor magnus (Doucette and Goble 1991), strengthening the muscles of the inner

thigh may help pull the kneecap into alignment. For the inner thigh pillow squeeze (figure 14.13e), have your client hold or pulse the squeeze for 15 to 20 seconds, repeating 3 to 5 times.

Hamstring Strain

The hamstring muscle, located on the posterior thigh, comprises the semimembranosus, semitendinosus, and biceps femoris (figure 14.14). The hamstrings are biarticular (two-joint) muscles producing extension of the hip and flexion of the knee. As with other frequently injured biarticular muscles, the hamstrings are subject to stretching at more than one point. Injuries to this muscle complex usually affect the common origin on the ischial tuberosity, and may affect the insertion behind the knee or the belly of the muscle.

Symptoms include tenderness and, usually, a large area of swelling. An injured person feels discomfort when gentle resistance is applied against knee flexion and hip extension.

Hamstring strains are described in three grades. Grade I sufferers complain of tightness at the end range of hip flexion and some pain or palpation. People with Grade II strains usually have adjusted their gaits, perhaps landing flat-footed with limited swing-through. Knee flexion and hip extension may cause moderate to severe pain with noticeable weakness. Recovery takes between one and three weeks. Grade III hamstring strains usually require the use of crutches and require a three- to twelve-week rehabilitation period (De Palma 1994).

Cause and Prevention

Hamstring strains are common with sprinters, gymnasts, and athletes in soccer, football, and basketball. They can result from a quick, explosive contraction

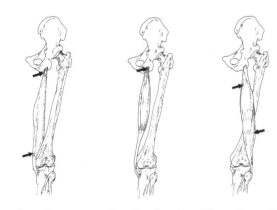

Semimembraneous   Semitendinosis   Biceps femoris

Figure 14. 14 Anatomy of the hamstrings. Arrows indicate most common sites of injury.

while the hip is in flexion and the knee is extending. The hamstring muscles decelerate the forward swing of the tibia, thus opposing the activity of the quadriceps. The imbalance of an overly strong quadriceps may cause the injury. Other causes may be hamstring fatigue, tight hamstrings, imbalance between the medial and lateral hamstrings, or improper running style.

The strong tendency for hamstring injuries to recur makes a solid case for a supplemental exercise prescription including stretching, strengthening, and cardiovascular maintenance. Best and Garrett (1996) report that following a hamstring injury, there is decreased flexibility and lower eccentric strength. Initial treatment typically consists of rest, ice, compression (elastic wrap), elevation, and pain relief (e.g., acetaminophen for 7 to 10 days). After the acute stages, heat (hot packs, whirlpool, or heating pad) may be used before the stretching exercises (Torg, Vegso, and Torg 1987). All activities should be followed by ice treatments to decrease inflammation and discomfort. Although someone with a grade I hamstring strain may continue to be active, a supplementary prescription for extra stretching and strengthening should begin immediately to avoid further injury.

Stretching Guidelines and Prescription

In addition to predisposing your client to a hamstring strain, tight hamstrings may cause low back pain. Because they attach to the back of the pelvis (see figure 14.14), tight hamstrings can prevent the pelvis from tilting forward when the spine flexes, forcing all movement to come from the lower back. Avoid stretches such as standing or sitting toe touches, where the lower body is static and the upper body is rounded and actively flexing.

The doorway hamstring stretch (figure 14.15a) promotes a static upper body with a lower body hip flexion. Your client lies on his back in a doorway with his buttocks close to the wall. One leg extends through the door while the other is raised up against the wall. The heel slides up the wall, gradually straightening the leg; after the client feels a comfortable, pleasant stretch, he holds his position for 30 to 60 seconds.

The straddle hamstring stretch (figure 14.15b) uses a table or chair for support. With feet pointing forward and one foot 3-4 feet behind the another, your client bends forward at the hips (not the waist) while holding the table for support. As the front leg stretches, she must avoid hyperextending the knee. She holds for 30 seconds, lowers slightly, and holds for another 15-30 seconds. Maintaining the lumbar lordotic curve in the lower back isolates the hamstrings and safeguards the back.

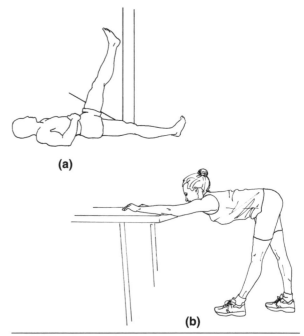

Figure 14.15   (a) Doorway hamstring stretch. (b) Straddle hamstring stretch.

You may need to delay these stretches until the second week for grade II hamstring strains. Active ROM movements in a prone or seated position can begin earlier or as soon as there is no pain (De Palma 1994). Work with a physician or physiotherapist for the timing on grade III strains; but your client should be pain-free.

Strengthening Guidelines and Prescription

You can begin resistive strengthening exercises immediately for a grade I strain, after about 3-6 days for grade II, and after 10-14 days of treatment in a grade III strain (De Palma 1994).

Avoid resistance exercises using a machine (such as knee flexion in a prone position), since the hamstrings are less efficient in a shortened position. However, knee flexion from a seated position allows the hamstrings to start stretched at the buttocks, improving their mechanical advantage in working through a full ROM. An added advantage with some machines is the ability to change the lever arm and torque by adjusting the position of the lower leg pad. A straight leg hip extension machine is also safe for strengthening hamstrings. If such a machine is not available, substitute elastic tubing or bands (figure 14.16).

Isokinetic exercises, such as with an electronic Cybex knee flexion machine, are effective in conjunction with isotonic and isometric exercises. Progressions to faster speeds may be more sport-specific for athletes.

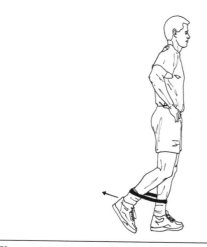

Figure 14.16 Straight leg hip extension with tubing.

In later phases of all three grades of hamstring strains, educate your clients to perform light-weight squats—foot fixed on the ground, and the lower body joints forming a kinetic chain (closed).

If your client is pain-free, have him swim or bike to maintain cardiovascular condition. Add jogging a few days later if appropriate. Simulate sport-specific activities for athletes, gradually introducing those skills that involve eccentric contraction of the hamstrings.

Lower Back Pain

Back pain usually arises in the soft tissues such as ligaments, fascia, and muscle, and with most clients should last no longer than three weeks. Ninety percent of clients with back pain should lose their symptoms within six weeks (Waddell 1987). People whose pain persists beyond six weeks, or who have exacerbated a previous injury, usually have not removed the stresses that created the original injury.

General Considerations for Prescription

Be aware of the stage of the injury. Gradually introduce appropriate exercises, following the acute treatment stage of the therapist (mainly modality treatment and pain relief). Be sure that your clients ask their therapists or physicians for any precautions or advice that will help you design a safe and effective exercise plan.

Base your exercise prescription goals for back rehabilitation on the specific diagnosis, history, and evaluation your client receives from his physician or therapist:

- Which structures/muscles need stretching?
- Which structures/muscles need strengthening?
- What deviations in posture, alignment, and stabilization need attention (see chapter 5)?

- What faults are present in movement mechanics in daily life, work environment, sport, or exercise routine (see chapter 13)?

Back pain can result from one or a combination of problems (Hooker 1994). See the brief descriptions, with implications for exercise, in table 14.1 on page 236. Then study figures 14.18 through 14.31 to learn a variety of exercises that will increase both the strength and the flexibility of the back.

Rotator Cuff Tendinitis (Impingement Syndrome)

Impingement in the shoulder is common because the space between the top of the humerus and the bottom of the acromion (the "roof" of the shoulder) is not particularly large (figure 14.17). Under certain circumstances, any of the structures running through the space—the supraspinatus tendon, the tendon of the long head of the biceps, or the shoulder bursa—can be impinged upon. Impingement usually occurs between the greater tubercle and either the acromion or the shoulder ligaments.

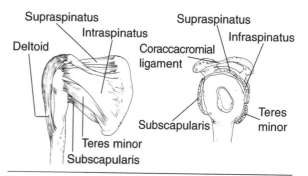

Figure 14.17 Anatomy of the shoulder rotator cuff.

Impingement syndrome often originates with soft tissue trauma that sets up a cycle of pain, biomechanical changes, and weakness. Swelling of the tissues makes the space even smaller, further irritating the tendons. There also may be reduced blood supply and the start of tendon degeneration. Pain may occur when the shoulder is abducted while internally (medially) rotated. Any movement that calls for raising the arm overhead while internally rotated has the potential to impinge on the tendons and bursa and cause injury.

Cause and Prevention

In clients without a history of trauma, repetitive overhead motion is usually the causative factor. As the muscles fatigue, tendon degeneration occurs. This is evident in activities with rapid eccentric contraction of

Table 14.1 Low Back Conditions and Exercise Implications

CONDITION	DESCRIPTION/CAUSE	EXERCISE IMPLICATION
(1) Muscular strain	Clients report a history of sudden or chronic stress that initiates pain in a muscular area during the workout. Pain is provoked by contraction or stretching of the involved muscle.	Mild contraction followed with a stretch (figures 14.18, 19, 20). Progress with intensity. Include abdominal strengthening (figures 14.26, 29, 30) and active extension exercise (figures 14.24, 28, 31).
(2) Piriformis or quadratus lumborum myofascial pain or strain	The Piriformis muscle refers pain to the posterior sacroiliac region and buttocks. It is a deep ache that worsens when sitting with hips flexed or adducted or during weight-bearing stops, and starts involving hip rotation. Pain from the quadratus lumborum is an aching or sharp pain in the lateral back area and upper buttock. Pain is felt on moving from sitting to standing, prolonged standing, or sneezing.	Stretching is the main component in changing any myofascial pain. Exercises should include stretching exercises such as figures 14.19, 14.20 and 14.23. They should also include strengthening exercises such as figures 14.25, 27, 30, 31).
(3) Lumbar facet joint sprains	The client will report a specific event that caused the problem, or a series of repetitive stresses that progressively got more painful. Pain gets sharper with certain movements. The pain feels deep and localized near the spinous process.	Stretching in all directions (figure 14.24, 26, 28, 29) should be within a comfort range (figures 14.18, 19, 21). Exercises should involve joint mobility, trunk stabilization, and posture control. Pain-free abdominal and back strengthening is important.
(4) Disc-related back problems	Pain is usually central but radiates across the back of one side. The client may describe a sudden or gradual onset after a workout that becomes more severe during resumption of activity. Forward bending and sitting increase pain, and a postural analysis may reveal a shifted hip and slightly flexed posture.	Unless working with a therapist, prescribe only gentle mobilization and postural exercises until the client is pain-free (figures 14.18, 21, 22). At this point, abdominal and back extensor strengthening should be emphasized with an eye to preventing re-injury (figures 14.24, 26, 27, 28).
(5) Sacroiliac (SI) joint dysfunction	The client will describe a dull, achy back pain near the bone prominences of the SI joint. The pain may radiate to the buttocks or thigh particularly during hip flexion, side bending to the painful side, or during the stance phase of walking. Pain may also be felt during trunk rotations, landing heavily on one leg, kicking, jumping, etc.	If one side of the back is tight, stretching is important (figures 14.19, 20, 23). Exercises that help (re)gain alignment and stability of the pelvis are important. Appropriate exercises may include figures 14.25, 14.26, 14.27, 14.28.

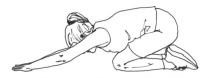

Figure 14.18 Kneeling back stretch. Tuck head and reach forward. Round the back and move the chest toward the floor.

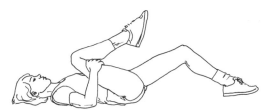

Figure 14.19 Single knee to chest. Lie supine with lower back pushed down. Pull one knee to the chest—enough to feel a comfortable stretch in the lower back.

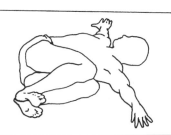

Figure 14.20 Lying knee rocking. Lie supine with knees bent 90 degrees. Allow knees to slowly rock from side to side through a pain-free range of motion. The back will rotate slightly.

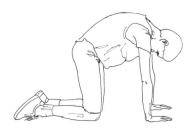

Figure 14.21 Mad cat stretch. Arch back while tucking your chin and tightening the stomach.

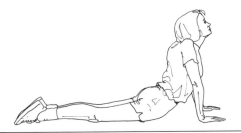

Figure 14.22 Prone press-up. From a prone position, extend elbows to raise upper body. Hips stay on the floor and the back is relaxed.

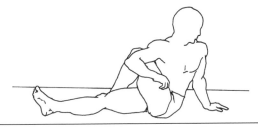

Figure 14.23 Spinal twist. Sit with right leg straight and left leg bent and on the outside of the right knee. Place the right elbow on the outside of the upper left thigh. Slowly turn head to look over the left shoulder.

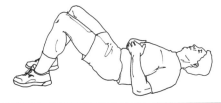

Figure 14.24 Back press. Lying on back with knees bent, tighten stomach by pressing elbows to floor.

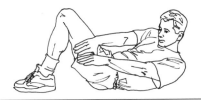

Figure 14.25 Diagonal curl-up. Lying on back with knees bent at 90 degrees and pelvis stabilized, raise head and shoulders while rotating to one side, reaching with arms at sides.

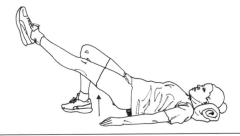

Figure 14.26 Hip lift bridge. Lying on back with both knees bent 90 degrees, lift buttocks from the floor and extend one knee, keeping stomach tight.

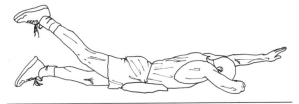

Figure 14.27 Opposite arm and leg lifts. From a prone position (or on all fours) raise opposite arm and leg 4 to 6 inches from the floor. Firm pillows or rolled towels should be under the pelvis and forehead.

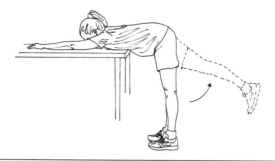

Figure 14.28   Supported hip extension. With the torso leaning flat over a table, raise legs alternately from the floor.

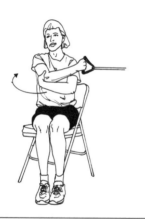

Figure 14.29   Seated trunk rotation with tubing. Hold band tight to chest (taut) and gently rotate away with pelvis and knees in place and back straight. Do only a pain-free range of motion.

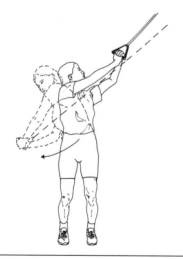

Figure 14.30   Diagonal downward rotation with tubing. Standing with feet shoulder-width apart, pull tubing with both hands downward across the body.

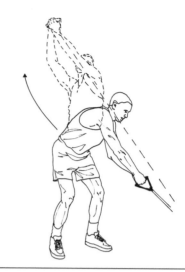

Figure 14.31   Diagonal upward rotation with tubing. Standing with feet shoulder-width apart, pull tubing with both hands, straightening the body and rotating away from the door/anchor.

the external (lateral) rotators such as throwing, swimming the butterfly, and serving in tennis. For example, someone doing an upright row exercise rotates his shoulder internally as he raises it. Raising the elbows high magnifies the danger of impingement. Another cause of impingement is muscle imbalance. The potential for muscle imbalance is high: major muscles such as the pectoralis major and latissimus dorsi rotate internally, countered only by small muscles such as the infraspinatus and teres major (chapter 5). Proper biomechanics requires a fine balance between joint mobility and stability. Overlooking such common causes may lead to progression of the impingement.

Modification of activities or of the workplace is critical for prevention and treatment. You can modify some activities to allow limited participation. Suggest swimming with fins and kicking only, or avoiding overhead serving when playing tennis or volleyball. Monitor your client's technique for faults such as upright rowing or lateral flies with the thumbs pointing down. To promote circulation in the shoulder area, prescribe upper body aerobics such as cross-country skiing, rowing, or arm ergometry.

Stretching Guidelines and Prescription

After testing for postural alignment and muscle tightness (chapter 5), address muscle imbalance with static stretches or PNF stretches (chapter 11). Demonstrate proper execution of shoulder exercises, including ROM exercises as in figure 14.32. Be sure that your client performs stretches with relaxed shoulder girdles and proper alignment, and with elbows below shoulder height in order to avoid entrapment of the supraspinatus tendon. Figures 14.33 and 14.34 illustrate specific stretches for internal and external rotators, designed to maintain muscle balance.

Overdevelopment or overtightness of the pectoralis major and anterior deltoid can force the shoulder into internal rotation. Figures 14.35 and 14.36 show exercises designed to stretch these muscles as well as the long head of the biceps.

Strengthening Guidelines and Prescription

Before progressing to specific shoulder joint resistive exercises, your clients should be able to lift their humerus (thumbs down) to 90 degrees while maintaining

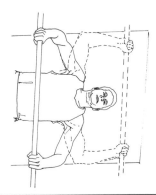

Figure 14.32 Lying wand shoulder rotations. Lying on table or floor, move wand toward head, then down toward waist through a pain-free range of motion.

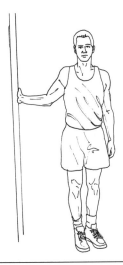

Figure 14.33 Doorway internal rotator stretch. With shoulder abducted 60 degrees and externally rotated, turn body gently away from doorway and hold.

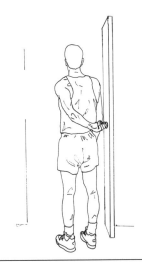

Figure 14.34 Doorway external rotator stretch. With shoulder abducted 60 degrees and externally rotated, turn body gently away from doorway and hold.

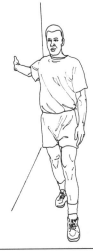

Figure 14.35 Wall pectoralis stretch. With the arm horizontally abducted against a wall, turn your body away from the wall. Repeat with elbow bent.

the scapula stabilized in retraction (adduction). The exercise for this involves actively stabilizing the scapula in retraction while actively abducting the arms with elbows flexed. Figure 14.37 illustrates another exercise for this training as well as for strengthening the scapular retractors.

A shoulder strengthening program for prevention/treatment of rotator cuff tendinitis centers around two activities: (1) strengthening the external rotators to maintain muscle balance, and (2) strengthening the supraspinatus because of its role in impingement syndrome.

Figures 14.38 and 14.39 show resistive exercises for strengthening the external rotators. Use of tubing or dumbbells can strengthen the supraspinatus and deltoids.

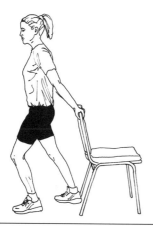

Figure 14.36 Anterior deltoid/biceps stretch. Reach behind you with a straight arm and grasp the top of a chair. Move your body forward and downward with arm directly back.

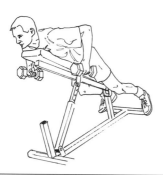

Figure 14.37 Scapular retraction with dumbbells.

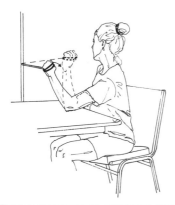

Figure 14.38 Shoulder external rotation with tubing. Pull tubing away from anchor point. Keep elbow bent at 90 degrees.

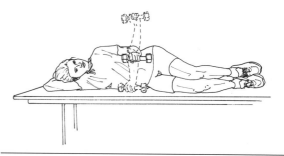

Figure 14.39 Sidelying flies with dumbbells.

The strengthening program should progressively increase repetitions, and then resistance, to build a strength and endurance base. Free weight exercises train proprioception and stabilization and should always be present. Tubing, machines, and isokinetics help movement in various positions and speeds.

Always keep in mind the impingement zone and the stage of rehabilitation. Clients should continue on a maintenance program of core exercises several times per week, and continue applying ice after workouts.

Highlights

- Inflammation such as tendinitis should be controlled by practicing **PRICE** (Prevention, Rest, Ice, Compression, Elevation).

- For the following injuries, this chapter describes cause/prevention, stretching guidelines, and strengthening guidelines: plantar fasciitis, Achilles tendinitis, shin splints, patellofemoral syndrome, hamstring strain, low back pain, and rotator cuff tendinitis.

- Exercises are described for treatment and prevention of all the above-mentioned problems.

Exercise Prescription for Special Populations

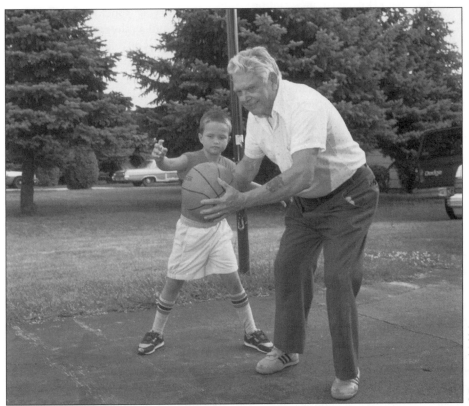

© Raymond J. Malace

- Arthritis
- Diabetes
- Exercise-Induced Asthma
- Hypertension

We often encounter clients with special health conditions. Although it is beyond our abilities to make diagnoses or to provide medical advice, our role is significant. People with health conditions are increasingly involved in physical activity. We must understand their conditions and acquire the knowledge necessary to write appropriate exercise prescriptions. When PAR-Qs or personal health histories reveal significant health problems, we should refer clients to their physicians for medical clearance before we prescribe exercise programs. We should communicate with our clients' physicians concerning limitations, effects of medications, progressions, and signs/symptoms to monitor. We must be understanding, educated about the disease, able to modify exercises appropriately, and motivated to create a friendly and optimistic atmosphere.

Specifically modified exercise prescriptions can dramatically improve our clients' health and quality of life. But because certain types of physical activity can aggravate health conditions, we must recognize those inherent risks. This chapter presents both (1) "red flag responses" to exercise, and (2) exercise prescription considerations.

Arthritis

Approximately one in six persons will have this disorder. It afflicts all ages but is more common in those over the age of 50 (CDC 1990).

Rheumatoid arthritis is a chronic, systemic inflammatory disease primarily involving small synovial joints (e.g., knuckles, wrist, and feet). The inflammation gradually destroys the joint surface (cartilage and bone) and weakens the joint capsule and ligaments. Acute stages are characterized by flare-ups or exacerbation with increased pain and inflammation.

Osteoarthritis is a progressive degenerative joint disease characterized by abrasion of the articular cartilage and formation of new bone at the joint surface (Ike, Lampman, and Castor 1989). Osteoarthritis strikes most of the weightbearing joints such as the facet joints of the spine, hip and knee, as well as the interphalangeal joints of the fingers.

Either kind of arthritis can cause pain, decreased ROM, joint instability, joint deformity, muscle weakness, and diminished cardiovascular endurance.

Red Flag Responses to Exercise

First, determine if the arthritis is in the acute or chronic stage. Rheumatoid arthritis often fluctuates between stages, and your exercise design for a chronic stage of rheumatoid arthritis would be similar to that for osteoarthritis. Pre-exercise medical evaluation is a necessary precaution—exercise must never worsen your client's condition. Follow these guidelines for arthritis sufferers:

- Pain lasting longer than two hours after exercise indicates the activity was too strenuous (Samples 1990).
- Any pain beyond temporary muscle soreness should be respected and reported.

- Fatigue is a side effect of rheumatoid arthritis. Clients with extreme fatigue at the beginning of the exercise session should not exercise that day (Sol 1991).
- Pain from rheumatoid arthritis tends to be worse in the morning, whereas pain from osteoarthritis may worsen as the day goes on. Plan the timing of your client's exercises accordingly.
- Certain joint angles and movements may be abnormally painful. Work within your client's *functional* range of motion, not the full ROM.
- Never prescribe excessive loads (e.g., lifting, carrying, shoulder bags) or high-impact activities (e.g., jogging).
- During flare-ups, prescribe adequate rest periods between sets of activity and between workouts.

Exercise Prescription Considerations

The major goals of exercise programs for people with arthritis are to achieve symptom-free movement and function, and to add some enjoyment to life. Your client's natural tendency to protect arthritic joints only weakens the supporting muscles and makes movement even more difficult. Design exercises to regain lost movement, maintain muscle strength, prevent further damage to the joint, and maintain adequate cardiovascular efficiency.

Flexibility

Flexibility exercises help to prevent contractures (shortening of muscle fibers) and to reduce pain where a contracture has already occurred. The exercise design should stretch the connective tissue around the joint, beginning with about 10 minutes of cardiovascular warm-up and large joint movements. Then select or adapt some of the following static stretches (figures 15.1 to 15.3) to suit your client and his condition. The

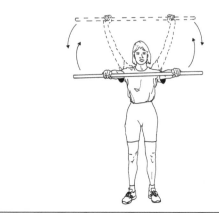

Figure 15.1   Shoulder flexion.

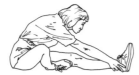

Figure 15.2   Modified hurdler's stretch.

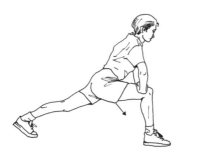

Figure 15.3   Front lunge stretch.

stretches deal with common functional movements of three large areas of the body (select other suitable stretches from chapter 14). Your client should do three to five repetitions of these exercises everyday, using slow fluid movements that lead into a static hold for at least 15 seconds (unless pain occurs).

Strength and Endurance

Functional mobility requires both strength and muscular endurance. Whereas excessive weight training can cause an inflammatory response, isometric exercises minimize pain and inflammation and should be part of most prescriptions. Have your clients hold the isometric contractions for six seconds, and after a brief rest, repeat three to five times. The least painful joint position is usually in the middle range of motion—but if possible, have your client work through an entire ROM emphasizing the development of muscular endurance (i.e., lighter resistance, more repetitions). Prescribe isometrics three times a week on alternate days (Gordon 1993). Depending on your client's needs, select or adapt some of the following exercises (figures 15.4 to 15.7).

Cardiovascular

Clients with rheumatoid arthritis often experience flare-ups of inflammation and are bedridden for several weeks. Take advantage of remissions to get them back to adequate levels of aerobic fitness.

Use of a whirlpool, massage, or hot pack before the warm-up and use of an ice pack or cold shower after the cooldown may relieve minor symptoms. Modify your prescription depending on your client's pain or other signs of inflammation.

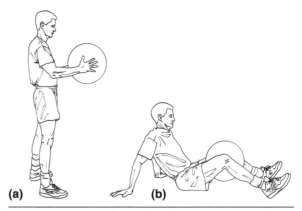

(a)   **(b)**

Figure 15.4   Beach ball squeeze.

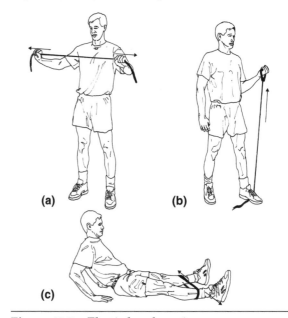

(a)   **(b)**

(c)

Figure 15.5   Elastic band routine.

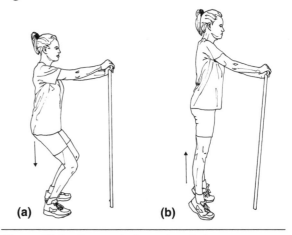

(a)   **(b)**

Figure 15.6   Supported squat and rise.

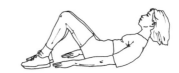

Figure 15.7   Curl and hold.

Mode

Exercising in water is one of the best modalities for training clients with arthritis (Levin 1991). The buoyancy of the water reduces the stress load on the joints and helps your client feel more relaxed. Use water temperatures around 85 to 90 degrees F (30 to 32 degrees C). Other activities that do not place excessive stress on damaged joints include the bicycle ergometer, rowing, cross-country machine, and walking (insist on shoes with good shock absorption). Your client may be able to tolerate an aerobic dance program with low-impact exercises and slower movements. Interval training and cross-training can vary the routine and provide periods of rest for the joint.

Intensity

It is best to start at 40 to 50% of heart rate reserve (HRR) (see chapter 7) and gradually increase to 60 to 75% HRR if no complications occur. Starting levels should elicit a perceived exertion of "fairly light," or 11-12 on the Borg scale.

Duration

Gordon (1993) suggests a system based on the number of calories people expend. A weekly goal for a beginner would be 10 calories per kilogram (2.2 pounds) of body weight per week. So a 75 kg (165 pound) client should burn 750 calories over at least three workouts to meet the recommended quota. A daily 20-minute walk will satisfy this goal.

Frequency

Frequency of activity can be fairly high, ranging from five to seven days per week, since the intensity and the total work done per session are usually moderate. Once the duration is up to 30-45 minutes, your client should be better able to tolerate exercising three or four days a week with a rest or with cross-training. For many clients, it may be advisable to separate days of cardiovascular and strength activities.

Additional Prescription Considerations

In addition to the usual factors of mode, intensity, duration, and frequency, consider the following for your clients with arthritis:

- Clients with arthritis need more time within a comprehensive warm-up and cooldown. Allocate at least 15 minutes for each period.
- Prescribe home activities for clients who cannot get to the fitness center or clinic on a daily basis.

- Having your client keep his legs straight with the knees supported while watching television can help prevent contractures and potential deformities (Rimmer 1994).
- Relaxation techniques, modified yoga, and even listening to music while exercising can alleviate pain and contractures that result from attempts to protect the damaged joint.
- Emphasize the use of good body mechanics to ensure proper alignment, good posture, and reduction in joint stress. Short lectures or illustrated handouts can prove helpful (see Gordon 1993).

Diabetes

Diabetes mellitus is a chronic disorder of glucose metabolism. It is secondary to malfunction of the beta cells located in the islets of Langerhans of the pancreas, whose function is the production and release of insulin (Miller and Keane 1987)

In diabetics, ingestion of glucose causes blood glucose to rise significantly. Because the kidneys cannot reabsorb all the excess glucose, sugar moves into the urine and causes the kidneys to retain water. The resulting excretion of large amounts of fluid and glucose lead to dehydration and subsequent malfunction of certain brain cells.

The two primary types of diabetes are type I, or insulin-dependent diabetes mellitus (IDDM); and type II, or non-insulin-dependent diabetes mellitus (NIDDM) (table 15.1).

Whether your client has Type I or II diabetes, you should help her accomplish three goals:

- Return and maintain blood sugar metabolism at optimal levels.
- Take special precautions against specific risks by (1) stabilizing blood pressure, cholesterol levels, and weight; (2) stopping smoking; (3) caring for the feet; and (4) exercising.
- Develop a healthy lifestyle and practical outlook on life (Gordon 1993).

Red Flag Responses to Exercise

Although exercise is a useful therapy for diabetics, it can exacerbate the condition when the disease is not under control. Pre-exercise medical evaluation is a necessary precaution. Be aware of the following:

- Signs of an insulin reaction may include headache, blurred vision, numbness of the lips, loss

Table 15.1 Classification of Diabetes

TYPE I	TYPE II
• Insulin-dependent diabetes mellitus (IDDM)	• Non-insulin-dependent diabetes mellitus (NIDDM)
• Usually starts during early childhood or adolescence	• Usually occurs in middle-aged and older adults.
• Beta cells of the islets of Langerhans atrophy and disappear. Since these cells produce insulin, the person must inject insulin to survive.	• 85%-90% of those with diabetes are NIDDM.
	• Can be treated with diet, exercise, and medication

of motor control, or strong rapid pulse (Murphy and Sydney 1992).

■ Evening exercise is not recommended for Type I diabetics. Low blood sugar (hypoglycemia) is most evident at this time, and the person may not be aware of a nocturnal insulin reaction (Sherman and Allbright 1990).

■ Insulin should not be injected less than 40-60 minutes before exercise; to avoid increased absorption, it should not be injected into limbs that are about to exercise (Sol 1991; Spenser 1991).

■ Winter months are more difficult times to exercise because of holiday overeating. Encourage indoor physical activity to maintain stable blood glucose levels.

■ High quality footwear with good absorption is extremely important for prevention of foot ulcers. Check feet for blisters, red spots, or cuts.

■ Have easily digestible carbohydrates, juice, cola drink, or candy on hand for any hypoglycemic reactions.

■ It is important to increase fluid intake to avoid dehydration on warm days.

Exercise Prescription Considerations

An exercise specialist, dietitian, and physician are the ideal team for developing the most appropriate program. Exercise can significantly reduce insulin requirements, depending on the intensity and duration of the exercise, level of training, and the nutritional status

(Wallberg-Henriksson 1992). For overweight type II diabetics, maximize caloric expenditure.

Cardiovascular Conditioning Guidelines

Warm-ups should be gradual and at least 10 minutes long, with no breath-holding. A gradual 10 minute cooldown will decrease the chances of arrhythmias and assist recovery (Vitug, Shchneider, and Ruderman 1988).

Mode

Prescribe aerobic exercises involving submaximal contractions of large muscle groups, such as swimming, cycling, and brisk walking. Activities such as basketball and racquet sports, even jogging, may injure the feet. Anaerobic exercises such as weightlifting may increase blood pressure (Sherman and Allbright 1992).

Intensity

Modify cardiovascular intensity to around 50 to 60% of heart rate reserve for older clients or those with other risks. For younger clients in good condition, an intensity of 60 to 85% maximum $\dot{V}O_2$ (HRR) may be acceptable (Vitug, Schneider, and Ruderman 1988). With some diabetics, heart rate is not always accurate, so use perceived exertion or MET equivalents for these clients.

Duration

Guidelines for duration depend on your client's fitness level and the intensity chosen. Apply the guidelines from chapter 7, except that the beginner may start at only 5-10 minutes, and durations longer than 40 minutes may promote overuse injuries.

Frequency

Frequency plays a more significant role with those with diabetes. Daily "doses" of activity are good preferably at the same time each day(Sherman and Allbright 1990). Pre-breakfast exercise may be preferable for some individuals with IDDM (type I) (Sherman and Allbright 1990).

Additional Prescription Considerations

Regular exercise, weight loss, and reduced calorie intake may be enough to achieve blood glucose control in clients with type II diabetes. Contact various national associations and pharmaceutical companies for client-centered print and audiovisual resources on exercise and diet (CDA 1995).

General Considerations

Older clients who may also have arthritis, cardiovascular diseases, or osteoporosis can benefit from 30 minutes of walking, swimming, or water exercise once they have obtained medical clearance. Closely monitor your clients during the initial stages of the program.

Dietary Considerations

Eighty percent of type II diabetics are obese. More than one-third could control the disease with diet alone. Always work with a nutritionist, and follow these guidelines:

- Weight loss should not exceed one to two pounds a week. Monitor blood glucose levels carefully.

- Modest weight losses (10-15 pounds) can improve metabolic control. Set realistic goals.

- Make specific recommendations for clients who travel frequently, eat out, or have ethnic food preferences.

- Many diabetes specialists recommend three smaller meals a day, along with a mid-afternoon and a bedtime snack.

- Be familiar with the necessary increases in food intake prior to different types (intensity and duration) of exercise (Rimmer 1994).

Exercise-Induced Asthma

Asthma afflicts about 1 to 2% of adults and 7% of the children in the United States. Although asthma can start at any age, its onset is most common before the age of 15 or after the age of 45. In the 1984 Olympics, 11.2% of American athletes had exercise-induced asthma. Asthma is caused by constriction of the airways into and out of the lungs (Weinstein 1987). It may be triggered by allergic reactions, temperature, infection, psychological stimuli, or physical exertion (exercise-induced asthma). It is believed that exercise triggers an attack because heat and water are drawn away from the lower respiratory tract to warm and humidify the air entering the lungs (Stamford 1991). The severity is determined by the intensity of the exercise.

Red Flag Responses to Exercise

Exercise—particularly high intensity exercise—can trigger asthmatic symptoms. Establish a working relationship with your clients' physicians so you will be able to recognize symptoms and help guide your clients in using their medications. For example, prescriptions may call for use of inhalers anywhere from 15 to 45 minutes prior to exercise; but physicians advise other people to "work through" tightness in the chest without using medication (Rimmer 1994). Be aware of the following:

- Symptoms usually develop around 6-12 minutes into the exercise session, and often get worse 5-10 minutes after exercise. Individualize your prescriptions accordingly.

- Clients should take their medications and use their inhalers if they can't work through initial chest tightness, in accordance with their doctors' directions.

- You may have to modify or cancel outdoor activities for asthmatic clients under environmental conditions such as heavy air pollution, high pollen count, or very cold temperatures.

- Clients should try to keep nasal passages clear for warm, humid air exchange. They should also stay well-hydrated to decrease mucous secretions (Sol 1991).

Exercise Prescription Considerations

Many adults with exercise-induced asthma (EIA) are becoming more active. You need to understand asthma and its implications for exercise to be able to prescribe effectively.

Warm-up is critical for the asthmatic. It should last a minimum of 10-15 minutes and consist of low-intensity aerobic activity (such as brisk walking), followed by stretching, and then a gradual increase in intensity up to the lower end of the prescribed training zone.

Cooldowns are also important. Asthma attacks often occur after exercise. Light exercise, stretching, and relaxation should continue for 10-15 minutes after the core program.

Cardiovascular Conditioning Considerations

With some experimentation, you can suggest appropriate prescription factors to avoid attacks.

Mode

Swimming is the exercise least likely to cause asthmatic attacks (Stamford 1991), since the temperature and humidity in pool areas keep the airways warm and moist. Once an asthmatic client becomes more fit, she may tolerate programs such as jogging. Interval training and circuit training are effective methods to improve aerobic and anaerobic systems, since the rest periods between exertions help prevent attacks. Be sure to monitor the lengths of the rest intervals, and prolong the recovery and/or reduce the work intensity if you note any respiratory distress.

Intensity

Intensity should begin at 40 to 60% and progress to 60 to 75% of HRR. Endurance athletes with asthma can often tolerate higher intensity levels.

Duration

Some clients respond positively to short, interval-type workouts. Afrasiabi and Spector (1991) describe a 4-6 minute aerobic routine repeated two to three times with a 5-minute rest between each set. For clients with mild to moderate asthma who have taken their medication, a duration of 20-35 minutes should be fine. Balance reduced intensity with increased duration in order to maintain total work per session yet avoid asthmatic symptoms.

Frequency

Frequency can range from 3-7 days per week depending on your client's condition, response to the exercise, and interest.

Additional Prescription Considerations

Exercise-induced asthma need not sideline your client, provided that you monitor the factors that affect her and follow these additional considerations:

- Circuit training can improve aerobic and anaerobic systems. As with cardiovascular interval training, the rest periods between exertions are essential and afford an excellent opportunity to monitor breathing, heart rate, perceived exertion, etc.
- In cold or dry air, your client should wear a scarf or surgical mask over her nose and mouth to decrease heat loss and warm the inspired air.

- Exercise can improve respiratory performance and strengthen respiratory muscles by encouraging people to breathe fully, exhale more forcefully, and optimize their breathing patterns (Bouchard, Shephard, and Stephens 1993).

Hypertension

Hypertension, the "silent killer," is an enormous problem. The Heart and Stroke Foundation (Ontario, Canada) recently reported that, compared with their 35- to 49-year-old counterparts of 20 years ago, only 75% compared to 84% now have healthy blood pressures (Carey 1996).

The U.S. National High Blood Pressure Program outlines categories of hypertension in Table 15.2 on the following page.

Red Flag Responses to Exercise

Because the body sends extra blood to working muscles, exercise typically raises BP temporarily. If clients have very high BP, their doctors may want to lower it with drugs before authorizing an exercise program. Exercise is generally safe for clients with mild to moderate hypertension (Franklin and Wappes 1996). Note the following:

- Inappropriate responses during exercise include systolic pressure above 250 mm Hg, diastolic pressure above 110 mm Hg, failure of systolic pressure to rise with increased workload, or a significant drop (10 mm Hg) in diastolic blood pressure (Sol 1991).
- Monitor BP during the first five workouts of a hypertensive client. Measure it before the workout, at peak load of the workout, and at the end of the workout.
- For severe hypertensives, discourage competitive games and the use of saunas or whirlpools.
- When engaging in strength and calisthenic exercises, hypertensive clients should avoid the following:
  1. Placing the head lower than the feet, such as an incline sit-up or a decline bench press.
  2. Holding the breath or straining. This creates the Valsalva Phenomenon which increases pressure within the chest cavity and prevents blood from returning to the heart.
  3. Lifting heavy weights.
  4. Performing arm exercises above shoulder level, such as shoulder presses or lateral arm raises.

Table 15.2 CLASSIFICATION OF HYPERTENSION

CATEGORY	SYSTOLIC BP (mm Hg)	DIASTOLIC BP (mm Hg)
Normal	< 130	< 85
High normal	130-139	85-89
Hypertension: Stage 1 (mild) Stage 2 (moderate) Stage 3 (severe) Stage 4 (very severe)	140-159 160-179 180-209 ≥ 210	90-99 100-109 110-119 ≥ 120

Reprinted, by permission from National High Blood Pressure Program, 1993. *Report of the Joint National Committee on Detection, Evaluation, and Treatment of High Blood Pressure*, 102.

5. "All out" exertions such as sprinting.

6. Isometrics.

- Clients who are serious about lifting weights should keep resistance below 60% of 1RM and monitor blood pressure between sets every few weeks.

- Clients on diuretics may experience dehydration and loss of electrolytes, which may cause muscle cramps or arrhythmias (Tanji and Batt 1995).

- Clients on beta-blockers experience little increase in exercise heart rate, and therefore should monitor intensity with the RPE scale (rating of perceived exertion—table 7.3). They may also experience reduced exercise capacity (Tanji and Batt 1995).

- Clients doing upper body work such as with the arm ergometer will achieve higher heart rates and BP values at lower workloads. Monitor these activities to determine your client's reaction.

Exercise Prescription Considerations

Research strongly suggests that regular exercise lowers BP in hypertensive individuals and reduces the risk of developing hypertension. The American College of Sports Medicine (1995) makes the following recommendations:

- Provide lifestyle counseling for clients with elevated exercise BP.

- Encourage endurance training for clients who are at high risk for developing hypertension.

- Endurance training will elicit an average reduction of 10 mm Hg from both systolic and diastolic blood pressures in people with mild to moderate hypertension (140-180/90-105 mm Hg).

- Exercise training at somewhat lower intensities—e.g., 40% to 70% $\dot{V}O_2$max (HRR)—appears to lower BP as much, or more, than higher intensities. This may be especially important for elderly or obese clients.

- Exercise should be part of the initial treatment strategy for mild to moderate hypertension.

- Individuals with marked elevations in BP should add endurance exercise only after initiating pharmacological therapy; the exercise may allow them eventually to decrease their medications.

- Do not use resistance training as the primary form of exercise for hypertensive clients. If performed as part of a balanced exercise prescription, it should involve low resistance with high reps, such as with circuit training. Avoid isometrics.

General Guidelines

First, decide on an appropriate type of moderate-level aerobic exercise. Then tailor other safe, effective prescription factors to suit your client's tastes and needs.

Mode

Brisk walking is an excellent choice for moderate aerobic exercise. Depending on your client's fitness level, jogging, stationary or outdoor cycling, swimming, stair-stepping, or low-impact aerobics may be appropriate. Most active people with mild to moderate but controlled hypertension may participate in sports with moderate to high dynamic demands and low static demands. Examples are soccer, tennis, distance running, baseball, and perhaps basketball. Hypertensives generally should avoid sports with higher static demands such as football, wrestling, sprinting, and contact hockey (Anders 1992).

Intensity

Use a perceived exertion rating of perhaps 10-12 (light exercise), particularly for clients on beta-blocking drugs that lower the maximum heart rate. Intensity levels should begin at 40% and need progress only up to 70% $\dot{V}O_2$max (HRR).

Duration and Frequency

Frequencies of five to six times per week and durations of 30-40 minutes allow significant volume (total work done) to the training (ACSM 1993).

Additional Prescription Considerations

Keep in mind these useful guidelines when prescribing for hypertensive clients:

- Three benefits of exercise that assist in reduction of blood pressure are (1) weight loss; (2) relaxation and anti-stress effect; and (3) reduction of resting heart rate, reflecting reduced cardiac output (Tanji 1990)

- Perform a graded exercise assessment to obtain systolic and diastolic BP at corresponding heart rate levels. With this information, you can instruct clients not to exceed a particular heart rate and consequently a particular blood pressure.

- Warm-ups and cooldowns should be easy and relatively long, with inclusion of relaxation techniques in the cooldown.

Highlights

- Always establish close communication with the physicians of clients whose health is compromised by such disorders as arthritis, diabetes, asthma, and hypertension.

- Modify your exercise prescription to take into account (1) special considerations presented by your clients' physicians and (2) the needs and desires you learn about in close consultation with your clients.

- Your first job is to be certain that your exercise prescription does not exacerbate your client's disorder.

References

Chapter 1

American College of Sports Medicine. 1991. *Guidelines for Exercise Testing and Prescription*. 4th ed. Philadelphia: Lea & Febiger.

Åstrand, P.O., and K. Rodahl, eds. 1977. *Textbook of Work Physiology*. New York: McGraw-Hill.

Buckley, R., and J. Caple. 1991. *One-to-One Training and Coaching Skills*. San Diego: Pfeiffer.

Canadian Society for Exercise Physiology. 1996. *The Canadian Physical Activity, Fitness, and Lifestyle Appraisal: CSEP's Plan for Healthy Active Living*. Ottawa: CSEP.

Dishman, R.K. 1990. Determinants of participation in physical activity. *J. Appl. Sport Sci.* 8:104-13.

Egan, G. 1990. *The Skilled Helper*. Pacific Grove, CA: Brooks/Cole.

Jones, A.P. 1991. Communication and teaching techniques. In *Program Design for Personal Trainers*. San Diego: IDEA.

Kizilos, P. 1991. The power of suggestion: How to get patients up and running. *Physician and Sp. Med.* 19 (3):167-69.

Orme, M. 1977. Teaching strategies and consultation skills: Probing techniques. In *Innovation in School Psychology*, ed. S. Miezitis and M. Orme, 70-83. Toronto: OISE.

Prochaska, J.O., C.C. DiClemente, and J.J. Norcross. 1992. In search of how people change: Applications to addictive behaviours. *American Psychologist* 47 (9).

Quinney, H.A., L. Gauvin, and A.E.T. Wall, eds. 1994. *Toward Active Living*. Champaign, IL: Human Kinetics.

Skinner, J.S. 1987. General principles of exercise prescription. In *Exercise Testing and Exercise Prescription for Special Cases*, ed. J.S. Skinner. Philadelphia: Lea & Febiger.

Trottier, M. 1988. Client-driven programming. Keynote address: Fit Rendezvous. Edmonton, Canada.

Wilmore, J.H. 1982. *Training for Sport and Activity*. Boston: Allyn & Bacon.

Chapter 2

Canadian Society for Exercise Physiology. 1996. *The Canadian Physical Activity, Fitness, and Lifestyle Appraisal: CSEP's Plan for Healthy Active Living*. Ottawa: CSEP.

Clark, J., and S. Clark. 1992. *Prioritize Organize: The Art of Getting it Done*. Shawnee Mission, KS: National Press.

DeBusk, R.F., U. Stenestrand, and M. Sheehan. 1990. Training effects of long versus short bouts of exercise. *American Journal of Cardiology* 65(15):1010-1013.

Dishman, R.K. 1990. Determinants of participation in physical activity. *Journal of Applied Sports Science* 8:104-13.

Dishman, R.K. 1994. *Advances in Exercise Adherence*. Champaign, IL: Human Kinetics.

Egan, G. 1990. *The Skilled Helper*. Pacific Grove, CA: Brooks/Cole.

Francis, L. 1990. Setting goals. *IDEA Today* May:8-10.

Gelatt, H.B. 1989. Positive uncertainty: A new decision making framework for counseling. *J. Counseling Psychology* 36:252-256.

Goldfine, H., A. Ward, P. Taylor, D. Carlucci, and J.M. Rippe. 1991. Exercising to health—What's really in it for your patients? *The Physician and Sportsmedicine* 19 (6):81-93.

Gray, J. 1992. *Men Are from Mars, Women Are from Venus*. NY: Harper Perennial.

King, A.C. 1991. Principles of adherence and motivation. In *Program Design for Personal Trainers*. San Diego: IDEA.

Patrick, K., B. Long, W. Wooten, and M. Pratt. 1994. A new tool for encouraging activity. Project PACE. *The Physician and Sportsmedicine* 22 (11):45-55.

Pronk, N.P., R.R. Wing, and R.W. Jeffery. 1994. Effects of increased stimulus control for exercise through use of a personal trainer. *Annals of Behavioral Medicine* 16:SO77.

Strachan, D., and J. Kent. 1985. *Long and Short Term Planning (skills program)*. Gloucester, Ont.: Tyrell Press.

Trottier, M. 1988. Client-driven programming. Keynote Address: Fit Rendezvous. Edmonton, AB.

Weylman, C.R. 1995. *Reaching the Potential Client*. Atlanta: The Achievement Group.

Chapter 3

Canadian Society for Exercise Physiology. 1996. *The Canadian Physical Activity, Fitness, and Lifestyle Appraisal: CSEP's Plan for Healthy Active Living*. Ottawa: CSEP.

Pronk, N.P., R.R. Wing, and R.W. Jeffery. 1994. Effects of increased stimulus control for exercise through use of a personal trainer. *Annals of Behavioral Medicine* 16:SO77.

Chapter 4

American Alliance for Health, Physical Education, Recreation and Dance. 1988. *Physical Best: American Alliance Physical Education & Assessment Program*. Reston, VA: AAHPERD.

American College of Sports Medicine. 1995. *Guidelines for Exercise Testing and Prescription*. 5th ed. Philadelphia: Lea & Febiger.

Borg, G.A.V. 1970. Perceived exertion as an indicator of somatic stress. *Scandinavian Journal of Rehabilitation Medicine* 2:92-98.

Canadian Society for Exercise Physiology. 1993. *Certified Fitness Appraiser Resource Manual.* Ottawa: CSEP.

Canadian Society for Exercise Physiology. 1996. *The Canadian Physical Activity, Fitness, and Lifestyle Appraisal: CSEP's Plan for Healthy Active Living.* Ottawa: CSEP.

Getchell, B., and W. Anderson. 1982. *Being Fit: A Personal Guide.* NY: Wiley.

Heyward, V.H. 1998. *Advanced Fitness Assessment and Exercise Prescription.* 3rd ed. Champaign, IL: Human Kinetics.

Heyward, V.H., and L.M. Stolarczyk. 1996. *Applied Body Composition Assessment.* Champaign, IL: Human Kinetics.

Jackson, A.S., and M.L. Pollock. 1985. Practical assessment of body composition. *The Physician and Sportsmedicine* 13:76-90.

Jequier, E. 1987. Energy, obesity, and body weight standards. *American Journal of Clinical Nutrition* 45:1035-1047.

Kendall, F.P., E.K. McCreary, and P.G. Provance. 1993. *Muscles: Testing and Function.* Baltimore: Williams & Wilkins.

Larsson, B., B. Svardsudd, L. Weilin, L. Wilhelmsen, P. Bjorntorp, and G. Tibbin. 1984. Abdominal adipose tissue distribution, obesity, and risk of cardiovascular disease and death: 13-year follow-up of participants in the study of men born in 1913. *British Medical Journal* 288:1401-1404.

Nieman, D.C. 1990. *Fitness and Sports Medicine: An Introduction.* Palo Alto: Bull Publishing.

Pollock, M.L., J.H. Wilmore, and S.M. Fox. 1978. *Health and Fitness Through Physical Activity.* NY: Wiley.

Shephard, R.J. 1988. PAR-Q, Canadian home fitness test and exercise screening alternatives. *Sports Medicine* 5:185-195.

Skinner, J.S. 1987. General principles of exercise prescription. In *Exercise Testing and Exercise Prescription for Special Cases,* ed. J.S. Skinner. Philadelphia: Lea & Febiger.

Wilmore, J.H., and D.L. Costill. 1994. *Physiology of Sport and Exercise.* Champaign, IL: Human Kinetics.

Wilson, D.M.C., and D. Ciliska. 1984. Lifestyle assessment: Development and the use of the FANTASTIC Checklist. *Canadian Family Physician* 30.

Chapter 5

Canadian Society for Exercise Physiology. 1996. *The Canadian Physical Activity, Fitness, and Lifestyle Appraisal: CSEP's Plan for Healthy Active Living.* Ottawa: CSEP.

Canadian Society for Exercisee Physiology. 1993. *Certified Fitness Appraiser Resource Manual.* Ottawa:CSEP.

Griffin, J.C. 1989. *All the Right Moves.* An unpublished manual.

Heyward, V.H. 1998. *Advanced Fitness Assessment and Exercise Prescription.* 3rd ed. Champaign, IL: Human Kinetics.

Kendall, F.P., McCreary, E.K., and Provance, P.G. 1993. *Muscles: Testing and Function.* Baltimore: Williams and Wilkins.

Nieman, D.C. 1990. *Fitness and Sports Medicine: An Introduction.* Palo Alto: Bull Pub.

Sale, D. and MacDougall, J.D. 1981. Specificity in strength training: A review for the coach and athlete. *Canadian Journal of Applied Sport Science* 6, 87-92.

Skinner, J.S. 1987. General principles of exercise prescription.

In *Exercise Testing and Exercise Prescription for Special Cases,* ed. By J.S. Skinner. Philadelphia: Lea and Febiger.

Chapter 6

American College of Sports Medicine. 1990. The recommended quantity and quality of exercise for developing and maintaining fitness in healthy adults. *Medicine and Science in Sports and Exercise* 22:265-274.

American College of Sports Medicine. 1995. *Guidelines for Exercise Testing and Prescription.* 5th ed. Philadelphia: Lea & Febiger.

Åstrand, P.O., and K. Rodahl, eds. 1977. *Textbook of Work Physiology.* New York: McGraw-Hill.

Blair, S.N., H.W. Kohl III, R.S. Paffenbarger Jr., D.G. Clark, K.H. Cooper, and L.W. Gibbons. 1989. Physical fitness and all-cause mortality: a prospective study of healthy men and women. *Journal of the American Medical Association* 262 (17):2395-2401.

Bouchard, C. 1994. Physical activity, fitness, and health: Overview of the Consensus Symposium. In: *Toward Active Living,* ed. H.A. Quinney, L. Gauvin, and A.E.T. Wall. Champaign IL: Human Kinetics.

Brooks, D., and C. Copeland-Brooks. 1991. Are you ready for the next step in circuit training? *IDEA Today* November-December:34-39.

Burfoot, A. 1995. How much should you run? *Runner's World* September: 66-67.

Canadian Society for Exercise Physiology. 1995. *The Canadian Physical Activity, Fitness, and Lifestyle Appraisal:CSEP's Plan for Healthy Active Living.* Ottawa: CSEP.

De Busk, R.F., U. Stenestrand, and M. Sheehan. 1990. Training effects of long versus short bouts of exercise. *American Journal of Cardiology* 65 (15):1010-1013.

Dishman, R.K. 1990. Determinants of participation in physical activity. *Journal of Applied Sports Science Research* 8:104-13.

Ebisu, T. 1985. Splitting the distance of endurance running: On cardiovascular endurance and blood lipids. *Japanese Journal of Physical Education* 30 (1):37-43.

Fair, E. 1992. Have equipment, will travel. *IDEA Today* May:57-61.

Gledhill, N., and V. Jamnik. 1996. Figure 4-1. In *The Canadian Physical Activity, Fitness, and Lifestyle Appraisal:CSEP's Plan for Healthy Active Living.* Ottawa: CSEP.

Goldfine, H., A. Ward, P. Taylor, D. Carlucci, and J.M. Rippe. 1991. Exercising to health—What's really in it for your patients? *The Physician and Sportsmedicine* 19 (6):81-93.

Hagan, R.D. 1988. Benefits of aerobic conditioning and diet for overweight adults. *Sports Medicine.* 5:144-155.

Haskell, W.L. 1985. Physical activity and health: Need to define the required stimulus. *American Journal of Cardiology* 55:4D-9D.

Haskell, W.L. 1995. Resolving the exercise debate: More vs. less. *IDEA Today* October:40-47.

Iknoian, T. 1992. 10 equipment trends that changed fitness. *IDEA Today* July-August:33-36.

International Federation of Sports Medicine Position Statement 1990. Physical Exercise: An important factor for health. *The Physician and Sportsmedicine* 18 (3):155-156.

Kuipers, H., and Keizer, H.A. 1988. Overtraining in elite athletes. *Sports Medicine* 5:79-92.

Paffenbarger, R.S. Jr., R.T. Hyde, A.L. Wing, and C. Hsieh. 1986. Physical activity, all-cause mortality, and longevity of college alumni. *New England Journal of Medicine* 314 (10):605-613.

Pate, R.R., M. Pratt, S.N. Blair, et al. 1995. Physical activity and public health: A recommendation from the Centers for Disease Control and Prevention and the American College of Sports Medicine. *Journal of the American Medical Association* 273 (5):402-407.

Pollock, C.L. 1992. Does exercise intensity matter? *The Physician and Sportsmedicine* 20 (12):123-126.

Quinney, H.A., L. Gauvin, and A.E.T. Wall., eds. 1994. *Toward Active Living*. Champaign IL: Human Kinetics.

Robinson, J. P., and G. Godbey. 1993. Has fitness peaked? *American Demographics* September:36-42.

Rotwein, R.E. 1995. Obsessed with exercise. *IDEA Today* September:57-60.

Sapega, A.A., T.C. Quedenfeld, R.A. Moyer, and R.A. Butler. 1991. Biophysical factors in range-of-motion exercise. *The Physician and Sportsmedicine* 9 (12):57-65.

Scotti, P. 1985. Fitness equipment: Keeping your club in shape. *IRSA Club Business* June:61.

Sillery, B. 1996. Essential technology guide to exercise and fitness. *Popular Science* January:65-68.

Skinner, J.S. 1987. General principles of exercise prescription. In *Exercise Testing and Exercise Prescription for Special Cases*, ed. J.S. Skinner. Philadelphia: Lea & Febiger.

Smith, E.L., W. Reddan, and P.E. Smith. 1981. Physical activity and calcium modalities for bone mineral increase in aged women. *Medicine and Science in Sports and Exercise* 13:60-64.

Stone, M.H., S.J. Fleck, N.T. Triplett, and W.J. Kraemer. 1991. Health- and performance-related potential of resistance training. *Sports Medicine* 11 (4):210-231.

Stone, M.H., R.E. Keith, J.T. Kearney, S.J. Fleck, G.T. Wilson, and N.T. Triplett. 1991. Overtraining: A review of the signs, symptoms and possible causes. *Journal of Applied Sports Science Research* 5 (1):35-50.

Turner, J. 1996. Exercise in futility. *Toronto Star* April 15:E1.

Wenger, H.A., and G.J. Bell. 1986. The interactions of intensity, frequency, and duration of exercise training in altering cardiorespiratory fitness. *Sports Medicine* 3:346-356.

Westcott, W.L. 1989. When more isn't better. *IDEA Today* February:24.

Westcott, W.L. 1991. Strength training: How much is enough? *IDEA Today* February:33-35.

Wilmore, J.H., and D.L. Costill. 1994. *Physiology of Sport and Exercise*. Champaign, IL: Human Kinetics.

Wolkodoff, N. 1995. Equipment of choice. *Fitness Management* July:34-37.

Chapter 7

Allen, D., and L. Goldberg. 1986. Physiological comparison of two cross-country ski machines. Paper presented at the annual meeting of the American College of Sports Medicine, Indianapolis. May.

American College of Sports Medicine. 1990. The recommended quantity and quality of exercise for developing and maintaining fitness in healthy adults. Medicine and Science in Sports and Exercise 22:265-274.

American College of Sports Medicine. 1995. *Guidelines for Exercise Testing and Prescription*. 5th ed. Philadelphia: Lea & Febiger.

Åstrand, P.-O., and K. Rodahl. 1986. *Textbook of Work Physiology* 3rd ed. New York: McGraw-Hill.

Baechle, T.R., ed. 1994. *Essentials of Strength Training and Conditioning*. Champaign, IL: Human Kinetics.

Birk, T.J., and C.A. Birk. 1987. Use of ratings of perceived exertion for exercise prescription. *Sports Medicine* 4:1-8.

Blair, S.N., H.W. Kohl, R.S. Paffenbarger, D.G. Clark, K.H. Cooper, and L.W. Gibbons. 1989. Physical fitness and all-cause mortality. *Journal of the American Medical Association* 262 (17):2395-2401.

Brynteson, P., and W.E. Sinning. 1973. The effect of training frequencies on the retention of cardiovascular fitness. *Medicine and Science in Sports and Exercise* 5:29-33.

Camaione, D.N. 1993. *Fitness Management*. Dubuque, IA: Brown & Benchmark.

Fox, E.L. 1979. *Sports Physiology*. Philadelphia: Saunders.

Fox, E.L., R.L. Bartels, J. Klinzing, and K. Ragg. 1977. Metabolic responses to interval training programs of high and low power output. *Medicine and Science in Sports and Exercise* 9(3):191-196.

Fox, E.L., and D.K. Mathews. 1974. *Interval Training: Conditioning for Sports and General Fitness*. Philadelphia: Saunders.

Gettman, L.R., and M.L. Pollock. 1981. Circuit weight training: A critical review of its physiological benefits. *The Physician and Sports Medicine* 9:44-60.

Haskell, W.L. 1985. Physical activity and health: Need to define the required stimulus. *American Journal of Cardiology* 55: 4D-9D.

Haskell, W.L. 1995. Resolving the exercise debate: More vs. less. *IDEA Today* Oct.:40-47.

Heyward, V.H. 1998. *Advanced Fitness Assessment and Exercise Prescription*. 3rd ed. Champaign, IL: Human Kinetics.

Horswill, C.A., C.L. Kien, and W.B. Zipf. 1995. Energy expenditure in adolescents during low intensity, leisure activities. *Medicine and Science in Sports and Exercise* 27(9):1311-1314.

Howley, E.T., and B.D. Franks. 1997. *Health Fitness Instructor's Handbook*. 3rd. ed. Champaign, IL: Human Kinetics.

Kosich, D. 1991. Exercise physiology 4(4). In *Personal Trainer Manual*. San Diego: American Council on Exercise.

Londeree, B.R., and S.A. Ames. 1976. Trend analysis of the %$\dot{V}O_2$max-HR Regression. *Medicine and Science in Sports and Exercise* 8:122-125.

MacDougall, J.D., and D.G. Sale. 1981. Continuous vs. interval training: A review for the athlete and the coach. *Canadian Journal of Applied Sport Science* 6(2):93-97.

MacDougall, J.D. 1977. The anaerobic threshold: Its significance for the endurance athlete. *Canadian Journal of Applied Sport Science* 2:137-140.

MacDougall, J.D., G.R. Ward, D.G. Sale, and J.R. Sutton. 1977. Muscle glycogen repletion after high-intensity intermittent exercise. *Journal of Applied Physiology* 42:129-132.

Marion, A., G. Kenny, and J. Thoden. 1994. Heart rate response as a means of quantifying training loads: Practical considerations for coaches. *Sports* 14(2):Part 1.

McArdle, W., F. Katch, and V. Katch. 1991. *Exercise Physiology: Energy, Nutrition, and Human Performance.* 3rd ed. Philadelphia: Lea & Febiger.

Murray, B. 1977. Interval training and specificity. *Swimming Technique* 14(1):2539-2540.

Nieman, D.C. 1990. *Fitness and Sports Medicine: An Introduction.* Palo Alto, CA: Bull Publishing.

Pollock, M., and J.H. Wilmore. 1990. *Exercise in Health and Disease.* Philadelphia: Saunders.

Pollock, M., L. Gettman, C. Milesis, M. Bah, L. Durstine, and R. Johnson. 1977. Effects of frequency and duration of training on attrition and incidence of injury. *Medicine and Science in Sports and Exercise* 9:31-36.

Powers, S.K., and E.T. Howley. 1990. *Exercise Physiology.* Dubuque, IA: Brown.

Sharkey, B.J. 1984. *Physiology of Fitness.* 2nd ed. Champaign, IL: Human Kinetics.

Sillery, B. 1996. Essential technology guide to exercise and fitness. *Popular Science* January:65-68.

Stewart, G.W. 1995. *Active Living.* Champaign, IL: Human Kinetics.

Wilmore, J.H., and D.L. Costill. 1994. *Physiology of Sport and Exercise.* Champaign, IL: Human Kinetics.

Wolf, M. D., and D.H. Richie. 1991. Selecting equipment, apparel, and footwear. In *Program Design for Personal Trainers.* San Diego, CA: IDEA.

Yacenda, J. 1995. *Fitness Cross-Training.* Champaign, IL: Human Kinetics.

Chapter 8

Bean, A. 1996. The truth about fat-burning. *Runner's World* September:46-50.

Blackburn, G.L., G.T. Wilson, B.S. Kanders, L.J. Stein, and P.T. Lavin. 1989. Weight cycling: The experience of human dieters. *American Journal of Clinical Nutrition* 49:1105-1109.

Brehm, B.A. 1996. Fat-burning: Getting down to the basics. *Fitness Management* March:25-26.

Brownell, K.D., and S.N. Steen. 1987. Modern methods of weight control: The physiology and psychology of dieting. *The Physician and Sportsmedicine* 15 (12):122-137.

Campbell, W.W., M.C. Crim, V.R. Young, and W.J. Evans. 1994. Increased energy requirements and changes in body composition with resistance training in older adults. *American Journal of Clinical Nutrition* 60:167-175.

Dattilio, A. 1992. Dietary fat and its relationship to body weight. *Nutrition Today* 27:13-19.

Dusek, D.E. 1989. *Weight Management The Fitness Way.* Boston: Jones and Bartlett.

Forbes, G. 1994. Body composition: Influence of nutrition, disease, growth, and aging. In *Modern Nutrition in Health and Disease,* ed. M. Shils, et al. Philadelphia: Lea & Febiger.

Garfinkel, P., and D. Coscina. 1990. Discussion: Exercise and obesity. In *Exercise, Fitness and Health,* ed. C. Bouchard, R.J. Shepard, T. Stephens, J.R. Sutton, and B.D. McPherson. Champaign, IL: Human Kinetics.

Health and Welfare Canada. 1988. Promoting healthy weights: A discussion paper. Ottawa, Ontario.

Heyward, V.H. 1998. *Advanced Fitness Assessment and Exercise Prescription.* 3rd ed. Champaign, IL: Human Kinetics.

Hodgetts, V., et al. 1991. Factors controlling fat metabolism from human subcutaneous adipose tissue during exercise. *Journal of Applied Physiology* 71:445-451.

Klesges, R., et al. 1993. Effects of television on metabolic rate: Potential implications for childhood obesity. *Pediatrics* 91:281-286.

Marks, B.L., A. Ward, D.H. Morris, J. Castellani, and J.M. Rippe. 1995. Fat-free mass is maintained in women following a moderate diet and exercise program. *Medicine and Science in Sports and Exercise* 27 (9):1243-1251.

McArdle, W.D., F.I. Katch, and V.L. Katch. 1991. *Exercise Physiology: Energy, Nutrition, and Human Performance.* Philadelphia: Lea & Febiger.

Miller, W.C. 1991. Diet composition, energy intake and nutritional status in relation to obesity in men and women. *Medicine and Science in Sports and Exercise* 23 (3):280-284.

Nieman, D.C. 1990. *Fitness and Sports Medicine: An Introduction.* Palo Alto, CA: Bull Publishing.

Report of a Joint FAO/WHO/UNU Expert Consultation. 1985. *Energy and Protein Requirements.* World Health Organization.

Romijn, J., et al. 1993. Regulation of endogenous fat and carbohydrate metabolism in relation to exercise intensity and duration. *American Journal of Physiology* 265:E380-E391.

Simopoulos, A., ed. 1992. *Metabolic Control of Eating, Energy Expenditure and the Bioenergetics of Obesity.* Basel, Switzerland: Karger.

Tremblay, A., et al. 1989. Impact of dietary fat content and fat oxidation on energy intake in humans. *American Journal of Clinical Nutrition* 47:799-805.

Walberg, J.L. 1989. Aerobic exercise and resistance weight training during weight reduction. *Sports Medicine* 47:343-356.

Williams, M.H. 1995. *Nutrition for Fitness and Sport.* 4th ed. Dubuque, IA: Brown & Benchmark.

Yarian, R., ed. 1995. *Health: Annual Editions 95/96.* Guilford, CT: Dushkin/Brown & Benchmark.

Chapter 9

American College of Sports Medicine. 1995. *Guidelines for Exercise Testing and Prescription.* 5th ed. Philadelphia: Lea & Febiger.

Howley, E.T., and B.D. Franks. 1997. *Health Fitness Instructor's Handbook.* 3rd. ed. Champaign, IL: Human Kinetics.

Chapter 10

Batman, P., and M. Van Capelle. 1992. *Exercise Analysis Made Simple.* 2nd ed. Arncliffe, NSW: F.I.A.

Edman, K.A.P. 1992. Contractile performance of skeletal muscle fibres. In *Strength and Power in Sport.* Boston: Blackwell Scientific.

Ellison, D. 1993. *Advanced exercise design for lower body.* San Diego: Movement That Matters.

Griffin, J.C. 1986a. A system for: Exercise analysis. *Canadian Association for Health, Physical Education, and Recreation Journal* 52(1):30-31.

Griffin, J.C. 1986b. A system for: Exercise design. *Canadian Association for Health, Physical Education, and Recreation Journal* 52(2):38-39.

Hamill, J., and K.M. Knutzen. 1995. *Biomechanical Basis of Human Movement.* Media, PA.: Williams & Wilkins.

Komi, P.V. 1992. Stretch-shortening cycle. In *Strength and Power in Sport.* Boston: Blackwell Scientific.

Lockridge, A. 1990. How to scrutinize exercises. *The Network* 3(12):1-2.

Moritani, T. 1992. Time course of adaptations during strength and power training. In *Strength and Power in Sport.* Boston: Blackwell Scientific.

Shier, D., J. Butler, and R. Lewis. 1996. *Hole's Human Anatomy and Physiology.* 7th ed. Dubuque, IA: Brown.

Stamford, B. 1986. Leverage and strength. *The Physician and Sportsmedicine* 14(12):206.

Wilmore, J.H., and D.L. Costill. 1994. *Physiology of Sport and Exercise.* Champaign, IL: Human Kinetics.

Wirhed, R. 1991. *Athletic Ability and the Anatomy of Motion.* Orebro, Sweden: Wolfe Medical.

Chapter 11

Alter, M.J. 1996. *Science of Stretching.* 2nd ed. Champaign, IL: Human Kinetics.

American College of Sports Medicine. 1990. The recommended quantity of exercise for developing and maintaining cardiorespiratory and muscular fitness in healthy adults. ACSM Position Statement. *Medicine and Science in Sports and Exercise* 22:265-274.

Baechle, T.R. 1994. *Essentials of Strength Training and Conditioning.* Champaign, IL: Human Kinetics.

Brooks, D. 1993. Where does PNF fit into a training program? In *Program Design for Personal Trainers.* San Diego: IDEA.

Burnside, M.G. 1990. Progressive stretching for fitness and health. *Canadian Association for Health, Physical Education, and Recreation Journal* 56: 20-24.

Calder, A.W., P.D. Chilibeck, C.E. Webber, and D.G. Sale. 1994. Comparison of whole and split weight training routines in young women. *Canadian Journal of Applied Physiology* 19(2):185-199.

Camaione, D.N. 1993. *Fitness Management.* Dubuque, IA: Brown & Benchmark.

Chu, D.A. 1992. *Jumping Into Plyometrics.* Champaign, IL: Leisure Press.

Eitner, E. 1982. Loosening. In *Physical Therapy for Sports.* W. Kuprian, ed. Philadelphia: Saunders.

Fair, E. 1992. Have equipment, will travel. *IDEA Today* May:57-61.

Fitness Ontario. 1983. A handbook for trainers of fitness leaders. Ministry of tourism and recreation. Toronto, ON:34-39.

Fleck, S.J., and W.J. Kraemer. 1987. *Designing Resistance Training Programs.* Champaign, IL: Human Kinetics.

Francis, L.L., P.R. Francis, and K. Welshons-Smith. 1985. Aerobic dance injuries: A survey of instructors. *The Physician and Sportsmedicine* 13(2):105-111.

Griffin, J.C. 1987. Fitness Injury Survey: Fitness Assessors and Programmers. *Canadian Association for Health, Physical Education, and Recreation Journal* 53(1):15-17.

Hamill, J., and K.M. Knutzen. 1995. *Biomechanical Basis of Human Movement.* Meida, PA: Williams and Wilkins.

Hartley-O'Brien, S.J. 1980. Six mobilization exercises for active range of hip flexion. *Research Quarterly for Exercise and Sport* 51 (4):625-635.

Heyward, V. 1998. *Advanced Fitness Assessment and Exercise Prescription.* 3rd ed. Champaign, IL: Human Kinetics.

Hoffman, S., and L. Francis. 1992. Is balance missing from your workout? *IDEA Today* March: 55-57.

Kendall F.P., E.K. McCreary, and P.G. Provance. 1993. *Muscles: Testing and Function.* Baltimore: Williams & Wilkins.

Knott, M., and Voss, P. 1985. *Proprioceptive Neuromuscular Facilitation.* 3rd ed. New York: Harper & Row.

Kuprian, W., ed. 1982. *Physical Therapy for Sports.* Philadelphia: Saunders.

McArdle, W., F. Katch, and V. Katch. 1991. Exercise Physiology: Energy, *Nutrition, and Human Performance.* 3rd ed. Philadelphia: Lea & Febiger.

McAtee, R.E. 1993. *Facilitated Stretching.* Champaign, IL: Human Kinetics.

O'Hagan, F.T., T.G. Sale, J.D. MacDougall, and S.H. Garner. 1995. Comparative effectiveness of accomodating and weight resistance training modes. *Medicine and Science in Sports and Exercise.* 27(8):1210-1219.

Osternig, L.R., R.N. Robertson, R.K. Troxel, and P. Hanson. 1990. Differential responses to PNF stretching techniques. *Medicine and Science in Sports and Exercise* 22:106-111.

Reid, J.G., and J. Thompson. 1985. *Exercise Prescription for Fitness.* Englewood Cliffs, NJ: Prentice-Hall.

Riley, D.P. 1982. *Strength Training by the Experts.* Champaign, IL: Leisure Press.

Sapega, A.A., T.C. Quendenfeld, R.A. Moyer, and R.A. Butler. 1991. Biophysical factors in range of motion exercise. *The Physician and Sportsmedicine* 9(12):57-65.

Stamford, B. 1995. How to warm up and cool down your workout. *The Physician and Sportsmedicine* 23(9):97-98.

Sudy, M. 1991. *Personal Trainer Manual (ACE).* Boston: Reebok University Press.

Voight, M., and S. Tippett. 1994. Plyometric exercise in rehabilitation. In *Rehabilitation Techniques in Sports Medicine*. 2nd ed. W.E. Prentice, ed. St. Louis: Mosby.

Voss, D., M. Ionta, and B. Myers. 1985. *Proprioceptive Neuromuscular Facilitation: Patterns and Techniques*. 3rd ed. Philadelphia: Harper & Row.

Wolkodoff, N.E. 1989. Building strength. *IDEA Today* July/August:17-22.

Chapter 13

Almekinders, L.C. 1993. Anti-inflammatory treatment of muscular injuries in sports. *Sports Medicine* 15 (3):139-145.

Baker, B.E. 1984. Current concepts in the diagnosis and treatment of musculotendinous injuries. *Medicine and Science in Sports and Exercise* 16 (4):323-327.

Clement, D.B., J.E. Taunton, and G.W. Smart. 1984. Achilles tendinitis and peritendinitis: Etiology and treatment. *American Journal of Sports Medicine* 12 (3):179-184.

Clippinger, K. 1990. Exercise analysis: A guide to injury prevention. *IDEA* Independent Study Course:1-10.

Francis, L. 1985. Aerobic dance injuries: A survey of instructors. *The Physician and Sportsmedicine* 13 (2):105-111.

Garrick, J. 1986. Epidemiology of aerobic dance. *American Journal of Sports Medicine* 14(1): 67-72.

Grana, W.A., and T.C. Coniglione. 1985. Knee disorders in runners. *The Physician and Sportsmedicine* 13 (5): 127-133.

Griffin, J.C. 1987. Fitness injury survey: Fitness assessors and programmers. *Canadian Association for Health, Physical Education and Recreation Journal.* 53(1):15-17.

Griffin, J.C. 1989. *All the Right Moves: A Self Assessment Guide to Safe Exercise Design.* Toronto: George Brown College.

Hamill, J. 1991. Muscle soreness. *Nike Sp. Research Review* Dec./Mar: 1-4.

Hess, G.P., W.L. Cappiello, R.M. Poole, and S.C. Hunter. 1989. Prevention and treatment of overuse tendon injuries. *Sports Medicine* 8 (6):371-384.

Lachmann, S. 1988. *Soft Tissue Injuries in Sport.* Oxford, England: Blackwell Scientific.

Marti, B. 1988. On the epidemiology of running injuries. *American Journal of Sports Medicine* 16 (3):285-294.

Messier, S. 1988. Etiologic factors associated with selected running injuries. *Medicine and Science in Sports and Exercise* 20 (5):501-505.

Nirschl, P.R. 1988. Prevention and treatment of elbow and shoulder injuries in the tennis player. *Clinical Sports Medicine* 7(2):289-308.

Nosaka, K., and P.M. Clarkson. 1995. Muscle damage following repeated bouts of high force eccentric exercise. *Medicine and Science in Sports and Exercise* 27:990, 1263-1269.

O'Connor, F.G., J.R. Sobel, and R.P. Nirschl. 1992. Five-step treatment for overuse injuries. *The Physician and Sportsmedicine* 20 (10):128-142.

Prentice, W.E. 1994. *Rehabilitation Techniques in Sports Medicine.* St. Louis: Mosby–Year Book.

Richie, D.H., S.F. Kelso, and P.A. Bellucci. 1985. Aerobic dance injuries: A retrospective study of instructors and participants. *The Physician and Sportsmedicine* 13(2):130-140.

Rothenberger, I. 1988. Prevalence and types of injuries in aerobic dancers. *American Journal of Sports Medicine* 16(4):403-407.

Styf, J. 1988. Diagnosis of exercise-induced pain in the anterior aspect of the lower leg. *American Journal of Sports Medicine* 16(2): 165-171.

Vetter, W. 1985. Aerobic dance injuries. *The Physician and Sportsmedicine* 13(2):114-120.

Wanhol, M.J., A.J. Siegel, W.J. Evans, and L.M. Silverman. 1985. Skeletal muscle injury and repair in marathon runners after competition. *American Journal of Pathology* 118:331-339.

Chapter 14

Andrish, J., and J.A. Work. 1990. How I manage shin splints. *The Physician and Sportsmedicine* 18 (12):113-114.

Batt, M.E., and J.L. Tanji.1995. Management options for plantar fasciitis. *The Physician and Sportsmedicine* 23 (6):77-86.

Best, T.M., and W.E. Garrett. 1996. Hamstring strains. Expediting return to play. *The Physician and Sportsmedicine* 24 (8):37-44.

Curwin, S., and W.D. Stanish. 1984. *Tendinitis: Its Etiology and Treatment.* Lexington, MA: Collamore.

De Palma, B. 1994. Rehabilitation of hip and thigh injuries. In *Rehabilitation Techniques in Sports Medicine.* 2nd ed. W.E. Prentice, ed. St. Louis: Mosby.

Doucette, S.A., and E.M. Goble. 1992. The effect of exercise on patellar tracking in lateral patellar compression syndrome. *American Journal of Sports Medicine* 20 (4):434-440.

Fick, D.S., J.P. Albright, and B.P. Murray. 1992. Relieving painful "shin splints". *The Physician and Sportsmedicine* 20 (12):105-113.

Galea, A.M. and J.M. Albers. 1994. Patellofemoral pain. Beyond empirical diagnosis. *The Physician and Sportsmedicine* 22 (4):48-58.

Hooker, D. 1994. Back rehabilitation. In *Rehabilitation Techniques in Sports Medicine.* 2nd ed., W.E. Prentice, ed. St. Louis: Mosby.

Myerson, M.S., and K. Biddinger. 1995. Achilles tendon disorders. Practical management strategies. *The Physician and Sportsmedicine* 23 (12):47-54.

Prentice, W.E. 1994. *Rehabilitation Techniques in Sports Medicine.* 2nd ed. St. Louis: Mosby.

Rizzo, T.D. 1991. Plantar fasciitis. Overcoming a nagging pain in the arch. *The Physician and Sportsmedicine* 19 (4):129-130.

Tanner, S.M., and J.S. Harvey. 1988. How we manage plantar fasciitis. *The Physician and Sportsmedicine* 16 (8):39-47.

Tauton, J.E., D.B. Clement, G.W. Smart, and K.L. McNicol. 1987. Non-surgical management of overuse knee injuries in runners. *Canadian Journal of Sports Science* 12 (1):11-18.

Torg, J.S., Vegso, J.J., and Torg, E. 1987. *Rehabilitation of Athletic Injuries: An Atlas of Therapeutic Exercise.* Chicago: Yearbook Medical Pub.

Waddell, G. 1987. A new clinical model for the treatment of low back pain. *Spine* 12 (7):632-644.

Chapter 15

Afrasiabi, R, and S.L. Spector. 1991. Exercise-induced asthma. It needn't sideline your patients. *The Physician and Sportsmedicine* 19 (5):49-60.

American College of Sports Medicine. 1995. *Guidelines for Exercise Testing and Prescription*. 5th ed. Philadelphia: Lea & Febiger.

American College of Sports Medicine. 1993. Physical activity, physical fitness, and hypertension. Position stand. *Medicine and Science in Sports and Exercise* 25:i-x.

American Heart Association. 1989. *Heart facts*. Dallas: American Heart Association.

Anders, D.L. 1992. Sound treatment strategies for active hypertensives. *The Physician and Sportsmedicine* 20 (11):108-118.

Bouchard, C., R.J. Shephard, and T. Stephens, eds. 1993. *Physical Activity, Fitness, and Health*. Champaign, IL: Human Kinetics.

Canadian Diabetes Association. 1995. *Exercise and Diabetes*. Ottawa: National Publications Committee.

Carey, E. 1996. Boomers pudgy and out of shape, new study finds. *Toronto Star* January 31:D1

Centers for Disease Control. 1990. Prevalence of arthritic conditions—United States, 1987. *Journal of the American Medical Association* 263:1758-1759.

Ekblom, B., and R. Nordemar. 1987. Rheumatoid arthritis. In *Exercise Testing and Exercise Prescription for Special Cases*, ed. J.S. Skinner. Philadelphia: Lea & Febiger.

Franklin, B.A., and J.R. Wappes. 1996. Taking the pressure off. How exercise can lower high blood pressure. *The Physician and Sportsmedicine* 24 (6):101-102.

Gordon, N.F. 1993. *Arthritis. Your Complete Exercise Guide*. Champaign, IL: Human Kinetics.

Gordon, N.F. 1993. Diabetes. *Your Complete Exercise Guide*. Champaign, IL: Human Kinetics.

Ike, R.W., R.M. Lampman, and C.W. Castor. 1989. Arthritis and aerobic exercise: A review. *The Physician and Sportsmedicine* 17 (2):128-137.

Kaplan, N.M. 1986. *Clinical Hypertension*. 4th ed. Baltimore: Williams & Wilkins.

Levin, S. 1991. Aquatic therapy. A splashing success for arthritis and injury rehabilitation. *The Physician and Sportsmedicine* 19:119-126.

Miller, B.F., and C.B. Keane. 1987. *Encyclopedia and Dictionary of Medicine, Nursing, and Allied Health*. Philadelphia: Saunders.

Murphy, R.J.L., and K. Sidney. 1992. Diabetes and physical activity: What the physical educator and coach should know. *Bulletin of the Cnadian Association for Health, Physical Education, and Recreation* Summer:7-11.

Report of the Joint National Committee on Detection, Evaluation, and Treatment of High Blood Pressure. 1993. *Archives of Internal Medicine* 153:154-183.

Rimmer, J.H. 1994. Fitness and Rehabilitation *Programs for Special Populations*. Dubuque, IA: Brown & Benchmark.

Samples, P. 1990. Exercise encouraged for people with arthritis. *The Physician and Sportsmedicine* 18 (1):123-127.

Sherman, W.M., and A. Allbright. 1990. Exercise and type I diabetes. *Sports Science Exchange,* 3:1-5.

Sherman, W.M., and A. Allbright. 1992. Exercise and type II diabetes. *Sports Science Exchange* 4:1-5.

Sol, N. 1991. Modifications for health conditions and special populations. In *Personal Trainer Manual*, ed. M. Sudy. San Diego: American Council on Exercise.

Spenser, M.L. 1991. Your health care plan: Individualized for your lifestyle. In *Learning to Live Well with Diabetes*, ed. M.J. Franz, et al.. Minneapolis: DCI.

Stamford, B. 1991. Exercise-induced asthma. Taking the wheeze out of your workout. *The Physician and Sportsmedicine* 19 (8):139-140.

Tanji, J.L. 1990. Hypertension. Part 1: How exercise helps. *The Physician and Sportsmedicine* 18 (7):77-82.

Tanji, J.L., and M.E. Batt. 1995. Management of hypertension. Adapting new guidelines for active patients. *The Physician and Sportsmedicine* 23 (2):47-53.

Taunton, J.E. and L. McCargar. 1995. Managing activity in patients who have diabetes. *The Physician and Sportsmedicine* 23 (3):41-52.

Vitug, A., S.H. Schneider, and N.B. Ruderman. 1988. Exercise and type I diabetes mellitus. In *Exercise and Sport Sciences Reviews,* ed. K.B. Pandoff. New York: Macmillan.

Wallberg-Henriksson, H. 1992. Exercise and diabetes mellitus. In *Exercise and Sport Sciences Reviews,* ed. J.O. Holloszy. Baltimore: Williams & Wilkins.

Weinstein, A.M. 1987. *Asthma*. New York: McGraw-Hill.

Index

Credits

Figure icon 10.5, figures 11.5, 14.9, 14.19, 14.21, and 14.22 reprinted, by permission, from V. Heyward 1998, *Advanced Fitness Assessment and Exercise Prescription, third ed.*, Champaign, IL, Human Kinetics, 57, 58, 62, 128, 303, 304, 307.

Figure 10.4 reprinted, by permission, from G. Carr, 1997, *Mechanics of Sport*, Champaign, IL, Human Kinetics, 177.

Figure icons 11.1a,b, 3a, 4a,b, 5a and 6a reprinted, by permission, from T.R. Baechle and R.W. Earle, 1995, *Fitness Weight Training*, Champaign, IL, Human Kinetics, 144, 148, 150, 151, 152, 155.

Figure 10.9 and 10.10 reprinted, by permission, from T. O'Brien, 1997, *The Personal Trainers Handbook*, Champaign, IL, Human Kinetics, 90 and 103.

Figure icon 10.4, figures 5.4a,b, 5.5, and 11.7 reprinted, by permission, from E.T. Howley and B.D. Franks, 1997, *Health Fitness Instructor's Handbook*, Champaign, IL, Human Kinetics, 258, 259, 261, 310.

Figure icons 10.3 and 12x.7 and figures 10.3, 10.7b, 10.16, and 15.7 reprinted, by permission, from B.B. Cook and G.W. Stewart, 1996, *Strength Basics*, Champaign, IL, Human Kinetics, 72, 90, 91, 112, 113, 135, 149.

Figure 14.2 reprinted, by permission, from L. Jozsa and P. Kannus, 1997, *Human Tendons*, Champaign, IL, Human Kinetics, 42 and 47.

Figure icons 12xx.1, 12xx.3, 12xx.5 and figures 11.8, 14.2a,b, 14.13a, 14.20, 14.23, and 15.3 reprinted, by permission, from M. Alter, 1997, *Sports Stretch*, Champaign, IL, Human Kinetics, 89, 90, 129, 139, 145, 164, 165, 200, 201.

About the Author

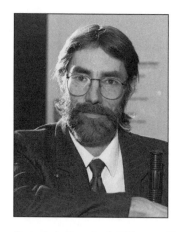

John C. Griffin is a professor and coordinator of the Fitness and Lifestyle Management Program at George Brown College in Toronto, Ontario. He has guided the program's growth by initiating exercise prescription, club management, and musculoskeletal rehabilitation streams; creating a personal training post-diploma certificate; and developing an internship program with the industry and fitness associations.

As a private consultant, speaker, and writer for public and private sector organizations around the globe, Griffin has authored over forty publications, given more than fifty presentations, and served as an advisor for Canadian national and provincial standards for personal trainers and fitness practitioners. His numerous awards and honors include the Mall Peepre Memorial Award for an outstanding contribution to fitness leadership in Canada (1991), the New South Wales Fitness Industry Association and VicFit Australian lecture award (1991), Ontario's Provincial Fitness Citation (1993), and the Ontario Association of Sport and Exercise Sciences (OASES) honorary award (1997).

A member of OASES's board of directors; the National Fitness Leadership Advisory Council; the Canadian Association of Health, Physical Education, Recreation and Dance; and the Canadian Society for Exercise Physiology, Griffin received his MSc in exercise physiology from the University of Alberta in 1974. He and his wife, Mary, live in Etobicoke, Ontario. In his free time Griffin enjoys hiking, camping, jogging, in-line skating, and adventure travel.